GASTRO-INTESTINAL
X-RAY DIAGNOSIS

GASTRO-INTESTINAL X-RAY DIAGNOSIS

A Descriptive Atlas

D. H. CUMMACK

MB ChB DMR FRCSE FFRRCSI

Consultant Radiologist in Administrative Charge
Western General Hospital, Edinburgh
Member of Clinical Teaching Staff, University of Edinburgh

Foreword by

SIR JOHN BRUCE

CBE TD DSc FRCSE FRSE

Regius Professor of Clinical Surgery
University of Edinburgh

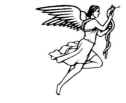

E & S LIVINGSTONE LTD

EDINBURGH & LONDON

1969

SBN 443 00629 6

Printed in Great Britain

FOREWORD

Until little more than a quarter of a century ago, the gastro-intestinal tract was the Cinderella of clinical medicine. Its physiological and pathological foundations, to say the least of it, were fragile: its disorders were ill-understood, their investigations relatively crude and their management largely empirical.

The situation is now vastly different. There have been enormous accretions to our knowledge of the structure, functions, and dysfunctions of the digestive organs; an armoury of sophisticated apparatus and a battery of significant tests have given scientific precision to the study of alimentary diseases. Many disciplines have had a share in these striking advances; none more so than surgery which has provided a background of living pathology and radiology which in the hands of the experts of today has become a formidable diagnostic tool both in research and diagnosis.

It is a great privilege to commend this remarkable—indeed unique—atlas to all interested in the gastro-intestinal tract. It does not purport to be a textbook of gastro-intestinal radiology or a manual of technique; in fact, it transcends these functions most importantly. It is no less than the record of a lifetime of experience accumulated through the years by a dedicated colleague and distinguished friend, Hunter Cummack. In a sense, it is his testimony and his testament, and both he and his associates may well be proud of his achievement.

The author has had a long and happy association since its beginnings with the Gastro-intestinal Unit in Edinburgh, and much of the material which has contributed to his remarkable experience stems from this fruitful and rewarding collaboration. Fortunately for us, his clinical colleagues, his interests did not end in the dark-room or at the viewing screen; he was a frequent visitor to the wards and to the operating room, and I believe that it is his intimate knowledge of living gastro-intestinal pathology that has made his radiological contribution so enlightened and so authoritative.

I believe that this monograph will fulfil a real need and that it is destined to become one of the classics of gastro-enterology. The selection and the reproduction of his beautiful illustrations have demanded a considerable sacrifice of time and leisure. A prodigious memory and loving care are other of the ingredients of such authorship, and it is a very great pleasure to congratulate him on a veritable magnum opus. It has taken his friends some time to persuade him to take up the pen. Now that he has done so he has placed all those interested in the alimentary tract and its disorders very greatly in his debt. His labours deserve all the success I am sure his book will command.

EDINBURGH 1969   JOHN BRUCE

PREFACE

This atlas stems from personal experience of the radiology of the gastro-intestinal tract at the Western General Hospital, Edinburgh, during the past 22 years. My interest was initially stimulated by Professor Sir John Bruce and Professor W. I. Card who founded the Gastro-intestinal Unit and who gave me every help and encouragement. I am deeply indebted to them and to their colleagues and successors who have also given me every assistance without which this work would have been impossible.

Since the foundation of the Gastro-intestinal Unit an important feature has been weekly 'grand rounds' involving joint participation by clinicians and radiologists. In addition I have had almost daily contact with its members and with consultants from other departments all of whom willingly provided me with clinical details of their patients.

The atlas is intended for all radiologists; for physicians and surgeons, particularly those interested in the gastro-intestinal tract, abdomen and associated organs; and for post-graduate students studying for higher qualifications.

I have deliberately omitted a chapter on the salivary glands because they are of limited interest to gastro-enterologists. I have included hiatus herniae in the chapter on the oesophagus and at the end of this chapter there are a few illustrations on the diaphragm. Most of the complications of the surgery of the stomach and duodenum are described in the chapter on the stomach. The two diseases which commonly affect both the small bowel and colon—Crohn's disease and tuberculosis—are chiefly discussed in the chapter on the small intestine, but also partly in the chapters on the colon and duodenum, with cross references.

Acute emergencies are mainly considered under the appropriate organ and are mentioned only briefly in the last chapter. Whenever possible the illustrations of each condition and disease are grouped together in the same order as in the text. There are no references to literature in the text—this being a record of personal experience.

There are so many people whom I would like to thank that it is not possible to name every one. However in addition to Professor Sir John Bruce and Professor W. I. Card, I would like to mention Dr W. Sircus and Dr J. McManus, Physicians, and Mr C. W. A. Falconer, Mr W. P. Small, Mr A. N. Smith, Surgeons, to the Gastro-intestinal Unit, Western General Hospital, and their present and past Senior Registrars and Registrars. I am also most grateful to Dr Eric Samuel, Radiologist-in-Charge of the Radio-diagnostic Department, Royal Infirmary, Edinburgh, and Reader in the Department of Diagnostic Radiology, University of Edinburgh, for much help and advice. Within my own staff I am indebted to Dr W. A. Copland and Dr G. M. Fraser, Consultants in the X-ray Department, who provided me with films of their cases; to my various Senior Registrars and Registrars, who have all given an immense amount of their time in helping to check the illustrations and read the proofs; to Miss Fegan and Miss Smith and their junior colleagues for helping with the preparation of the radiographs, etc.

I cannot praise my two secretaries, Mrs Jones (née Bertram) and Mrs Fraser, too highly. They gave me invaluable help.

The majority of the photographic prints were made by Mr Malcolm Liddle, to whom nothing was too much trouble; the excellence of his work can be seen in the quality of the illustrations.

I am greatly indebted to the staff of Messrs E. & S. Livingstone. Any success this book may have will be due in no small measure to their efforts. It has been a great pleasure working with them.

Finally I would like to thank Professor Sir John Bruce who so kindly agreed to write the foreword.

EDINBURGH, 1969   D. H. CUMMACK

CONTENTS

CHAPTER I

THE BARIUM MEAL

MOST experienced radiologists have developed a satisfactory method of their own. However, the author's technique is described in detail for the benefit of more junior colleagues and as an aid to the interpretation of many of the subsequent illustrations.

As a preliminary it is important that the radiologist should ask the patient a few questions such as his age, the duration of his symptoms, the number and nature of any operations. This is not merely to obtain further details which might help to plan the examination but also to gain the confidence of the patient.

The same type of barium should always be used so that normal and abnormal appearances are readily appreciated. Micropaque* suspension is most satisfactory and is recommended undiluted except in infants and children, when the addition of some water may be necessary to make it more palatable.

Fluoroscopy (screen examination), including the preliminary examination of the chest, should always be minimal to spare the patient unnecessary radiation and to prevent the eyes of the radiologist from becoming tired. Television equipment with image intensification is of great value because dark adaptation is unnecessary and more detail can be seen, but it has certain drawbacks. The apparatus is bulky and the procedure is thus physically more tiring for the operator. The assessment of the radiographic factors is also more difficult and therefore automatic exposure equipment is recommended.

As soon as an abnormality is detected on fluoroscopy, one or more films should be taken of this area to demonstrate the suspected lesion as clearly as possible. Alternatively, in the light of previous experience, a mental note should be made to examine this area carefully later in the supine or prone position.

It is never necessary to waste time in an attempt to make a precise diagnosis during fluoroscopy. The diagnosis is made after inspection of the films including any additional ones considered necessary. No efforts should be spared to get films of the highest quality. Kilovoltage (kV) in the range 70 to 90 (and 60 for babies) rather than at a higher level is recommended in an average patient. It is also recommended that the kV should be raised or lowered by 10 (which halves or doubles the exposure time) and not by intervening amounts as it is easier thereby to assess the exposure factors. It is a great advantage to have an assistant to alter these on the instructions of the radiologist.

An oral cholecystogram and barium meal can conveniently be performed at one examination. The films of the gall-bladder in the erect position are taken initially following its identification on fluoroscopy. This will be discussed later in the section on the biliary tract (p. 260). The barium meal examination is then carried out. It is not advisable to perform a cholecystogram, intravenous cholangiogram and barium meal at the same attendance except in special cases.

During the course of the meal attention is directed not merely to the detection of intrinsic lesions but also to displacement by enlarged neighbouring organs.

ROUTINE TECHNIQUE

Preliminary fluoroscopy of chest and diaphragm.

Patient erect in right anterior oblique position, holding the beaker of barium in his left hand.

Two mouthfuls of barium taken and its passage down the oesophagus carefully observed.

Particular attention paid to oesophago-gastric junction to note obstruction, splitting of the stream of barium, etc.

Attention now directed to the stomach.

Three or four more mouthfuls of barium taken

* Made by Damancy and Company Ltd., Slough, England.

A

with intermittent fluoroscopy and slow rotation of the patient so that the stomach is viewed from different angles.

No immediate palpation since pyloro-spasm sometimes provoked.

Females should hold up a pendulous right breast with the right hand.

Subsequent careful palpation of all areas with fluoroscopy. Films taken of any detected lesion or suspicious area.

Barium coaxed into the duodenum by palpation with the gloved hand.

One 12 in. × 10 in. (30·5 × 25·4 cm.) or 14 in. × 14 in. (35·6 × 35·6 cm.) film of the stomach and duodenum taken. Right anterior oblique position preferred as this shows the lesser curvature of the stomach and the duodenal bulb to the best advantage. Sometimes helpful to use compression by means of a pad between the screen and the patient.

Four spot films of the duodenal bulb unobscured by barium in distal duodenum and preferably also clear of the spine now taken with compression. These films should, if possible, include the incisura and the lower part of lesser curvature of stomach.

In all, less than 5 oz. of barium normally required. If stomach dilated, 10 oz. or more should be given.

Patient now takes as big a mouthful of barium as possible and retains it in his mouth.

Table is tilted to horizontal position. During tilting the patient turns to face the table as this not merely saves time but is easier for the patient.

When horizontal and in prone position, he is instructed to swallow the barium. If propulsion down oesophagus too slow, the table is inclined slightly raising the head.

Oesophagus should be examined with maximum distension as this more clearly shows indentation by enlarged glands, etc.

Stomach and duodenum then carefully viewed fluoroscopically.

Patient now turned on his back.

Stomach and duodenum inspected and palpated.

Even if no abnormality detected on fluoroscopy, supine films are taken after the following manœuvre.

Patient lies on his right side in order to fill the antrum and duodenum. Subsequently turns on left side until antrum and duodenal loop are opened out and clearly seen. This causes the gastric air bubble to distend the antrum and duodenal bulb which are

coated with barium giving excellent air contrast. To steady himself patient grasps with his right hand the side of the table or a hand-grip fixed opposite his left shoulder. One 12 in. × 10 in. (30·5 × 25·4 cm.) or 14 in. × 14 in. (35·6 × 35·6 cm.) film of the stomach and duodenum now taken, sometimes using compression, the optimum position being determined by fluoroscopy. Four spot films taken of duodenal bulb with variable rotation or compression. A difference of rotation of approximately 7° between each film may be employed so that pairs can be viewed stereoscopically.

Finally, the upper jejunum is inspected and palpated and films are taken if necessary.

The patient should not be dismissed until his films have been carefully scrutinised and found satisfactory. If they are inadequate or if a doubtful lesion is seen, he is re-examined immediately. If flocculation of the barium in the stomach has occurred it is an advantage for the patient to drink more barium before additional films are taken.

MODIFICATION OF ROUTINE TECHNIQUE

If the stomach empties slowly, a discussion about items of food which the patient particularly fancies may help to relax the pylorus.

More commonly it is advisable for him to wait for a quarter of an hour or so in his changing cubicle.

When a large fluid residue is present it is a waste of time to examine for a prolonged period, or to take films in the erect position except to show the size of the fluid residue and sometimes a lesser curve lesion. The prone and supine positions are of much greater value.

It is at this stage that the most reliable estimate of the degree of pyloric or duodenal obstruction is obtained. A six-hour film is a less accurate method of estimating this because the size of the gastric residue at that time depends on various factors, including what the patient has eaten in the interval.

In aged and infirm patients and others who cannot stand, four or five mouthfuls of barium should be given before the patient is placed on the X-ray table. This is time-saving and minimises discomfort to the patient. It cannot of course be done if the mode of emptying of the stomach following an operation, e.g. gastro-enterostomy, has to be studied.

EXAMINATION OF CERVICAL OESOPHAGUS

True lateral erect position centring on cervical oesophagus. Bolus of barium in patient's mouth.

Exposure factors set.

Patient swallows the barium and exposure made at that moment. With experience it is usually possible to get satisfactory views. At least one large and four spot films necessary.

Patient turned to postero-anterior (P.A.) position and further large and spot films taken.

Ciné films unnecessary except sometimes in study of motility disorders.

EXAMINATION FOR OESOPHAGEAL VARICES

Patient preferably supine with right side slightly elevated and head slightly lowered in moderate Trendelenburg position.

He swallows a mouthful of Micropaque, after which he is instructed to make no further movements of swallowing.

Films taken while patient is asked to perform the Valsalva manœuvre or preferably after he has held a deep breath as long as possible. In some cases varices are most obvious during quiet respiration. Optimum position determined by fluoroscopy and if possible the oesophagus should not be superimposed on the spine or heart.

EXAMINATION FOR HIATUS HERNIA

Prone position used initially with head lowered and pad beneath the stomach.

Films taken after patient has swallowed a large bolus of barium. First film a true antero-posterior (A.P.) even although the oesophagus is superimposed on the spine. Second film oblique with left side raised while patient still in prone position. These films are also excellent for demonstrating oesophagitis and ulceration. Sometimes the erect position after swallowing a bolus of barium shows an ulcer crater more clearly.

In some cases where there is a very short oesophagus and the hiatus hernia is stretched, the supine position with left side raised and pressure applied to the stomach frequently demonstrates the hernia clearly when other methods have failed. To steady himself the patient should clasp with his left hand the side of the table or a hand-grip placed at level of his right shoulder.

EXAMINATION FOR SCLERODERMA (SYSTEMIC SCLEROSIS)

Either prone or supine position satisfactory with head lowered. Careful fluoroscopy during barium swallow to note motility. Prone position most valuable for demonstration of any associated hiatus hernia.

EXAMINATION OF FUNDUS OF STOMACH

The following manœuvre is performed to coat the fundus with barium and to use the gastric air bubble to provide a double contrast effect.

Patient initially supine, table then tilted to the erect position.

Four spot films and/or one or two of larger size taken, with graduated rotation, particular attention being paid to the oesophago-gastric junction. True lateral position trying to touch toes sometimes valuable (p. 297).

If patient weak and unable to stand, he is turned from the supine to the prone position with table horizontal or head slightly raised. This is also the best method of demonstrating gastric varices.

EXAMINATION OF JUNCTION OF FUNDUS WITH BODY OF STOMACH

This difficult area can be examined in two ways. Particularly necessary in cup and spill deformity.

A. Erect position. Four spot films with graduated rotation centred on upper end of lesser curvature.

B. Four spot films and one or two large films as follows:

Patient lying on right side.

Table then tilted raising the head until most of barium is in the antrum and a good *en face* view obtained following fluoroscopic control. Only minimal amount of barium should be used.

EXAMINATION OF BODY OF STOMACH

In addition to erect, prone and supine views, the supine position with the left side raised, i.e. L.A.O., is excellent for demonstrating some lesions, especially ulcers *en face*.

EXAMINATION OF INCISURA, ANTRUM AND PREPYLORIC REGION

Difficult in erect position in some cases unless firm compression or palpation applied.

Prone position excellent, especially in presence of large fluid residue. Otherwise supine position best of all—with left side slightly raised and with some compression for the incisura—with right side raised for the antrum and prepyloric region.

EXAMINATION OF DUODENUM

Procedure for examination planned at an early stage of the barium meal. The four spot films of the bulb in erect position omitted if bulb inadequately filled.

Films in prone position valuable in stenosis of the bulb.

Sometimes prone view with some obliquity is the only satisfactory position to show the junction of first and second parts.

In most cases, however, the supine position with the right side slightly raised is far superior to the erect or prone for all parts of the duodenum. This view is also the most important for the detection of an enlarged duodenal loop in tumours of the head of the pancreas. In these cases compression should be omitted as it tends to exaggerate the size of the loop.

In all cases of jaundice, four spot films centred on the ampulla of Vater are necessary to detect an early ampullary or pancreatic tumour, or sometimes a finely calcified stone impacted at the lower end of the common bile duct.

EXAMINATION FOR TUMOUR OR CYST OF BODY OF PANCREAS

Sometimes suspected in the erect and horizontal positions by forwards lateral and occasionally downwards displacement of the stomach. Palpable mass may also be present.

Confirmation as follows.

Stomach well filled with barium. Patient lies on right side and table tilted to angle of 45° to 50° until barium has partially run from the fundus into the antrum. Precise angle determined by fluoroscopy. Posterior aspect of stomach lies against pancreatic tumour causing a 'wedge' effect—the thin end of the wedge being posterior. Stomach also displaced forwards.

AIR CONTRAST EXAMINATION

Particularly important when there is doubt following a conventional barium meal.

Tube with end opening passed into the stomach. A Levine tube cut off at proximal side opening is satisfactory.

Fifty millilitres undiluted Micropaque injected with patient supine.

Patient turned to prone position then back to supine position in order to coat the stomach with barium.

Air injected down the tube under fluoroscopic control. Patient positioned to show the part under investigation to best advantage.

For the fundus, the films are taken in the prone position with the head of the table slightly elevated if necessary.

To examine the duodenum a longer tube is employed.

Particularly valuable in cases of suspected enlargement of the head of the pancreas or indentation of the duodenal loop by other space-occupying lesions. Thirty milligrams Buscopan* injected intravenously to cause relaxation when end of tube is in second part of duodenum.

Micropaque injected down tube followed by as much air as is necessary to distend the duodenum.

EXAMINATION IN THE LATE POST-OPERATIVE CASE

General principles same as in routine meal, but less barium should be used, especially after a partial gastrectomy.

Careful fluoroscopy following initial mouthful to note mode of filling of jejunum after gastroenterostomy.

One large film preferably with compression and four spot films centred on anastomosis in erect and supine positions and others as considered necessary.

EXAMINATION IN HAEMATEMESIS

Patient must be handled with care. Decision as to when he is fit rests with the clinician. Otherwise no contra-indication to a barium meal at the earliest moment.

Television of great value, especially as most patients present as emergencies.

* Manufactured by Boehringer, Ingelheim Ltd., Isleworth, England.

Naso-gastric tube should be withdrawn into the upper oesophagus and reintroduced into the stomach at the end of the examination.

Two mouthfuls of undiluted Micropaque are swallowed.

Patient turned on his right side with table horizontal or with head slightly elevated.

One 12 in. by 10 in. film of stomach and four spot films of duodenal bulb taken with patient in this position.

He is then turned on his back.

Further films of oesophagus, stomach and duodenum are taken as suggested below. It is usually necessary for a mouthful or two more of barium to be taken but as little as possible should be given.

In bleeding from the oesophagus, characteristic streaky filling defects are seen slopping up and down as blood clot does not mix with barium. Adequate films of oesophagus in these cases are necessary to determine precise nature of the lesion.

Fresh unclotted blood in the stomach causes irregular fluffy filling defects and creates difficulty in examination and diagnosis.

Clotted blood in the stomach causes a more regular and clear-cut filling defect and this fortuitously forms around the lesion which is causing the haemorrhage, drawing attention to it. Therefore adequate films of this area must be taken.

When bleeding is from a duodenal ulcer without significant stenosis, the oesophagus and stomach are usually reasonably free from blood but it is present in the duodenum. In the presence of duodenal stenosis, on the other hand, there is usually considerable blood in the stomach. Adequate films are taken of duodenum to show a possible ulcer. Sometimes the round filling defect due to an artery in the base of the ulcer can be seen.

Thus the nature and position of the blood direct the attention of the radiologist at an early stage of the barium meal to the site of the bleeding, and films of this suspected area are taken and subsequently scrutinised.

THE GASTROGRAFIN* MEAL

Erect and supine films of the abdomen are essential before a Gastrografin meal.

Forty to fifty millilitres are usually sufficient.

Detail using Gastrografin is poorer than with barium, and the mucosal pattern sometimes appears coarser. Because of its high osmotic pressure Gastrografin should not be given to dehydrated babies.

However, it has the great advantage of not producing any complications should it leak into the peritoneal cavity.

A Gastrografin meal is mainly used in the investigation of early post-operative complications and in certain acute abdominal emergencies.

EARLY POST-OPERATIVE COMPLICATIONS

The purpose of a Gastrografin meal is:

(*a*) To demonstrate or exclude a leak, especially at an anastomosis. An adequate number of films, especially spot films of the stomal region, must be taken.

(*b*) To differentiate between a loculated effusion and a loop of bowel. Gastrografin outlines the lumen of the bowel. A loculated effusion is not opacified unless a fistula is present.

(*c*) To determine the nature and degree of an obstruction.

When stomal obstruction follows a Polya gastrectomy or a Billroth I gastrectomy, raising the left side of the patient and tilting the table slightly towards the vertical, frequently results in the remnant starting to empty.

A Gastrografin meal becomes progressively of less value the further down the small bowel an obstruction occurs.

ACUTE ABDOMINAL EMERGENCIES

At the beginning of the examination the movements of the diaphragm are studied. Impairment of movement of one dome suggests an inflammatory process adjacent to it.

Gastrografin is of particular value in the diagnosis of a perforation, acute cholecystitis and acute pancreatitis.

PERFORATION

In a suspected perforation particular attention must be paid to the duodenal bulb for the presence of a duodenal ulcer, and to detect any extra-luminal streaks or bubbles of gas. Gastrografin may leak into the peritoneal cavity confirming the diagnosis but it is surprising how infrequently this occurs even in a proved perforation. Following such a leak the Gastrografin is absorbed and ultimately the urinary bladder may be opacified.

ACUTE CHOLECYSTITIS

The duodenal bulb and the loop immediately distal to it are carefully examined with the patient in the supine and prone positions to note any obstruction. This is discussed later in the section on the biliary tract (p. 265).

ACUTE PANCREATITIS

When acute pancreatitis is suspected an adequate number of films should be taken to demonstrate any displacement of the stomach and duodenum as already described in the barium meal. The left dome of the diaphragm must also be carefully examined since disease affecting the tail and body of pancreas commonly causes impaired motility. Sometimes a trace of fluid is seen at the left costophrenic angle.

PERFORATION OF THE OESOPHAGUS

Films of the neck and chest should always be taken in the first instance in cases of suspected perforation. To determine its site a tube with an end opening should be introduced as far as the lower oesophagus. A Levine tube cut off at the proximal side opening is satisfactory. Gastrografin is injected down the tube which is gradually withdrawn until the leak is demonstrated. Films must also be taken at appropriate intervals. When the end of the tube is in the upper oesophagus or pharynx it tends to be regurgitated. Under these circumstances an ordinary Levine tube with side openings is more readily manipulated and better tolerated by the patient since a greater length is in the oesophagus.

* Manufactured by Schering A. G. Berlin.

CHAPTER II

THE OESOPHAGUS

RADIOLOGICAL METHODS OF INVESTIGATION

Plain films of the chest and neck are required in cases of suspected perforations and swallowed foreign bodies. In patients with dysphagia a chest film is also of value in estimating the presence and extent of inflammatory changes at the lung bases from inhalation of oesophageal content. Occasionally the soft-tissue shadow caused by a hiatus hernia or dilated oesophagus may be seen, sometimes containing a fluid level.

A barium meal is the standard method of examination and must include the stomach and duodenum.

A Gastrografin meal is the procedure of choice in the investigation of leaks and fistulae when the suspected site is known with reasonable certainty, e.g. at a suture line. When the site is unknown, the Gastrografin should be injected down a tube, which is gradually withdrawn (p. 6).

Instillation of Iodised Oil. In cases of congenital atresia a soft rubber catheter is introduced through the mouth into the upper blind segment. Two to three millilitres of iodised oil (Neo-hydriol* is satisfactory) are injected. As Gastrografin is somewhat irritant it is not used in case some should inadvertently enter the trachea or bronchi. Usually only an A.P. view and a lateral view are necessary. At the end of the examination as much of the oil as possible is sucked out.

CLINICAL RADIOLOGY

NORMAL APPEARANCES

In the upper oesophagus the contractions of the crico-pharyngeus are so fleeting that it is difficult to show a contraction on a film.

* Manufactured by May and Baker Ltd., Dagenham, England.

Subsequently the bolus of barium is propelled into the stomach by peristaltic or stripping waves even with the patient in the Trendelenburg position. Occasionally, in particular if thick barium is used, and especially in the elderly, fine tertiary contractions may be seen causing a ripple border.

The mucosal pattern normally consists of four or five fine parallel folds. The pattern may be interrupted by round translucencies due to air bubbles or swallowed saliva.

The vestibule is a normal fusiform dilatation of the lower end of the oesophagus commonly having a slight constriction in its middle. This constriction was formerly considered to be caused by the attachment of the phreno-oesophageal ligament, but is now thought to be due to a prominent ridge of mucosa at the junction of the upper squamous and lower columnar epithelium. The radiological appearances of both these types of epithelium are similar. There is a slight narrowing at the upper end of the vestibule due to the inferior oesophageal sphincter. When a normal stripping wave passes down the oesophagus it stops at this sphincter. The dilated vestibule then collapses and some barium refluxes up the oesophagus.

CONGENITAL ANOMALIES

Congenital short oesophagus is rare. Many cases previously considered as such were probably acquired as a result of an oesophagitis.

Congenital diverticula are usually found in the middle or lower oesophagus. Characteristically they are flask-shaped as opposed to the peaked or tented appearance of the rarer traction type.

Congenital Atresia. This condition usually becomes evident within 24 to 48 hours of birth. In the commonest type, the upper end is blind and the lower portion communicates with the trachea or left bronchus and thus air is present in the stomach and bowel. If there is no such communication, the stomach and bowel are collapsed and air is absent from the gut.

Dysautonomia. This is a familial condition characterised by autonomic imbalance and associated with difficulty in swallowing usually from birth. There is delay in relaxation of the crico-pharyngeus. Some general dilatation of the oesophagus also occurs due to the motility disorder and inadequate relaxation of the gastro-oesophageal sphincter.

SLIDING HIATUS HERNIA

In recent years many articles have been written about hiatus herniae, the oesophago-gastric junction, factors preventing or favouring regurgitation, etc., but there is still disagreement on the mechanism and anatomical details.

There is no doubt that absence of a hiatal valve caused by a low flat left dome of diaphragm, e.g. in emphysema, or by a high partial gastrectomy, facilitates gastro-oesophageal reflux.

When small, a hernia is sometimes difficult or impossible to differentiate from the vestibule, but when it is of even moderate size the diagnosis is comparatively easy. In the early stages a hernia may be present intermittently but ultimately it becomes permanent. The oesophageal hiatus of the diaphragm tends to become increasingly wider with time.

Mucosal Folds of Sliding Herniae. These can usually be traced without interruption from the body of the stomach through the oesophageal hiatus of the diaphragm to the top of the hernia. In addition, one large fold commonly runs from the anterior wall to the posterior wall immediately to the left of the oesophago-gastric junction. It is presumably caused by oblique fibres of the stomach which hook round the notch between the oesophagus and fundus. Sometimes there is a slight transverse constriction like a cap near the top of a hernia.

Shape and Behaviour. When a stripping wave passes down the oesophagus it stops immediately above the hernia, i.e. at the oesophago-gastric junction. It is not common to see reflux or collapse of the hernia at that moment. This is an important point in differential diagnosis from the vestibule (p. 7).

When barium has regurgitated from the body of the stomach causing distension of the hernia, reflux occurs up the oesophagus after a momentary delay at the oesophago-gastric junction.

The ease or difficulty of regurgitation from the body of the stomach into the hernia varies from patient to patient and at different times in the same patient. Distension of the stomach with barium usually facilitates regurgitation.

Even with careful technique it is not always possible to demonstrate the hernia or to differentiate it from the vestibule. However, in many such cases this is of academic interest—the important findings being gastro-oesophageal reflux and the presence or absence of radiological changes caused by oesophagitis.

In all cases of hiatus hernia a careful search must be made for a peptic ulcer. Most commonly the ulcer will be duodenal but may be in the stomach especially at the point where it passes through the hiatus.

OESOPHAGITIS
Peptic Oesophagitis

This is most commonly associated with a hiatus hernia, especially of the sliding type. The earliest signs are spasm of the lower oesophagus with blurred and sometimes wavy mucosal folds. The barium may not adhere satisfactorily to the mucosa, in which case the lower oesophagus is not outlined. Oesophagoscopy is much more accurate than a barium meal in determining the presence, severity and extent of oesophagitis.

The detection of superficial erosions is difficult, but as ulcers become larger they cause irregular projections from the lumen and sometimes a beaded appearance. As the disease progresses the oesophagus may become smooth with an absent mucosal pattern and at this stage oesophagoscopy may reveal leukoplakia.

Oesophagitis may heal with a degree of stenosis, and a food particle may cause complete obstruction. The narrowed area may take the form of a localised stricture or may extend over a considerable length with significant shortening of the oesophagus. These cases merit special attention. The herniated pouch is markedly stretched, especially in the erect position, and at first sight can look remarkably like the normal oesophagus both as regards calibre and mucosal pattern. However, on careful examination the mucosal folds in the hernia are seen to be continuous with those in the body of the stomach. Furthermore, the oesophageal hiatus of the diaphragm is wider than normal and the hernia can be distended by reflux of barium from below the diaphragm. The best method of achieving this is to apply pressure to the stomach with the patient supine and his left side raised.

Differential Diagnosis of Peptic Oesophagitis. A carcinoma is the most important condition to be excluded, but its appearances generally are more persistent. It must be remembered that a narrow central channel with lateral shoulders ('bird on the wing' appearance) more characteristic of a carcinoma is occasionally seen in oesophagitis. In both cases a hiatus hernia may be present but is much more common in association with an oesophagitis.

Varices may cause difficulty in diagnosis. However, the radiological appearances are variable and the abnormalities disappear following a stripping wave and in the erect position except when the varices are gross.

Acute Corrosive Oesophagitis

The degree and extent depend on the nature and volume of swallowed corrosive. Radiology using opaque medium is not indicated in the acute phase. A stricture usually extending over a considerable length may subsequently occur in the lower oesophagus. In such cases a hiatus hernia usually develops as a result of the shortening.

Monilial Infection of the Oesophagus

This may occur in chronically ill patients on long-term antibiotics. Radiologically there is diffuse irregularity with superficial ulceration,

THE LOWER OESOPHAGUS LINED WITH COLUMNAR EPITHELIUM

This is not uncommon and the columnar epithelium may extend up as high as the middle of the oesophagus. Peptic oesophagitis may be present at the lower end of the squamous-lined segment. More commonly a Barrett's ulcer, i.e. a deep peptic ulcer, occurs in the segment lined with columnar epithelium and healing is commonly associated with considerable fibrosis resulting sometimes in stenosis. A hiatus hernia is usually also present.

PARA-OESOPHAGEAL HERNIA

This is less common than the sliding type—accounting for less than 10 per cent. of all herniae.

The oesophageal hiatus of the diaphragm is wide and it permits herniation of the fundus, and subsequently of the oesophago-gastric junction into the thorax. In the final stage, the stomach rotates so that the greater curvature is uppermost. The oesophagus is more or less of normal length and may pursue a somewhat tortuous course. As would be expected, it does not enter the stomach at the top of the hernia as in the sliding type and therefore reflux and oesophagitis are not such prominent features.

A para-oesophageal hernia may be seen on a chest film as an opacity with a fluid level behind the heart.

The hernia may be intermittent in the early stages. When large it is fixed except in very rare instances. Incarceration and strangulation are uncommon.

The diagnosis is easy, but it is essential in every case to look for another lesion—e.g. gastric ulcer, carcinoma, etc. The reason is that this hernia by itself may cause minimal symptoms and another lesion has often prompted the patient to seek advice.

VARICES

With careful technique these can be demonstrated radiologically in 70 to 80 per cent of cases. They are seen as tortuous changing filling defects, especially at the margins of the lower oesophagus. Except when gross they disappear in the erect position or after a stripping wave in the horizontal. This distinguishes them from superficial carcinoma, epidermolysis bullosa, oesophagitis, etc., which cause persistent deformity (it must be remembered, however, that even these lesions are usually more clearly demonstrated in the horizontal position). Following a severe bleed the varices and an enlarged spleen may temporarily become smaller.

In all cases, a careful search must be made for a peptic ulcer which is present in approximately 10 per cent. of cases. Only infrequently can a dilated azygos vein be shown, and even rarer is widening of the distance between the dorsal spine and pleural reflection on the left side caused by dilated varices. Following a successful porto-caval anastomosis, the varices gradually disappear.

Varices may occur in the presence of superior mediastinal venous obstruction. The blood flow is in the reverse direction, but of course this cannot be detected by a barium swallow.

DISPLACEMENT OF OESOPHAGUS

Many congenital and acquired respiratory and cardio-vascular abnormalities cause displacement, but attention is drawn only to the following:

(a) *An aberrant right subclavian artery* indents the oesophagus obliquely immediately above the level of the aortic arch usually on the posterior aspect but occasionally on the anterior aspect. At first sight the deformity may simulate a carcinoma.

(b) *A dilated descending aorta* may cause obstruction of the lower end of the oesophagus simulating achalasia or a carcinoma. The detection of the dilated aorta should prevent this error in diagnosis.

(c) *Pericarditis.* Occasionally a smooth narrowing is caused over a considerable length of the lower oesophagus but the mucosa remains intact.

(d) *Slipping or Wandering Oesophagus.* In some cases of mitral stenosis the oesophagus may slip from one side of the dilated left atrium to the other. An obstruction may be present when it is on one side and thus dysphagia may be intermittent.

(e) *Fibrosis of a lung*, especially of an upper lobe, displaces the oesophagus to the affected side.

(f) *Mediastinal fibrosis* may cause distortion, displacement and irregular narrowing of the oesophagus with proximal dilatation.

(g) *A bronchial carcinoma* can cause displacement and indentation and ultimately infiltration of the wall of the oesophagus.

(h) *Lymph node enlargement* causes displacement with smooth indentations best seen with maximum oesophageal distension.

MOTILITY DISORDERS

Achalasia

The earliest radiological signs are feeble, simultaneous contractions similar to tertiary contractions throughout the oesophagus with failure of relaxation of the gastro-oesophageal sphincter. There is also some dilatation of the oesophagus with slight stasis.

In an established case, there is gross dilatation with elongation, tortuosity, a fluid residue, and a tapering lower extremity. The oesophageal wall is thickened and there is almost complete atony. However, cholinergic drugs such as mecothane* in a dosage of 10 mg. given subcutaneously usually provoke vigorous contractions resulting in rapid

* Manufactured by Martindale, Samoore Ltd., London, England.

emptying of the oesophagus. The fluid-trap effect of the oesophageal residue prevents the formation of a gas bubble in the fundus of the stomach provided that the patient has been in the erect position for some time. The dilated oesophagus can sometimes be seen on a chest film as a soft-tissue shadow with a fluid level, slightly to the right of the midline.

In doubtful and early cases, motility studies help in diagnosis, but oesophagoscopy is usually necessary to exclude a carcinoma. Oesophagoscopy should also be carried out in established cases where there is a change in the character of symptoms and especially where there is an irregular obstruction or a long stricture at its lower extremity.

If adequate stretching of the gastro-oesophageal sphincter is carried out at an early stage of the disorder, the oesophagus ceases to dilate and the lower half may contract and resemble oesophageal spasm.

Following a successful Heller's operation, some dilatation may remain. Gastro-oesophageal reflux, however, may be a prominent feature.

Effect of Anticholinergic Drugs such as Atropine, Probanthine* or Buscopan on a Normal Oesophagus

These drugs markedly diminish or abolish movements, causing dilatation—the appearances mimicking those of diffuse systemic sclerosis (scleroderma). Thus, if a patient is being treated with an anticholinergic drug the radiologist must be informed otherwise an error in diagnosis can easily be made.

Cork-screw Oesophagus (curling)

This is more common in the elderly, and is seen particularly if thick barium is used. It is characterised by simultaneous contractions varying greatly in magnitude from a simple ripple in some patients to deep powerful contractions with pulsion diverticula in others—with pressures on motility studies up to 200 cm. of water. The site of the contractions varies. The diverticula are initially transient but ultimately become permanent. In all cases, a careful search must be made for a high gastric ulcer or an early oesophageal cancer or oesophagitis, as these can provoke this disorder.

In many cases the condition is symptomless, but in others pain is sometimes severe and difficult to

* Manufactured by G. D. Searle and Co. Ltd., High Wycombe, Bucks, England.

distinguish from cardiac angina. Dysphagia may be prominent.

The oesophageal wall in advanced cases becomes thickened by fibrosis and muscular hypertrophy which is most obvious on barium swallow using television or on cineradiography. The shortening of the oesophagus may induce a hiatus hernia.

This disorder is similar to diffuse oesophageal spasm which may represent a different phase of the same condition. Thus a patient may show features of one or the other at different times.

Diffuse Oesophageal Spasm

This is characterised by a prolonged powerful contraction of a long segment of lower oesophagus with proximal dilatation. In the late stages thickening of the oesophageal wall due to muscular hypertrophy is common and may be seen on films of good quality and on cineradiography. A hiatus hernia may also be present.

In rare instances muscular hypertrophy is present without pain or other symptoms.

Post-vagotomy Spasm

Rarely in the immediate post-operative period following vagotomy there is spasm of the lower two inches or so of the oesophagus causing a tapered uniform narrowing with proximal dilatation. Mild dysphagia is present, but the condition usually returns to normal in two to three weeks.

Crico-pharyngeal Indentation

It is virtually impossible to demonstrate the movements of the normal crico-pharyngeus on a film. If it fails to relax normally it causes a more persistent indentation of the posterior wall below the level of the cricoid cartilage. This is readily demonstrated on one or more spot films of the upper oesophagus and is differentiated from a carcinoma by being smooth and by the absence of a soft-tissue shadow. Occasionally in the stage of elevation during swallowing, there may be slight forwards displacement of the trachea.

This condition is usually associated with dysphagia located to the neck and may predispose to the development of a Zenker's diverticulum.

Cineradiography is of value in demonstrating the abnormally persistent contraction.

Spasm associated with Acute Infection

In severe pharyngeal and upper respiratory infections diffuse spasm causing a smooth uniform narrowing of the upper two to three inches of the oesophagus is sometimes present. This is usually associated with mild dysphagia.

Bulbar Palsy

The pharynx is dilated and there is inability to instigate movements of swallowing. Failure of relaxation of the crico-pharyngeus may also be observed.

Dystrophia Myotonica

The oesophagus is smooth, dilated and with diminished or absent motility throughout its entire length. Barium usually spills into the trachea.

Schatzki's Ring

This is a smooth localised narrowing of the oesophagus two to three inches above the cardia, but there is considerable confusion as to its nature. Some cases considered as such are more likely to be due to a hiatus hernia with localised oesophagitis. In all probability there are a number of different causes of this radiological abnormality including a ring of spasm, localised fibrosis due to a narrow band of oesophagitis and a rather prominent ridge at the junction between columnar and squamous epithelium.

Oesophagoscopy usually determines the precise aetiology.

Diffuse Systemic Sclerosis (Scleroderma)

The oesophagus is affected in this disease more frequently than was at one time thought. It is particularly important to examine the patient in the head-down position. In the early stages feeble simultaneous contractions appear in the middle of the oesophagus, and even although the gastro-oesophageal sphincter relaxes normally some dilatation with stasis is present.

As the disease progresses, impairment of motility becomes more marked and ultimately complete atony results. Reflux of gastric content is then unopposed causing oesophagitis which may be severe. A hiatus hernia commonly subsequently develops.

In suspected cases the rest of the alimentary tract

should be carefully examined for further evidence of this disease (pp. 128 and 201).

Dermatomyositis

The oesophagus may be affected in the late stage of the disease. It is characterised by smooth narrowing throughout its length with greatly diminished motility proceeding to atony.

Sideropenic Dysphagia (Plummer-Vinson syndrome)

In this condition a small shelf-like web may arise from the anterior wall of the cervical oesophagus. To demonstrate such a web it is advantageous to take four spot films—the X-ray exposure being made immediately after the barium has been swallowed and with the patient in the true lateral position.

There is some evidence that webs are occasionally present in normal individuals. They frequently escape detection since films of this part of the oesophagus are not taken as a routine. Sometimes the webs occur after partial gastrectomy—presumably associated with sideropenia.

Miscellaneous Neurological Disorders

In the aged, disordered movements are sometimes seen with dilatation and stasis.

In patients who have had a tracheo-oesophageal fistula or repair of atresia a curious motility disorder with irregular contractions and some stasis may be noted in the middle and lower oesophagus.

SIMPLE TUMOURS

These are rare. They cause smooth filling defects but the overlying mucosa is usually intact.

CARCINOMA

This is by far the commonest malignant tumour.

A barium meal is a very accurate diagnostic method. At an early stage a carcinoma produces a persistent localised irregularity of one wall—seen best with maximum oesophageal dilatation. Sometimes it is associated with feeble simultaneous contractions adjacent to the lesion simulating a cork-screw oesophagus and this might mislead the observer into diagnosing the more simple lesion. Unfortunately, by the time the patient comes for investigation, the disease is usually well advanced and presents the following radiological appearances:

Carcinoma of Cervical Oesophagus

Irregularity of the lumen with narrowing and a soft-tissue shadow displacing the trachea anteriorly are usually present. The barium readily coats the lesion so that films are easily obtained.

Carcinoma of the Middle and Lower Oesophagus

The most common radiological appearance is an irregular filling defect with narrowing of the lumen. There is slight dilatation proximally though not so marked as in most motility disorders. The tumour may show as a narrow central lumen with lateral shoulders ('bird on the wing' appearance), but this is not absolutely diagnostic of a carcinoma, and may occasionally be found in peptic oesophagitis. Only if the tumour is large can a soft-tissue swelling be detected.

Occasionally the lesion presents as a smooth stricture which at the lower end of the oesophagus mimics an oesophagitis or achalasia. In the middle of the oesophagus the stricture can be confused with a healed peptic ulcer in cases where the lower oesophagus is lined with columnar epithelium.

In other cases the tumour is bulky, causing an irregular filling defect in the oesophageal lumen. Sometimes such tumours extend over a considerable length and if situated in the lower half of the oesophagus may initially simulate oesophageal varices. The persistence of the defects, however, makes the diagnosis obvious.

Following radiotherapy the lumen may be smooth, but a waist-like narrowing usually remains.

In the late stages, a fistula to the trachea may develop, especially where there is a recurrence following radiotherapy.

In all cases a complete barium meal must be performed because a carcinoma in the lower oesophagus commonly arises as a direct extension from the fundus of the stomach. Occasionally also two tumours may be found. Oesophagoscopy is necessary for confirmation, to obtain biopsy material, and to make the diagnosis in a doubtful case. This is particularly so in long-standing cases of achalasia and peptic oesophagitis when it is suspected that a neoplasm might have supervened.

PERFORATION OF OESOPHAGUS

Preliminary films of the chest and neck must be taken and these show subcutaneous and mediastinal emphysema. If examination by a contrast medium is undertaken, Gastrografin and not barium must be used.

A perforation following oesophagoscopy is almost always posteriorly at the level of the sixth or seventh cervical vertebra. Perforation from retching and vomiting—the Mallory-Weiss syndrome—is uncommon. In such cases the tear is at the lower end of the oesophagus but its demonstration by Gastrografin is rarely possible.

FOREIGN BODIES IN THE OESOPHAGUS

To examine for a suspected foreign body in the oesophagus plain films of the neck and chest must always be taken initially. The presence of subcutaneous or mediastinal emphysema indicates a perforation. If the foreign body is opaque it can be detected on the films and no further examination is usually necessary except for the demonstration of the site of a possible perforation. If no foreign body is seen and there is no suspicion of a perforation a mouthful of barium should be swallowed under fluoroscopic control. The foreign body is usually coated with barium.

ACQUIRED DIVERTICULA

A Zenker's diverticulum originates posteriorly. It is preceded by failure of relaxation of the crico-pharyngeus and arises immediately above the attachment of this muscle to the pharynx. When large, barium initially enters the diverticulum and only when full does barium spill over into the oesophagus. The diverticulum may ultimately extend into the superior mediastinum.

Multiple diverticula arise as a result of a cork-screw oesophagus usually in the lower half. Initially they are transient but ultimately become permanent.

Occasionally a diverticulum is produced by traction from mediastinal lymph nodes.

HAEMATEMESIS

Varices and peptic ulceration are the commonest causes of a major haemorrhage from the oesophagus. Profuse bleeding from an oesophagitis is uncommon. The blood clot produces streaky filling defects in the column of barium readily seen moving up and down the oesophagus to a variable degree. When varices bleed they are usually large enough to be easily demonstrated by a barium meal. The radiologist, however, must not be satisfied with their detection and must search for a peptic ulcer in the stomach or duodenum which is not infrequently present and which may be the cause of the haematemesis.

STRICTURES OF THE OESOPHAGUS

Most fibrous stenoses are due to a chronic peptic oesophagitis. Others follow repair of perforations, tracheo-oesophageal fistulae, etc., and need no further description. Rarely a stricture follows vagotomy, presumably due to haemorrhage and/or trauma at the time of operation.

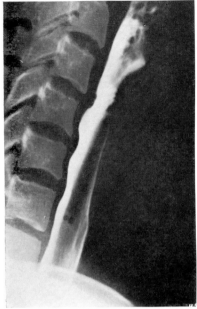

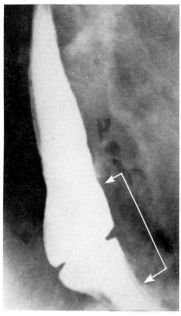

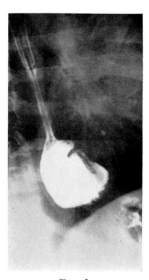

Fig. 3

Fig. 1

Fig. 2

Fig. 1. Normal cervical oesophagus. The posterior border of the oesophagus is parallel to the cervical spine and separated from it by only a few millimetres. **Fig. 2.** Normal lower oesophagus. The vestibule (arrowed)—a temporary fusiform dilatation of the lower end of the oesophagus—is clearly seen. Indentations in the middle of the vestibule now considered to be due to a prominent ridge of mucosa at the junction between squamous and columnar epithelium. The inferior oesophageal sphincter at upper end of the vestibule was relaxed at the moment the film was taken. **Fig. 3.** Normal oesophagus. Vestibule distended with barium and indented only on its anterior aspect—uncommon. Inferior oesophageal sphincter immediately above vestibule contracted at the moment the film was taken.

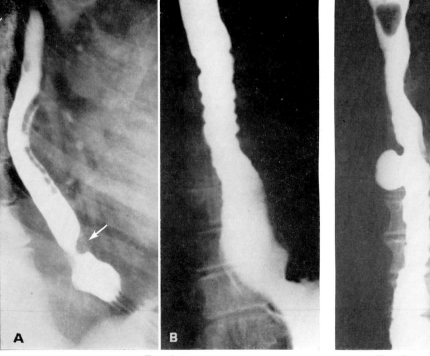

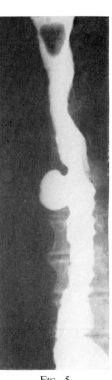

Fig. 6

Fig. 4

Fig. 5

Fig. 4. Tertiary contractions. Symptomless. A: Normal smooth outline. The translucencies are air bubbles. The inferior oesophageal sphincter (arrowed) was partially contracted at the moment the film was taken. The dilatation below this is the vestibule. B: A few seconds later. Ripple border due to fine synchronous contractions of the circular muscle. **Fig. 5.** Tertiary contractions involving the lower half of the oesophagus proceeding to a cork-screw oesophagus. Pulsion diverticulum present. The large translucency at the upper end of the oesophagus is an air bubble. **Fig. 6.** Senile oesophagus with disordered motility conforming to no definite pattern and resulting in stasis and dilatation. Female aged 85.

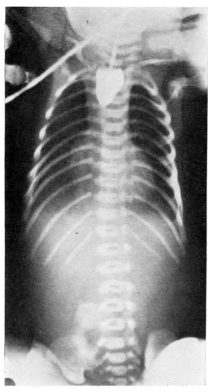

FIG. 7

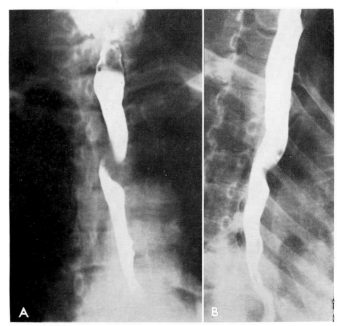

FIG. 8

Fig. 8. Bilateral pharyngocoele. Note air-filled pouches lateral to the spine and behind angle of mandible. The patient could distend them at will. Otherwise symptomless.

Fig. 7. Atresia of oesophagus. Fine catheter passed into proximal blind segment and a little Neo-hydriol injected demonstrating complete obstruction. Absence of gas in stomach and bowel indicating that there is no communication between the lower oesophageal segment and the left main bronchus or trachea. The Neo-hydriol is sucked out at end of examination.

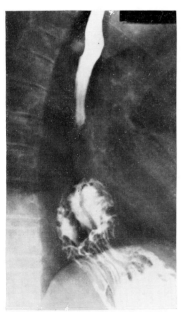

FIG. 9

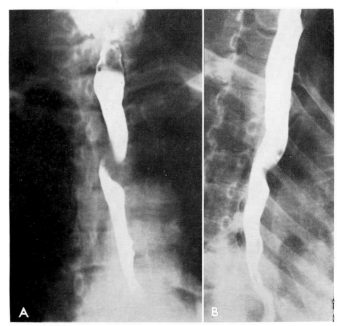

FIG. 10

Fig. 9. Aberrant right subclavian artery. Circular opacity causing indentation of the posterior wall of the oesophagus above the level of the carina—the common position. Sliding hiatus hernia also present with spasm of the lower oesophagus due to co-existing oesophagitis. Prone view. (Print reversed.) **Fig. 10.** Aberrant right subclavian artery anterior to the oesophagus —the less frequent position. A: P.A. view. Indentation of the oesophagus above the aortic arch at first sight suggesting a carcinoma. B: Oblique view—the indentation is on the anterior aspect.

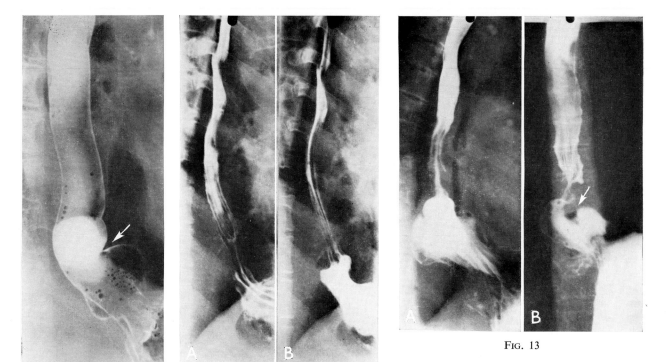

FIG. 11   FIG. 12   FIG. 13

Fig. 11. Sliding hiatus hernia with wide oesophago-gastric junction (arrowed) and free reflux. No obvious oesophagitis. Female, aged 80, with symptoms of heartburn and regurgitation, but with a low acid output. **Fig. 12.** Small sliding hiatus hernia. A: The mucosal folds from the body of the stomach extend proximally to the oesophago-gastric junction. A little spasm of the lower end of the oesophagus. B: The mucosal folds of the lower oesophagus are indistinct and wavy indicating a mild oesophagitis confirmed at oesophagoscopy. In spite of its small size the hernia required surgical repair because of the severity of the symptoms. **Fig. 13.** Sliding hiatus hernia. Localised chronic oesophagitis present with shoulders ('bird-on-the-wing' appearance) at the lower end of the oesophagus. A: Prone—oblique view. (Print reversed.) B: True A.P. Patient prone. (Print reversed.) Large mucosal fold (arrowed) running antero-posteriorly in the hernia immediately to the left of the oesophago-gastric junction. This fold is commonly seen in a hernia but is not seen in the vestibule.

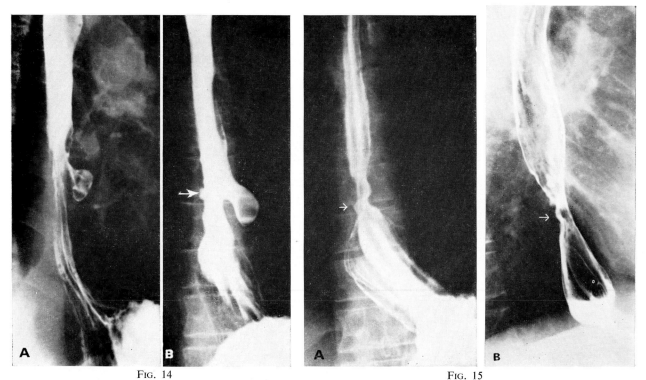

FIG. 14   FIG. 15

Fig. 14. Sliding hiatus hernia with oesophagitis and shortening of the oesophagus. A: The mucosal pattern of the fundal pouch when stretched and collapsed looks remarkably like oesophageal mucosa. B: The fundal pouch is distended showing clearly the presence of a hiatus hernia. Ulcer crater (arrowed) also seen at lower end of oesophagus. The congenital diverticulum containing food residue on the left side of the oesophagus acts as a convenient landmark for the study of the anatomy in both illustrations. **Fig. 15.** Sliding hiatus hernia with short oesophagus and ulcer (arrowed) at the lower end of the oesophagus. A: Prone view. (Print reversed.) The hernia is satisfactorily demonstrated with gastric-type mucosal folds extending up to the ulcerated area at the lower end of the oesophagus. B: Erect view. The hernia resembles the lower oesophagus. The narrowed ulcerated area at the lower end of the oesophagus is again clearly seen.

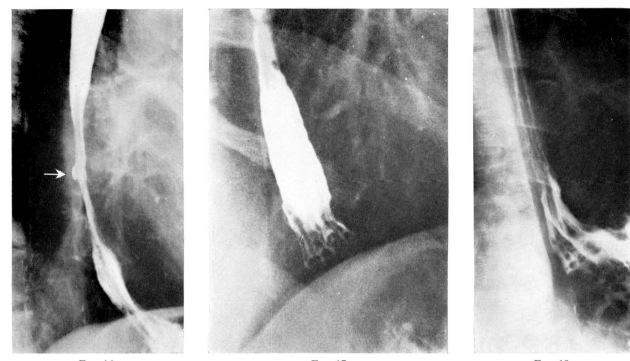

Fig. 16   Fig. 17   Fig. 18

Fig. 16. Sliding hiatus hernia with short oesophagus and long narrowed segment due to oesophagitis at the lower end of the oesophagus. Moderately large peptic ulcer (arrowed) also present. The herniated pouch of stomach is stretched and collapsed and looks remarkably like the lower oesophagus. Erect film. **Fig. 17.** Small sliding hiatus hernia. Obvious gastric type mucosal pattern above the diaphragm—the only suggestion of a hiatus hernia on this film. The hernia was more clearly demonstrated on other films. Complaint of heartburn and retro-sternal pain with some vomiting occasionally of a little blood. **Fig. 18.** Sliding hiatus hernia with short oesophagus. The prominent mucosal folds in the hernia are clearly seen to be continuous with those in the stomach below the diaphragm.

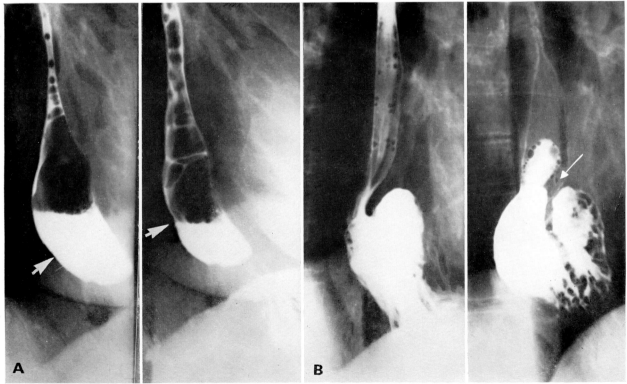

Fig. 19

Fig. 19. Sliding hiatus hernia. A: Erect films. A hiatus hernia cannot be diagnosed on these films alone. A point of change of motility (arrowed) was obvious on fluoroscopy indicating the probability of a hernia. B: Same case. Prone films. (Prints reversed.) Obvious hiatus hernia. In film on right typical large fold (arrowed) in the hernia running antero-posteriorly immediately to the left of the oesophago-gastric junction.

B

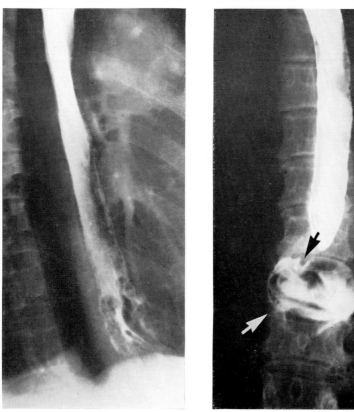

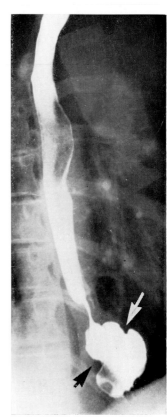

Fig. 20   Fig. 21   Fig. 22

Fig. 20. Sliding hiatus hernia with severe oesophagitis—indicated by failure of barium to adhere satisfactorily to the mucosa of the lower oesophagus causing a moth-eaten appearance and absent mucosal pattern. The prominent mucosal folds of the hernia are clearly depicted. Widely patent oesophago-gastric junction with free regurgitation. At oesophagoscopy gross oesophagitis with leukoplakia was found—more severe than the radiological appearance would have suggested. **Fig. 21.** Sliding hiatus hernia with indentations (arrowed) forming a cap at proximal part of hernia. The gastric mucosal folds obviously extend to the top of the cap. **Fig. 22.** Sliding hiatus hernia with persistent indentations (arrowed) causing a small pouch proximally like a cap.

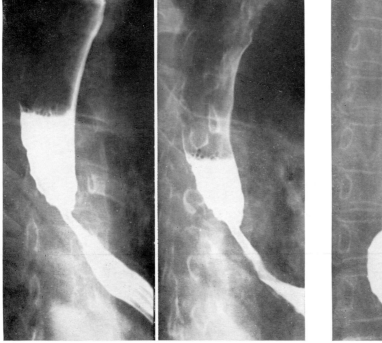

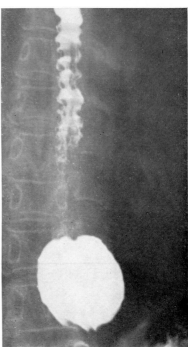

Fig. 23   Fig. 24

Fig. 23. Severe chronic oesophagitis with considerable narrowing at lower end of oesophagus causing some dilatation and stasis proximally. The oesophagus is short and a sliding hiatus hernia, which is stretched, is also present. Previous right pneumonectomy with subsequent compensatory emphysema on the left side. The depressed and flattened left dome of diaphragm obliterated the hiatal valve and permitted free regurgitation. **Fig. 24.** Tertiary contractions of oesophagus causing typical transverse ridging in a case of sliding hiatus hernia. Prone film. (Print reversed.)

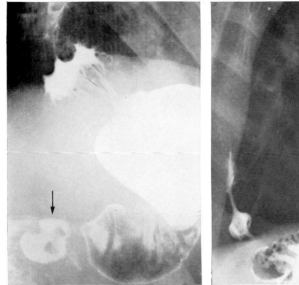

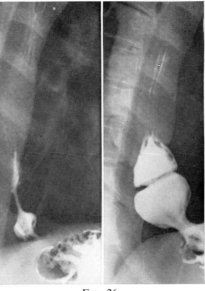

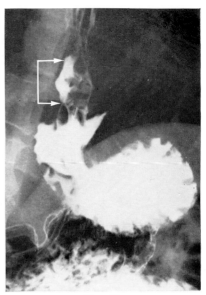

FIG. 25   FIG. 26   FIG. 27

Fig. 25. Sliding hiatus hernia associated with chronic oesophagitis and a duodenal ulcer (arrowed)—a common combination. In this case the inflammation affecting the lower end of the oesophagus is particularly severe—the swelling and oedema causing indentation of the fundus on each side of the oesophago-gastric junction. **Fig. 26.** Hiatus hernia and oesophagitis simulating Schatzki's ring. Interval of a few seconds between the two films. Oesophagoscopy revealed a hiatus hernia with leukoplakia and chronic oesophagitis. Duodenal ulcer also present. **Fig. 27.** Sliding hiatus hernia with large peptic ulcer (arrowed) of the Barrett type in the lower oesophagus. These ulcers originate in columnar type epithelium but may extend to involve the squamous epithelium. A few months previously the patient had had a severe bleed from this ulcer.

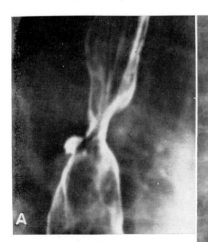

FIG. 28

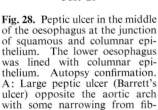

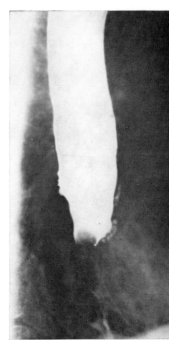

Fig. 28. Peptic ulcer in the middle of the oesophagus at the junction of squamous and columnar epithelium. The lower oesophagus was lined with columnar epithelium. Autopsy confirmation. A: Large peptic ulcer (Barrett's ulcer) opposite the aortic arch with some narrowing from fibrosis. B: After one month's treatment the ulcer has healed leaving a stricture. Small sliding hiatus hernia also demonstrated.

(By courtesy of the Editor of the *American Journal of Roentgenology*.)

FIG. 29

Fig. 29. Chronic oesophagitis causing a curious beaded appearance at the lower end of the oesophagus due to 'collar stud' type of ulceration. Stricture present at which a foreign body (a pea) had become impacted. Hiatus hernia also present—not clearly demonstrated because of the degree of oesophageal obstruction.

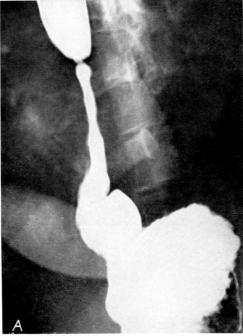
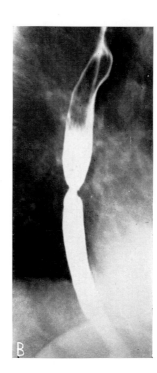

FIG. 30

Fig. 30. Lower oesophagus lined with columnar epithelium.   Narrowing from peptic ulceration a little below the level of the carina—proved at oesophagoscopy with biopsy to be at the junction of squamous and columnar epithelium.   Hiatus hernia also present.   A: Patient supine with the left side elevated and pressure applied to the stomach.   Hernia well demonstrated. B: Erect.   The stricture is clearly seen but the hernia is not demonstrated.

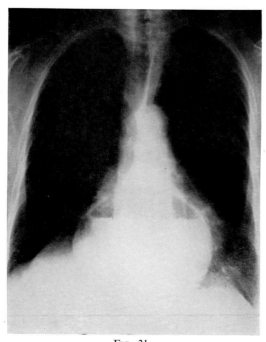
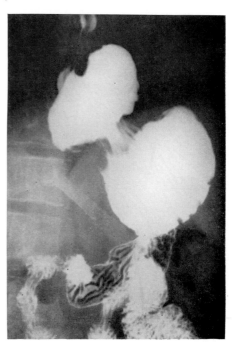

FIG. 31   FIG. 32

Fig. 31. Large para-oesophageal hiatus hernia containing a fluid level seen behind the heart.   This was an incidental finding on a chest film.

Fig. 32. Hiatus hernia due to a crush injury.   The hernia was initially of the para-oesophageal type, but an element of sliding subsequently occurred.   Normal appearance of remainder of stomach and duodenum.

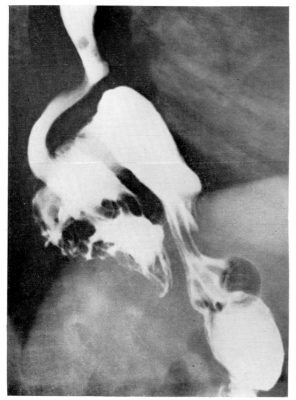

FIG. 33

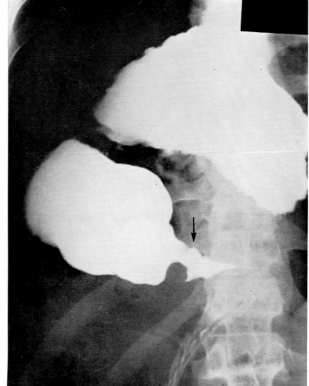

FIG. 34

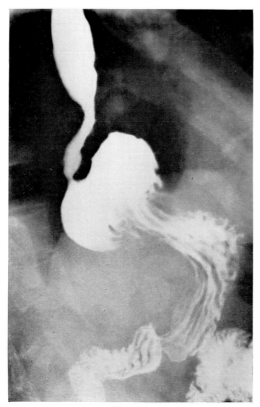

FIG. 35

Fig. 33. Para-oesophageal hiatus hernia—the oesophagus being of normal length. In spite of its size the hernia was symptomless and was an incidental finding.

Fig. 34. Large para-oesophageal hiatus hernia. The stomach has rotated so that the greater curvature is uppermost. Large duodenal ulcer also present (arrowed) which subsequently perforated.

Fig. 35. Para-oesophageal hiatus hernia with an element of sliding subsequently. Unusually severe oesophagitis causing narrowing and marginal irregularity due to ulceration in lower 4 in. to 5 in. (10 to 12 cm.) of oesophagus.

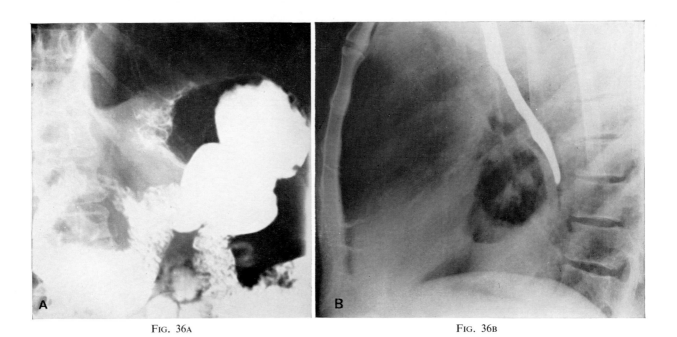

FIG. 36A

FIG. 36B

Fig. 36. Intermittent para-oesophageal hiatus hernia. A: Initial barium meal. No evidence of a hiatus hernia. B: Lateral chest film a few weeks later. Appearance suggests a large hiatus hernia. C: Second barium meal. Most of the stomach is in the hernial sac. Operation subsequently performed and presence of large hernia confirmed.

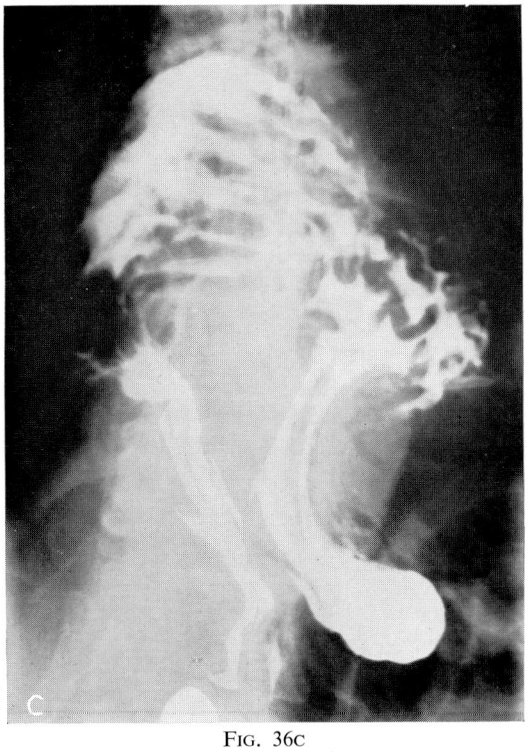

FIG. 36C

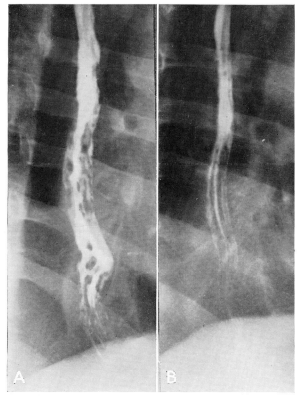

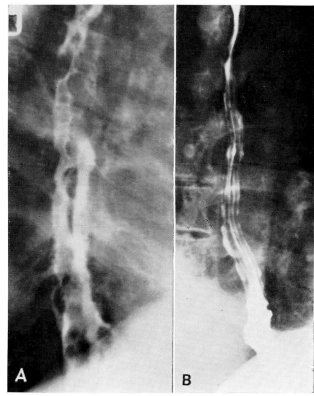

FIG. 37

FIG. 38

Fig. 37. Oesophageal varices involving the middle and lower oesophagus. A: Typical sinuous and marginal filling defects. B: After a peristaltic wave the varices are no longer seen. **Fig. 38.** Gross oesophageal varices. Supine oblique films. A: Large sinuous and marginal filling defects involving the lower two-thirds of the oesophagus. The oesophagus is also wider than normal to accommodate the large varices. B: The varices have disappeared following a successful porto-caval anastomosis.

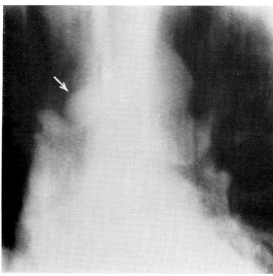

FIG. 39

Fig. 39. Dilatation of azygos vein (arrowed) in a case of gross oesophageal varices. Tomographic cut at level of carina.

Fig. 40. Oesophageal varices of moderate size. Characteristic sinuous filling defects seen in the middle of the oesophagus. In the lower oesophagus the varices are not seen because at the moment the film was taken the oesophagus was distended with barium which ironed out the varices. In addition a peristaltic wave seen near lower end had temporarily milked the blood from the varices.

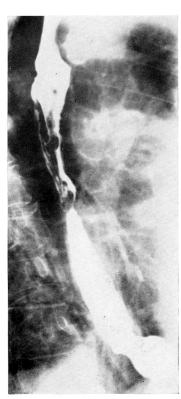

FIG. 40

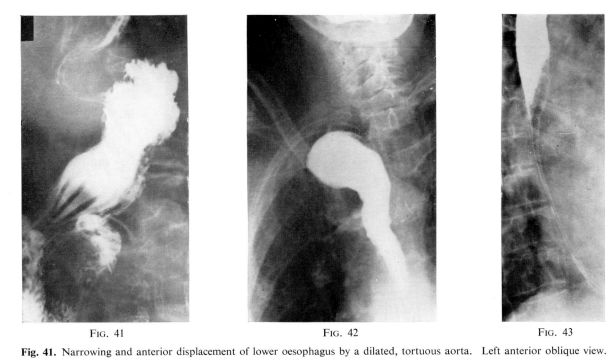

FIG. 41   FIG. 42   FIG. 43

Fig. 41. Narrowing and anterior displacement of lower oesophagus by a dilated, tortuous aorta.   Left anterior oblique view.

Fig. 42. Displacement of upper thoracic oesophagus to the right by chronic fibroid tuberculosis of the right upper lobe.

Fig. 43. Smooth narrowing of lower half of oesophagus due to involvement by fibrosis in a case of chronic pericarditis.   The mucosal pattern is intact.

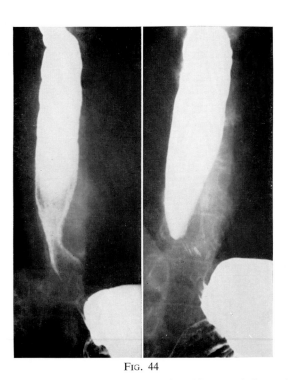

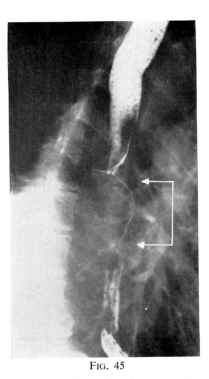

FIG. 44   FIG. 45

Fig. 44. Displacement and narrowing of lower end of oesophagus by a dilated atheromatous aorta.   Some dilatation proximally.   History of slight dysphagia.   Supine views.

Fig. 45. Bronchial carcinoma of right lower lobe causing oesophageal displacement and obstruction (arrowed).   Note also large soft tissue swelling posteriorly.   An intrinsic oesophageal carcinoma would not have caused such a degree of displacement.

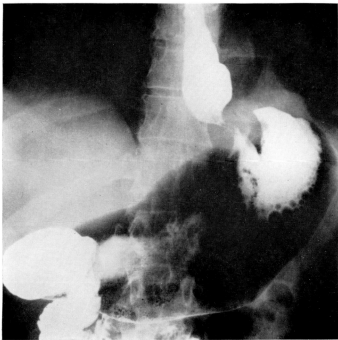

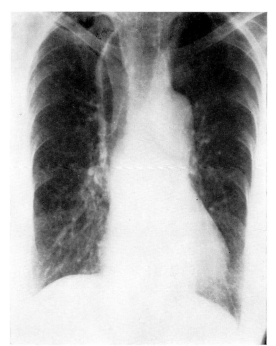

Fig. 46

Fig. 47

Fig. 46. Deformity of fundus of stomach due to fibrosis and a tight oesophageal hiatus following hiatus hernia repair. Distension of the stomach with gas from inability to belch.

Fig. 47. Achalasia of oesophagus. Routine chest film shows gross dilatation of oesophagus with thickening of its wall due to a stagnation oesophagitis. This is seen on the patient's right side opposite the superior mediastinum. Indistinct fluid level behind the heart. Dilatation of oesophagus to this degree is almost always due to achalasia.

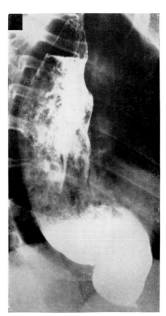

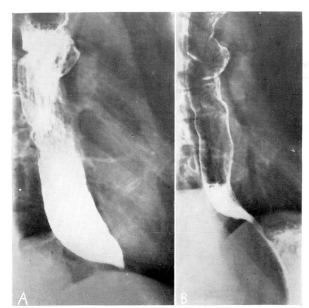

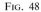

Fig. 48

Fig. 49

Fig. 48. Achalasia of the oesophagus—late stage. Characteristic appearance, viz. gross dilatation, large food and fluid residue, tortuosity, tapering lower extremity and absence of gastric air bubble.

Fig. 49. Achalasia of oesophagus. A: Gross dilatation with large residue and typical rat-tail narrowing of the lower extremity. Absence of gastric air bubble because the oesophageal fluid residue acts as a trap. B: Following mecothane (a cholinergic drug), rapid emptying confirming the diagnosis of achalasia.

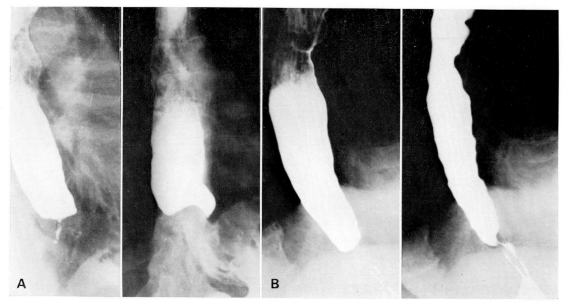

Fig. 50

Fig. 50. Achalasia of oesophagus with unusual radiological features causing difficulty in diagnosis. A: Two films showing irregular narrowing at the lower end of the oesophagus with dilatation proximally and a fluid residue. A carcinoma could not be excluded. No hiatus hernia demonstrated. Oesophagoscopy impossible because of osteo-arthritis of the cervical spine. Treated conservatively as the patient was a poor operative risk. B: Three years later. Some clinical improvement. Normal mucosal pattern clearly seen at the lower end of the oesophagus supporting the diagnosis of achalasia. Tertiary contractions also present in the oesophagus seen on the right hand film. A chronic duodenal ulcer was also present—a common association.

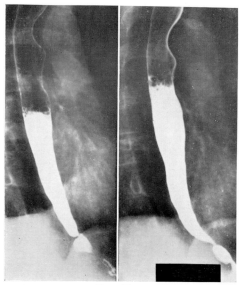

Fig. 51

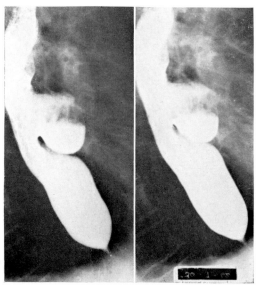

Fig. 52

Fig. 51. Achalasia of the oesophagus. Only minimal dilatation and stasis because of bouginage on numerous occasions at an early stage in the disease. Small diverticulum at lower end possibly congenital but might be the result of trauma. History of dysphagia for 20 years with regurgitation of undigested food. Heller's operation with relief of symptoms.

Fig. 52. Achalasia of oesophagus with stricture at lower end from stagnation oesophagitis. Persistent dilatation proximally with a food residue. Differentiation from a scirrhous type of carcinoma was not radiologically possible. No hiatus hernia demonstrated. At oesophagoscopy no evidence of a carcinoma. Treatment by dilatation. Patient alive and well six years later. Congenital diverticulum present—an incidental finding.

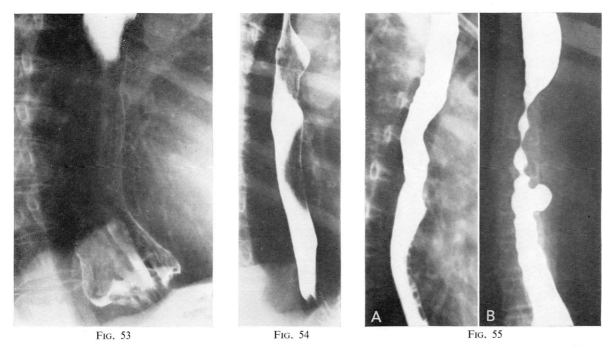

Fig. 53   Fig. 54   Fig. 55

Fig. 53. Achalasia of oesophagus following Heller's operation. Persistent dilatation—rather more than usual—but no thickening of the wall indicating absence of stagnation oesophagitis. The barium passed into the stomach without delay. Clinical cure. **Fig. 54.** Effect of atropine on a normal oesophagus. Dilatation with diminished motility and excellent mucosal coating due to absence of secretion. The appearances resemble diffuse systemic sclerosis (scleroderma)—in fact this was the radiological diagnosis until it was ascertained he was being treated with atropine for peptic ulcer type pain. **Fig. 55.** Tertiary contractions of oesophagus. A: Almost normal appearance. The translucencies present are due to swallowed air. B: A few seconds later. Classical synchronous contractions with one large diverticulum.

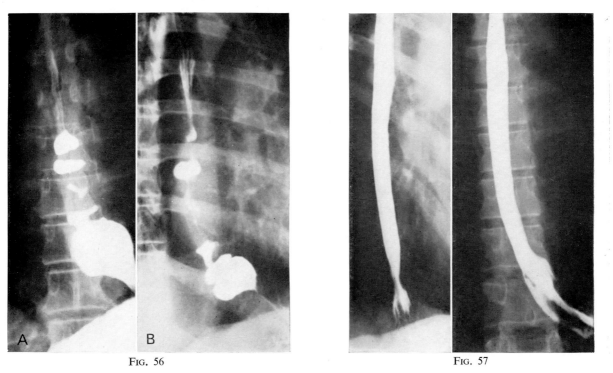

Fig. 56   Fig. 57

Fig. 56. Characteristic cork-screw oesophagus. A and B: Variable contractions of the circular muscle. Patient previously had a repair of a hiatus hernia. Now no symptoms referable to his oesophagus.

Fig. 57. Diffuse oesophageal spasm involving lower two thirds of oesophagus and with uniform narrowing of the lumen. Small hiatus hernia also present. Prolonged powerful contractions extending over a considerable length noted on fluoroscopy and on motility studies. Complaint of intermittent dysphagia with retro-sternal pain

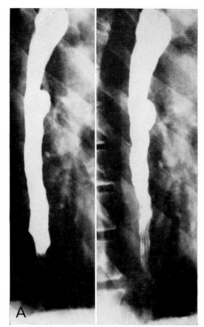

FIG. 58A

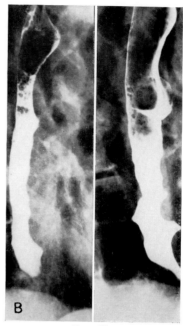

FIG. 58B

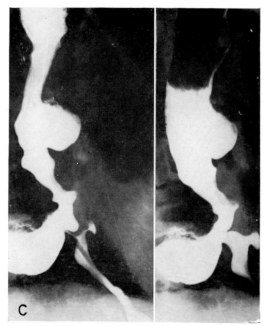

FIG. 58C

Fig. 58. Cork-screw oesophagus associated with diffuse oesophageal spasm—an extremely severe case. History of rheumatoid arthritis and Raynaud's phenomenon for 20 years. Kerato-conjunctivitis sicca of more recent onset. A: Barium swallow showing marked spasm of lower half of oesophagus with irregular synchronous contractions and tendency to formation of diverticula. B: Six months later—synchronous contractions more pronounced. Diverticula more obvious. Motility studies demonstrated pressures up to 200 cm. of water. C: Four years later—further progress of disease. Gross distortion of the oesophagus with the presence of numerous large persistent diverticula. Stasis in upper oesophagus. Pain and dysphagia now severe. Long myotomy performed and diverticula excised with considerable clinical improvement.

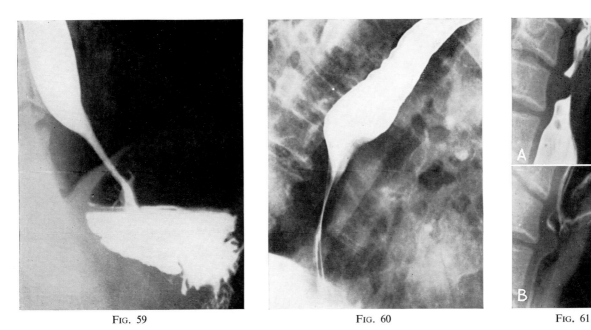

FIG. 59   FIG. 60   FIG. 61

Fig. 59. Post-vagotomy oesophageal spasm causing a smooth tapered narrowing of lower 3 in. (7 cm.) with a little dilatation proximally. Difficulty in swallowing for two weeks following vagotomy and partial gastrectomy for a duodenal ulcer. Subsequent complete recovery.

Fig. 60. Post-vagotomy fibrosis of oesophagus causing a long smooth stricture and dilatation proximally—a rare complication. Persistent dysphagia following vagotomy for duodenal ulcer.
(By courtesy of the Editor of the *Journal of the Royal College of Surgeons of Edinburgh*.)

Fig. 61. Crico-pharyngeal indentation due to failure of relaxation of crico-pharyngeus. A: Patient not actively swallowing. Typical smooth persistent indentation posteriorly. B: During the act of swallowing the indentation is still obvious. Approximation of crico-pharyngeus to the larynx. At this moment there is a soft tissue swelling anteriorly which must not be mistaken for a carcinoma.

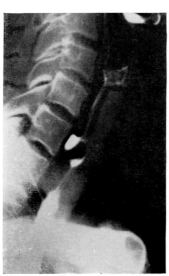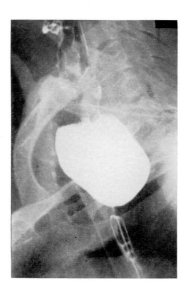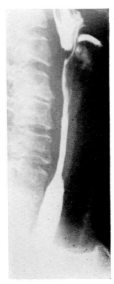

FIG. 62   FIG. 63   FIG. 64

Fig. 62. Crico-pharyngeal indentation with the subsequent development of a small pharyngeal diverticulum immediately above it. History of difficulty in swallowing for a few months with some regurgitation.

Fig. 63. Large pharyngeal diverticulum extending posteriorly and to the left—the usual position. On swallowing, barium initially entered the diverticulum. Only when it was full did barium spill over into the oesophagus.

Fig. 64. Diffuse spasm of upper 3 in. (7 cm.) of oesophagus due to acute pharyngeal and upper respiratory infection. Some difficulty in swallowing localised to the neck. Marked congestion of the pharynx. Complete recovery following penicillin.

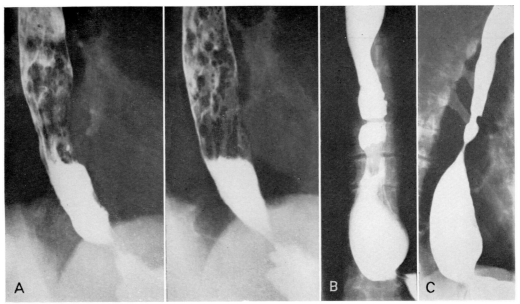

FIG. 65

Fig. 65. Motility disorder simulating achalasia in a case of congenital tracheo-oesophageal fistula treated surgically two years previously. Recent complaint of difficulty in swallowing with weight loss and vomiting. A: Two erect films showing persistent dilatation of oesophagus with a fluid residue and smooth narrowing of its lower end similar to achalasia. The motility studies were unusual with no sphincter zones and feeble contractions in the lower half. B. and C: Following mecothane, vigorous disordered movements developed with increase in the rate of emptying.

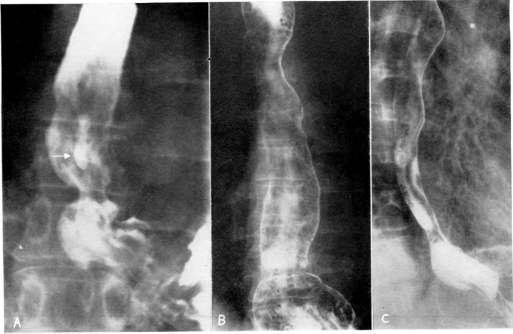

FIG. 66

Fig. 66. Diffuse systemic sclerosis with dilatation and almost complete atony. Hiatus hernia with free reflux also present. Case of chronic rheumatoid arthritis and Raynaud's phenomenon. A: Ulcer (arrowed) at lower end of oesophagus. Prone position. (Print reversed.) B: After treatment the ulcer has healed but the hiatus hernia and atony of oesophagus remain. Prone position. (Print reversed.) C: Erect film. Hiatus hernia and some oesophageal dilatation though not so marked as when horizontal. Obvious pulmonary fibrosis.

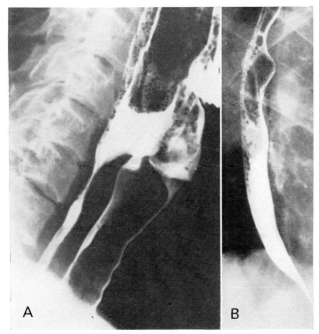
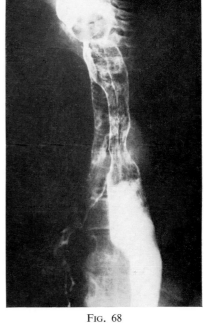

FIG. 67   FIG. 68

Fig. 67. Dermatomyositis. Characteristic smooth narrowing with rigidity and diminished motility. A: Cervical oesophagus. B: Thoracic oesophagus. On fluoroscopy inco-ordination of oesophageal movements with spillage of barium into the trachea. History of progressive dysphagia and weight loss for 10 months. Remainder of gastro-intestinal tract normal. Good response to dilatation and steroids.

Fig. 68. Dystrophia myotonica. Characteristic dilated atonic oesophagus with mucosal atrophy. Inco-ordination of movements of swallowing resulting in barium spilling into the larynx and down the trachea.

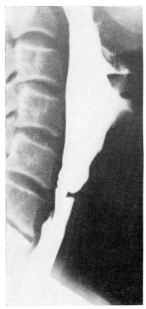
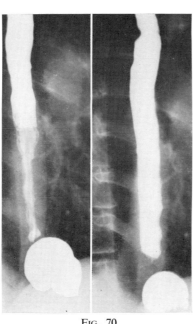
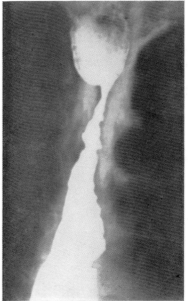

FIG. 69   FIG. 70   FIG. 71

Fig. 69. Oesophageal web. Narrow, sharp, shelf-like filling defect arising from the anterior wall of the cervical oesophagus. Case of sideropenic dysphagia (Plummer-Vinson's syndrome) in a female aged 50. Presence of web confirmed by oesophagoscopy.

Fig. 70. Diffuse muscular hypertrophy of oesophagus with spasm and a small hiatus hernia. The thickened oesophageal wall is clearly seen. Minimal symptoms referable to the oesophagus. Incidental finding on barium meal in case of carcinoma of head of pancreas.

Fig. 71. Fibrosis with stenosis of the oesophagus over a considerable length caused by leakage of thorotrast at the time of a carotid angiogram 20 years previously. Note thorotrast in the soft tissues around the barium-filled oesophagus.

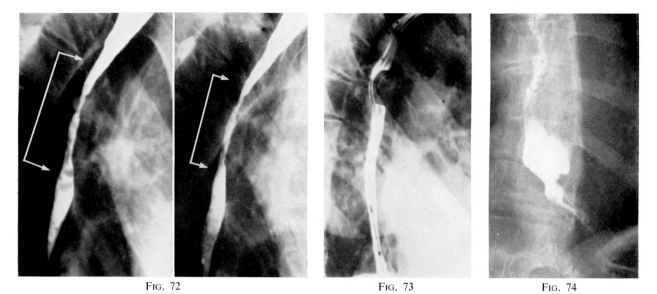

FIG. 72   FIG. 73   FIG. 74

Fig. 72. Epidermolysis bullosa. Narrowing of oesophagus (arrowed) with multiple indentations caused by superficial bullae.

Fig. 73. Benign tumour of oesophagus at level of carina with smooth outline and covered by mucosa with normal pattern. Confirmed at oesophagoscopy. Incidental finding.

Fig. 74. Carcinoma of lower oesophagus causing an irregular filling defect and partial 'bird-on-the-wing' appearance. Dilatation of the oesophagus proximal to the tumour.

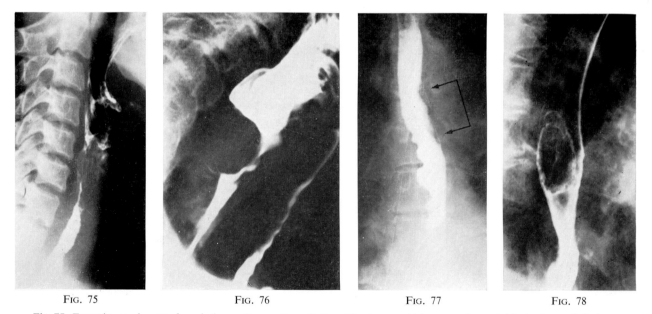

FIG. 75   FIG. 76   FIG. 77   FIG. 78

Fig. 75. Extensive carcinoma of cervical oesophagus. Irregularity of the lumen which was easily coated by barium. Soft tissue swelling especially anteriorly.

Fig. 76. Carcinoma of cervical oesophagus causing a large filling defect posteriorly—smoother than usual. It is easily differentiated from the crico-pharyngeal indentation by its size, persistence and the soft tissue swelling anteriorly causing slight forward displacement of the trachea. The oesophageal obstruction has caused some barium to spill over into the trachea.

Fig. 77. Carcinoma of oesophagus. Irregularity of left lateral border opposite the carina (arrowed). The tumour was visible only on maximum oesophageal dilatation. Initial biopsies were negative and only after one year was histological proof obtained. Mild cork-screw oesophagus also present—an occasional incidental finding.

Fig. 78. Localised fungating type of carcinoma of the middle of the oesophagus causing a bulky filling defect. This is an uncommon type of tumour.

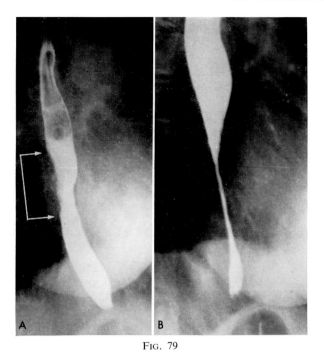

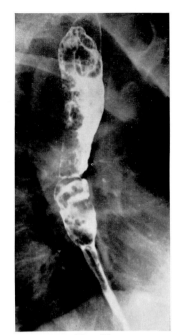

FIG. 79   FIG. 80

Fig. 79. Carcinoma of oesophagus.   A: Superficial irregularity (arrowed) only visible with maximal distension.   B: Six months later following radiotherapy.   Smooth residual narrowing of oesophagus due to fibrosis.

Fig. 80. Diffuse fungating carcinoma of oesophagus involving its upper two-thirds and with a large extrinsic mass posteriorly. This is a rare type of tumour.

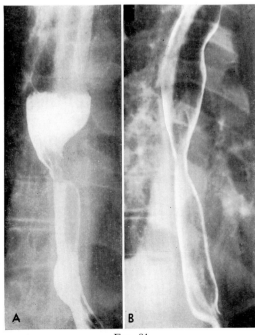

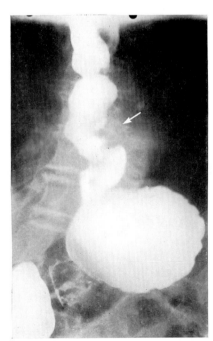

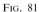

FIG. 81   FIG. 82

Fig. 81. Carcinoma of mid oesophagus—a common site.   A: Obstruction with dilatation proximally and a small fluid residue.   B: After radiotherapy, marked improvement with characteristic smooth waist-like narrowing at the treated site.   The calibre of the affected area rarely returns to normal.

Fig. 82. Large bulky carcinoma (arrowed) of lower oesophagus immediately above a sliding hiatus hernia which was demonstrated more clearly on other views.

C

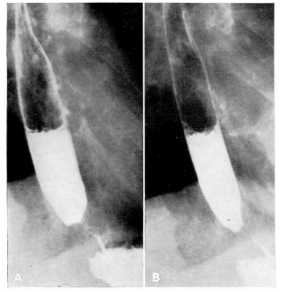

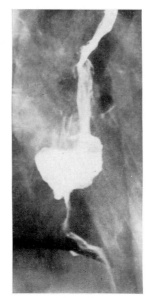

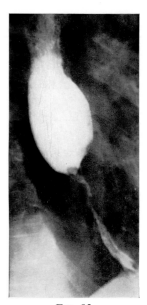

Fig. 83   Fig. 84   Fig. 85

Fig. 83. Carcinoma of lower end of oesophagus causing some difficulty in diagnosis. A: The obstruction is irregular and suggests a carcinoma. B: A few seconds later the narrowing is smoother and could be mistaken for achalasia.

Fig. 84. Carcinoma of oesophagus in a long-standing case of achalasia. Large irregular filling defect at lower end with gross dilatation and a large fluid residue proximally. The barium pouring down the dilated oesophagus forms a relatively narrow stream in front of the large fluid residue.

Fig. 85. Carcinoma of lower oesophagus causing an irregular stricture with multiple small filling defects. Case of hiatus hernia with chronic oesophagitis, shortening and dilatation proximally. Malignancy was suspected radiologically but oesophagoscopy was required for confirmation. The hiatus hernia is stretched and its mucosal pattern simulates normal oesophageal mucosa.

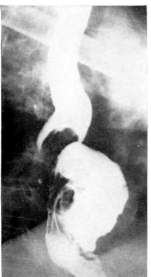

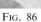

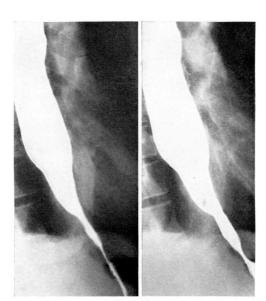

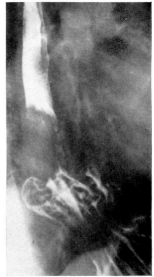

Fig. 86   Fig. 87   Fig. 88

Fig. 86. Fungating carcinoma of fundus of stomach involving lower oesophagus in a patient with a para-oesophageal hiatus hernia. Known case of hiatus hernia but recent history of increasing difficulty in swallowing and weight loss.

Fig. 87. Diffuse scirrhous carcinoma of lower end of oesophagus due to an extension from the stomach. On these two films a diffuse oesophageal spasm could not be excluded but examination of stomach made the diagnosis obvious.

Fig. 88. Carcinoma of the lower end of the oesophagus causing an irregular filling defect. Case of sliding hiatus hernia with chronic oesophagitis of many years duration. The degree of obstruction and eccentric channel suggest a carcinoma rather than a simple oesophagitis, but oesophagoscopy was necessary for confirmation.

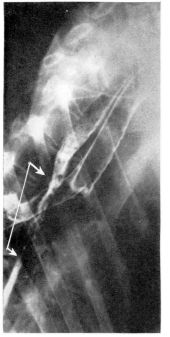
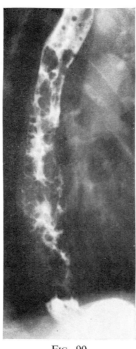
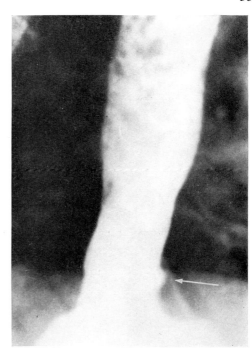

FIG. 89   FIG. 90   FIG. 91

Fig. 89. Perforation of a recurrence of a carcinoma of oesophagus. Treatment by radiotherapy one year previously. Gastrografin swallow shows a long irregular stricture (arrowed) opposite the carina. Some Gastrografin has entered the trachea through the fistula.

Fig. 90. Extensive recurrence of a gastric carcinoma in the oesophagus causing widespread filling defects. Partial gastrectomy two years previously.

Fig. 91. Ulcer (arrowed) in lower oesophagus causing massive haematemesis. Hiatus hernia also present—not shown on this film. Gross reflux of barium from stomach obvious on fluoroscopy. The filling defects seen in the column of barium in the lower oesophagus are due to blood clot. The patient was on steroids for severe ulcerative colitis and died two weeks later from toxic dilatation of the colon. Autopsy confirmation of hiatus hernia and bleeding ulcer.

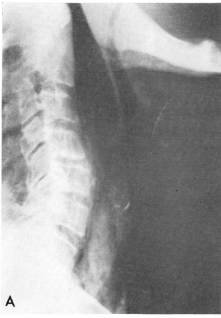
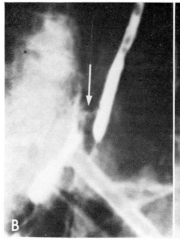
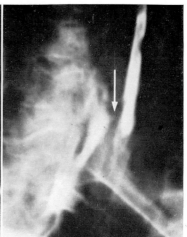

FIG. 92B

FIG. 92A

Fig. 92. Perforation of upper oesophagus following oesophagoscopy. A: Lateral view of neck. Gross surgical emphysema. B: Two films show leak of Gastrografin (arrowed) posteriorly from lower cervical oesophagus—the common site. Injection of Gastrografin down a Levine tube with side openings is preferable for examination of cervical oesophagus.

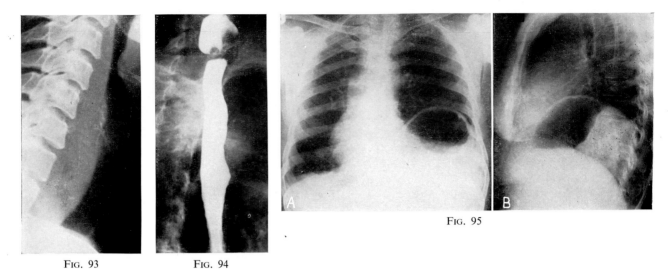

FIG. 93   FIG. 94   FIG. 95

Fig. 93. Retropharyngeal abscess following perforation of oesophagus.   Soft tissue swelling with traces of gas behind the trachea, displacing it forwards.

Fig. 94. Fibrous stricture of oesophagus following perforation in root of neck 16 months previously.   Successfully treated by bouginage.

Fig. 95. Eventration of diaphragm.   Elevation of left dome of diaphragm with paralysis indicated by paradoxical movements on fluoroscopy.   Large gastric air bubble.   A: P.A. view.   B: Lateral view.

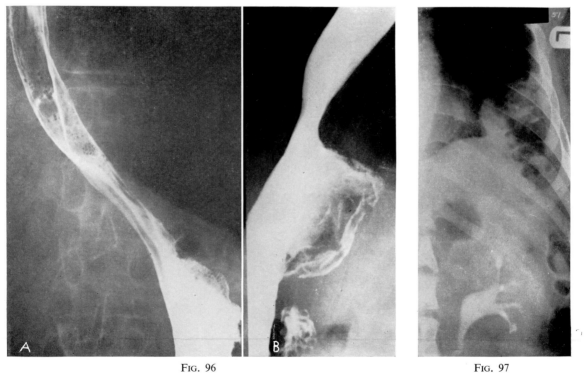

FIG. 96   FIG. 97

Fig. 96. Easy regurgitation due to low left dome of diaphragm and absence of the hiatal valve.   Emphysema of left lung following right pneumonectomy.   A: P.A. view.   B: Supine, oblique view with left side raised.

Fig. 97. Hernia through pleuro-peritoneal hiatus containing splenic flexure of colon, depicted by gas and faecal content. Incidental finding during an intravenous pyelogram.

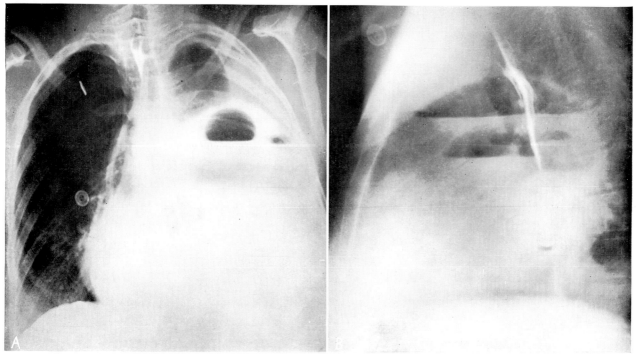

FIG. 98

Fig. 98. Large hernia through left dome of diaphragm containing small bowel. Multiple air-fluid levels present. A: P.A. view. B: Lateral view. Repair of hiatus hernia several years previously. Sudden development of severe upper abdominal and chest pain. At operation some loops of small bowel were ischaemic. Presumably the hernia had developed after the operation for hiatus hernia repair and had suddenly become strangulated.

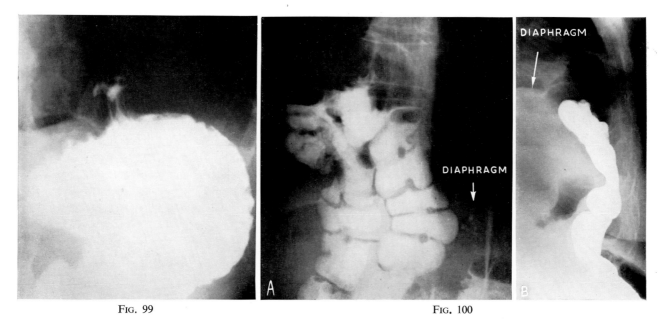

FIG. 99   FIG. 100

Fig. 99. Hernia of small part of fundus of stomach through a congenital foramen in left dome of diaphragm. On a chest film an opacity was seen suggesting a peripheral bronchial carcinoma.

Fig. 100. Hernia of transverse colon through foramen of Morgagni. Incidental finding on the follow-through of a barium meal. A: A.P. view. B: Lateral view showing the hernia situated anteriorly.

CHAPTER III

THE STOMACH

METHODS OF EXAMINATION

Plain erect and supine films are of limited value. They are necessary in acute abdominal emergencies especially when a perforation is suspected and may be taken in cases of pyloric or duodenal obstruction to show the degree of distension. They are also necessary if a swallowed foreign body is suspected and as a preliminary to the investigation of post-operative complications.

Sometimes a tumour may be shown as a filling defect when the stomach contains an adequate amount of gas. In particular, a fundal carcinoma can sometimes be seen on a film of the chest. Rarely a large simple ulcer may be detected by the translucency extending beyond the border of the stomach due to retained air in the crater.

A barium meal is the standard method of examination, including cases of massive haematemesis. For most conditions it is a very accurate diagnostic method. In certain parts of the stomach, particularly the body and proximal part of the antrum, gastroscopy and the gastro-camera are more valuable for the detection of the finer points of detail. It is however worth noting that a small lesion, e.g. ulcer or carcinoma, may not be detected at laparotomy without opening the stomach.

A Gastrografin meal is used in the investigation of acute abdominal emergencies and immediate post-operative complications.

CLINICAL RADIOLOGY

NORMAL APPEARANCES

It is not proposed to describe these at length but only to draw attention to the following points.

The distance between the fundus of the stomach and the base of the left lung is variable. Occasionally it represents only the thickness of the diaphragm but sometimes the left lobe of the liver extends across the midline and substantially increases this distance. In such cases differentiation from a tumour of the fundus in the form of a plaque may be difficult.

The normal retro-gastric space is also variable as it depends upon the build of the patient. It is usually less than the width of a normal vertebral body but in thick-set individuals may be greater.

The mucosal pattern of the fundus and most of the greater curvature is coarser and more irregular than elsewhere. On the lesser curvature aspect and in the antrum the folds tend to be parallel to the long axis of the stomach. At the junction of the lesser curve with the fundus care must be taken not to mistake the normal folds for an ulcer. Sometimes in the prepyloric region a fold runs transversely and may mimic an ulcer or a congenital diaphragm.

Occasionally the region of the cardiac orifice presents a funnelled appearance with radiating folds when seen *en face*—simulating early gastric varices. Another view at approximately right angles to the previous one is helpful in differentiation.

Cup and spill deformity is so common at least in a minor degree that it can be considered a normal variant. In the erect position barium initially enters the distended fundus which sags down posteriorly and only when the fundus is filled does barium spill over into the body of the stomach. By the end of the meal the stomach may have returned to a more usual shape. Care should always be taken not to miss a gastric ulcer at the junction of the fundus with the body.

CONGENITAL ANOMALIES

Congenital Hypertrophic Pyloric Stenosis. To save time and reduce irradiation, the examination should start about five minutes after the barium has been given to the baby. The baby is examined prone and gradually turned into the right lateral or almost right lateral position. Films are taken when the duodenal bulb is filled. The radiological appearances of this abnormality are characteristic and similar to the adult form of the disease—elongation and narrowing of the pylorus with intact mucosa, indentation of base of the bulb, etc. (p. 44). The stomach is dilated and the peristaltic waves are vigorous. If the myotomy is incomplete following a Ramstedt operation some deformity with narrowing remains.

Antral spasm may cause confusion but the prepyloric narrowing in this condition is not so marked and tends to be more conical. Following medical treatment and proper feeding, the appearances in antral spasm rapidly disappear and the pylorus returns to normal.

A gastric diverticulum almost always occurs on the postero-medial aspect of the fundus and should not be mistaken for an ulcer, especially as its size does not vary at different examinations. Characteristically it is flask-shaped and is lined with normal gastric type mucosa which can be readily demonstrated. Occasionally when filled with air, it causes a translucency which can also be detected on a plain film.

Duplication of the stomach is a very rare abnormality.

A congenital diaphragm in the antrum causes a sharp indentation of the lumen in the prepyloric region. It is usually symptomless but in some instances causes obstruction.

A cholecyst-duodenal band causes a smooth localised indentation of the lesser curvature aspect of the antrum and usually the greater curvature is unaffected. The mucosal pattern is normal and only rarely is an actual obstruction present.

Congenital absence of the muscular coat is very rare. Perforation of the stomach occurs shortly after birth.

Malrotation of the fore-gut is also very rare. The stomach lies on the right side behind the liver which is in its normal position. The small and large bowel are also normally situated.

GASTRIC ULCER

A gastric ulcer is the lesion most commonly found in the stomach. It appears as a projection beyond the normal border of the stomach in the profile view. When *en face*, the ulcer shows as a persistent localised barium residue which becomes more obvious when the surrounding barium is dispersed by compression or palpation.

The erect position is excellent for the demonstration of ulcers on the lesser curvature, especially towards its posterior wall—the most common site. This position is also satisfactory for showing ulcers on the greater curvature of the body and antrum. A fluid level is sometimes present in a large ulcer. Ulcers at the incisura may be difficult to detect with the patient erect, even when firm compression used.

The supine position with the left side slightly raised is best for demonstrating ulcers at the incisura. When the right side is raised ulcers in the antrum and prepyloric region are clearly demonstrated, and fortunately, the duodenum is also best seen in this position so that this supine-oblique film is most valuable.

Ulcers at the incisura and in the antrum may also be satisfactorily shown in the prone position, especially if a large fluid residue is present in the stomach.

The best method of confirming an ulcer high up on the posterior wall of the lesser curvature suspected in the erect position is to demonstrate it *en face* by the technique previously described (p. 3).

An ulcer may be difficult to detect in a hiatus hernia and the prone position is recommended with the fundus coated with barium and distended with air. These ulcers have a special tendency to bleed, sometimes severely.

Hour-glass deformity due to a chronic gastric ulcer is now rare in this country. Fibrosis from a chronic antral lesser curve ulcer causes shortening of the lesser curvature and bulging of the greater curvature— the 'scrotal' or 'tea-pot' stomach. This is more common presumably because an ulcer at this site is more likely to escape detection at any early stage and thus may remain untreated for a period.

A barium meal is an essential investigation in estimating the progress of an ulcer. When healing occurs radiating folds due to scarring are commonly seen. Sometimes a dimple may remain which, on a barium meal, cannot be differentiated from a small ulcer crater.

In the case of a prepyloric ulcer, healing can cause two different types of deformity—stenosis resembling an adult hypertrophic pyloric stenosis, or more commonly flattening of one aspect usually the lesser curvature adjacent to the pylorus. There is a variable fluid residue and dilatation of the stomach.

When a cup and spill deformity is present a careful

search must be made for an ulcer at the junction of the fundus with the body as previously described (p. 3).

Gastric stasis, e.g. from pyloric stenosis, duodenal stenosis, duodenal ileus, etc., predisposes to the development of a gastric ulcer. There is an interesting form of atony associated with a gastric ulcer where a large glutinous residue is present without any mechanical obstructive cause. On a barium meal this residue causes an appearance simulating polyposis of the stomach and masks the ulcer. The residue is also extremely difficult to wash out. In such cases healing of the ulcer is accelerated by drainage, e.g. gastro-enterostomy.

Perforation of a gastric ulcer is not nearly so common as in the case of a duodenal ulcer. The methods of investigation and radiological appearances are similar (p. 95).

The following appearances may occasionally cause difficulty and lead to over-diagnosis of an ulcer. Careful fluoroscopy and films at different angles usually clarify the position.

1. 'Furrowing' of the antrum due to peristaltic waves may simulate a greater curve ulcer. A fluoroscopic study of the waves easily prevents this erroneous diagnosis. Similarly, two peristaltic waves close together may simulate a lesser curve ulcer.

2. Coarse mucosal folds of the greater curvature emerging from behind the lesser curvature when viewed in the erect right anterior oblique position.

3. The summit of the duodeno-jejunal flexure when it extends just above the incisura.

4. Coarse mucosal folds at the junction of the lesser curvature with the fundus. Four 'spot' films of this area should be taken in the erect position and, if necessary, another series *en face* as previously described (p. 3). A careful study is then made of the course of these folds.

5. The posterior aspect of the fundus of the stomach commonly hangs down producing a 'fringe'. If the medial aspect of this fringe protrudes beyond the lesser curve, an ulcer may erroneously be diagnosed. Careful study shows that this projection is part of the 'fringe'.

6. On fluoroscopy a swallowed metallic foreign body or metallic clips at the suture line of a partial gastrectomy may closely resemble an ulcer. The improved detail on a film makes the diagnosis easy.

Differentiation between a Simple and Malignant Ulcer

This is a most important decision and fortunately the great majority of ulcers are and remain simple. Occasionally, however, the most innocent-looking ulcer ultimately turns out to be malignant. Thus, in all cases, healing should be checked gastroscopically or radiologically, and if complete, malignancy can be excluded except in very rare instances. The observation of complete healing is particularly important when mucosal atrophy is present.

An ulcer should always be looked upon as possibly malignant when it has a filling defect around its margins, producing the meniscus sign. When seen in profile such an ulcer may appear *en plateau*, i.e. not extending beyond what would be the normal border of the stomach. Many of these ulcers are in fact simple, the filling defect being due to oedema. Gastroscopy is usually more helpful provided that the ulcer can be clearly seen. Gastric cytology, however, in these cases is not of much value. A simple method of differentiation, though not completely foolproof, is re-examination after two or three weeks' medical treatment. Simple ulcers are then substantially reduced in size but malignant ulcers are relatively unchanged and in fact may present a more irregular appearance due to disappearance of oedema and inflammatory reaction.

Approximately two-thirds of ulcers on the greater curvature and in the fundus are malignant. Large prepyloric ulcers should also be considered suspicious especially if they show the meniscus sign.

SIMPLE TUMOURS

A simple tumour causes a smooth or lobulated filling defect and sometimes more than one is present. An adenomatous polyp arising in the antrum may prolapse into the duodenum. A leiomyoma is usually large by the time the patient comes for radiological investigation and characteristically it has a smooth outline with central ulceration due to necrosis—the target sign. These tumours may be locally malignant. Other less common simple tumours are lipomatoma and fibromatoma.

Multiple benign adenomata are sometimes seen causing smooth filling defects usually on the crests of the rugae. Radiologically, they are difficult to distinguish from mammillary gastritis.

DIFFERENTIAL DIAGNOSIS

1. Air bubbles may cause initial confusion. However, they are more translucent, can be broken up and alter their shape.

2. Food residue may simulate polyposis especially in gastric atony (p. 40).

CARCINOMA

Sometimes a carcinoma of the fundus of the stomach can be suspected on a chest film by a filling defect outlined by the gastric air bubble. Similarly attention may be drawn to a possible carcinoma of the body on a supine film of the abdomen.

A barium meal is the standard radiological procedure and is probably the most accurate single method of diagnosing a carcinoma.

Many carcinomata are associated with a low or absent acid output and with atrophic folds. In some instances when they occur in the antrum the acid output is normal or even high with normal or coarse folds proximally.

In the fundus the greatest difficulty may be encountered because the soft-tissue shadow indicated by the distance between the base of the left lung and the gastric air bubble is variable. The double contrast technique as previously described (p. 3) is of great value, showing in some carcinomata thickened, rigid folds and in others mucosal destruction. During fluoroscopy, a careful study should be made of the mode of entry of the barium into the stomach. Splitting of the stream of barium usually denotes a carcinoma at the oesophago-gastric junction. In addition, the lower oesophagus is commonly involved causing irregular obstruction and with some distension proximally.

Varices in the fundus should cause no difficulty as they are usually also present in the lower oesophagus and unless gross, disappear in the erect position.

Recurrence of malignant disease after partial gastrectomy commonly causes a collar-like filling defect around the stoma. As the disease progresses, the tumour extends particularly up the lesser curvature aspect, causing mucosal destruction with a filling defect.

RADIOLOGICAL TYPES

I. Malignant Ulcer

The difference between simple and malignant ulcers has already been described (p. 40). A malignant ulcer may grow extremely slowly and be present for years before its true nature is realised. A condition with which it is liable to be confused is *formation cavitaire d'origine dynamique de Moutier*. This is a transient appearance on the greater curvature caused by a circular area of contraction around an erosion. At first sight, this may closely simulate a malignant ulcer but it usually disappears before the end of the barium meal. Thus an erroneous diagnosis should not be made.

II. Scirrhous Carcinoma

A. Localised Type. The mucosal pattern overlying the tumour is absent giving a smooth appearance, and the stomach wall is rigid.

When localised to the posterior wall the tumour is almost impossible to detect unless ulceration occurs. Ultimately the tumour may extend around the stomach causing a napkin-ring or hour-glass deformity.

DIFFERENTIAL DIAGNOSIS

1. Adult hypertrophic pyloric stenosis (p. 44). The mucosal pattern can normally be traced through this lesion, but in many cases, the diagnosis remains in doubt. Both lesions may show indentation of the base of the duodenal bulb. Gastroscopy may help, but it is wise in doubtful cases to consider the lesion as malignant.

2. Pseudo-malignancy in pernicious anaemia. The narrowed area is presumably caused by spasm. It is usually in the prepyloric region and since the mucosa is atrophic, the lesion is usually considered malignant. In many cases, the diagnosis can be made only at laparotomy.

3. A healed gastric ulcer. A careful search should be made for radiating folds.

4. The narrowed antrum following gastroenterostomy.

B. Diffuse Type. This is more common and usually begins in the antrum. Initially it may cause dilatation proximally but ultimately the whole stomach becomes contracted. There is lack of pliability and the mucosal pattern is atrophic or even absent. In rare cases, calcification may occur. The pylorus is rigid so that barium passes readily into the duodenum. Even although the peristaltic waves are weak and ultimately become absent, the stomach empties rapidly. Sometimes the tumour extends diffusely up the oesophagus.

DIFFERENTIAL DIAGNOSIS

1. Prolonged anorexia may result in some generalised contraction and mucosal atrophy. The stomach, however, is pliable and peristalsis is normal.

2. Amyloidosis is associated with a smooth atrophic mucosal pattern and as some rigidity is also present, differentiation from a scirrhous carcinoma is radiologically impossible.

3. Oedema of the stomach wall in cases of reticulosis of the plasmacytosis group causes similar appearances. As the duodenum and small intestine are usually similarly affected, a generalised disorder rather than a purely gastric lesion should be suspected.

4. Syphilis of the stomach is very rare and is usually indistinguishable from a scirrhous carcinoma. Serological reactions, however, are helpful.

5. A diffuse lymphosarcoma can also give similar appearances.

6. The late stage following ingestion of a corrosive liquid.

7. Rare conditions—e.g. sarcoidosis and chronic non-specific inflammation. Some cases labelled as such ultimately turn out to be malignant.

8. Crohn's disease rarely affects the stomach and only when the duodenum and small bowel are extensively involved. It causes narrowing, irregularity and sometimes ulceration especially in the antrum.

III. Fungating or Encephaloid Type

This causes an irregular filling defect or fingerprinting—obvious on palpation during fluoroscopy as well as on the films. Ulceration may occur in such tumours. A large tumour of this type may be seen on a plain film of the chest or abdomen—the gas acting as a contrast medium.

In other cases the malignant infiltration produces extremely coarse irregular folds which at first sight resemble simple hypertrophic rugae. However, their rigidity and persistence, especially on fluoroscopy with palpation, make the diagnosis obvious.

Following treatment by cytotoxic drugs the appearances occasionally return almost to normal.

DIFFERENTIAL DIAGNOSIS

1. Indentation of the antrum by the lumbar spine, or greater curvature by the left ribs commonly causes some difficulty. The defect, however, is smooth and palpation during fluoroscopy makes the diagnosis obvious.

2. Menétrier's disease. The hypertrophied mucosal folds particularly affect the greater curvature and are more pliable than a carcinoma. Occasionally after a number of years, a carcinoma may supervene in this condition.

3. A bezoar causes no difficulty as it can readily be displaced by palpation and positioning. Even when it is large and fills the stomach barium can be spread around it.

4. A localised chronic subphrenic abscess may indent the fundus. It commonly causes some irregularity and as palpation is impossible it is difficult to differentiate from a carcinoma. Such an abscess may be evident several months after the original abdominal operation.

5. Faeces in the colon overlying the stomach occasionally cause some difficulty. This is resolved by rotating the patient and by palpation.

6. Reticulosis causes similar thickened rigid folds which however tend to be more extensive.

IV. Multifocal Superficial Carcinoma

This is a rare condition and is associated with thickened mucosal folds presumably due to a coexisting chronic gastritis. Superficial ulcers develop which heal with some fibrosis. The radiological diagnosis from simple chronic hypertrophic gastritis is not possible as the stomach distends normally, peristalsis is unaffected, and the mucosal folds are pliable.

RETICULOSIS

These tumours are often indistinguishable from carcinomata. They tend, however, to be bulkier and more extensive and when the mucosa is diffusely infiltrated the folds are commonly thicker and more irregular. Ulceration often occurs in lymphosarcomata, and perforation is more common than in carcinomata. Sometimes perforation occurs into the colon causing a gastro-colic fistula.

In rare instances a lymphosarcoma diffusely infiltrates the stomach producing a radiological appearance indistinguishable from a scirrhous carcinoma.

GASTRITIS

This is one of the most difficult conditions to interpret radiologically.

If excessive mucus is present, then it is safe to say that gastritis is present. In some cases the mucus causes long linear thread-like filling defects in the barium, in others a scalloped appearance. Frequently it prevents the barium from adhering satisfactorily to the mucosa and thus the pattern is indistinct.

NATURE OF FOLDS

The difficulty in the radiological assessment is that the size and prominence of the folds depend upon:

(a) The state of contraction of the muscularis mucosae which is variable.

(b) The presence or absence of mucosal oedema, congestion, and/or cellular infiltration.

(c) The thickness of the secreting mucosa.

Any abnormality is usually most obvious on the greater curvature aspect of the body and fundus. In some instances the folds vary greatly from one examination to another and at different times during the course of the same barium meal.

Fine or Absent Mucosal Folds

When the mucous membrane is atrophic, the folds are fine or even absent—particularly on the greater curvature and at the fundus. These appearances are found in 'atrophic gastritis', pernicious anaemia, long-standing iron deficiency anaemia, certain conditions associated with general alimentary mucosal atrophy, e.g. hypothyroidism, etc. The acid output is low or absent. In some cases a gastric ulcer is present and its detection is relatively easy. The peristaltic waves are more or less normal, and the walls of the stomach pliable.

A diffuse scirrhous carcinoma and certain other conditions—e.g. amyloidosis and occasionally reticulosis, are also associated with mucosal atrophy. In these cases, the peristaltic waves are weak or absent and the stomach walls tend to be rigid, but in some instances the differentiation from simple mucosal atrophy is not possible.

Coarse Mucosal Folds

These are found in a variety of conditions.

(a) As a general rule in cases of peptic ulceration the higher the acid output the coarser the mucosal folds. These coarse folds are most commonly associated with a duodenal ulcer and are particularly obvious in the Zollinger-Ellison syndrome. Less commonly they are associated with gastric ulceration in which case the ulcer may be difficult to detect. On the other hand barium between coarse folds may mimic a gastric ulcer.

(b) Increase in the parietal cell mass without a duodenal ulcer in some secreting adenomata of the pancreas.

(c) Certain cases of chronic gastritis, with hyposecretion or even achlorhydria. In spite of the fact that the folds are coarse, the mucous membrane is, in fact, atrophic. There may also be an excess of mucus.

(d) Menétrier's disease. The coarse folds are usually localised to the greater curvature and generally the acid output is low or absent.

(e) Mammillary gastritis, i.e. 'chronic gastritis' with multiple small nodulations particularly on the crests of the rugae. There may be a excess of mucus in the stomach. In some cases there is a low acid output while in others it is normal or high and a duodenal ulcer may be present.

(f) Biliary gastritis. Following a gastro-enterostomy or a Polya gastrectomy, reflux of bile into the stomach may occur and this sometimes causes oedema and swelling of the mucosa. The radiological appearances are in no way different from those of coarse mucosal folds from any other cause.

(g) 'Antral gastritis.' In this condition the coarse hypertrophied folds are restricted to the antrum.

The thickened rigid mucosal folds seen in some forms of carcinoma and reticulosis should not cause any confusion. The only exception is the rare instance of multifocal superficial carcinoma. It must be remembered that occasionally an antral carcinoma is associated with simple coarse mucosal folds in the proximal part of the stomach and with a high acid output.

GASTRIC VARICES

The recognition of varices by barium meal is difficult as they are easily confused with coarse mucosal folds. They occur at the fundus of the stomach and cause sinuous or lobulated filling defects and sometimes a soap bubble appearance. Occasionally the lesser curvature is indented by a large gastric vein. The varices substantially improve or disappear after a successful porto-caval anastomosis.

The patient should be examined in the prone position using an air contrast technique. Particular attention should be paid to the oesophago-gastric junction where the indentations are more obvious and may present a rosette appearance. A complete barium meal should be performed to search for oesophageal varices which are usually present and for a peptic ulcer which occurs in about 10 per cent. or even more of such cases.

Varices are usually well demonstrated by splenic venography.

ADULT HYPERTROPHIC PYLORIC STENOSIS

This is a dangerous diagnosis to make on one barium meal without contributory clinical evidence. The condition is not uncommon but the radiological appearances can closely simulate a prepyloric gastric ulcer with an inflammatory mass, or a carcinoma, or even a distended, inflamed gall-bladder adjacent to the antrum. Approximately one-third of cases have a gastric ulcer in the proximal part of the stomach. This condition can occur in pernicious anaemia, in which case the radiological diagnosis of a carcinoma is usually made.

The pylorus is elongated and narrowed and the the base of the duodenal bulb is indented by the hypertrophied muscle. The mucous membrane pattern is normal and the lumen in the area of stenosis is approximately midway between the greater and lesser curvature aspects. There may be a tiny localised dilatation in the middle of the affected part, presumably at the junction of the normal pylorus with the abnormal muscular hypertrophy of the antrum. Occasionally there is a slight kinking at this point.

DISPLACEMENTS

The stomach should be well filled with barium and fluoroscopic examination is most rewarding. A palpable mass can then be readily identified and its relationship to the stomach established. Thus it is easy to determine whether a mass is intrinsic or extrinsic as regards the stomach. The mode of displacement by the left lower ribs or by the kyphotic lumbar spine in a thin person is obvious.

An enlarged spleen usually displaces the stomach medially but occasionally downwards. Adhesions may occur between the spleen and the greater curvature of the stomach, causing deformity and irregularity which must not be mistaken for a carcinoma. In some cases when the spleen lies posteriorly, the body of the stomach is displaced forwards simulating a tumour or cyst of the body of pancreas but at a slightly higher level.

A ruptured spleen causes considerable displacement of the stomach with local indentations due to blood clot. Bulging of the left flank usually also occurs but the left psoas shadow may still be evident.

A tumour or cyst of the body of the pancreas usually displaces the body of the stomach forwards and downwards. Occasionally a pseudo-cyst and rarely a cyst or tumour displaces the stomach upwards and to the right.

A large liver displaces the stomach downwards and to the left and the duodenal bulb may also be indented from above.

VOLVULUS OF THE STOMACH

The most common form is on the cardio-pyloric axis when a large para-oesophageal hernia is present. Only rarely does it occur in the absence of such a hernia.

A volvulus on the transverse axis is rare and is usually associated with elevation and paralysis of the left dome of the diaphragm. It may simulate a carcinoma because of obstruction and deformity in the middle of the stomach.

HAEMATEMESIS

The method of examination has already been described (p. 4). When fresh, the blood appears as fluffy, irregular filling defects. Clot forms mainly adjacent to the lesion causing the haemorrhage and fortuitously draws attention to it. The clot has a circumscribed appearance which at first sight suggests a tumour. Sometimes as the examination proceeds the clot is displaced revealing the lesion more clearly.

The commonest cause of bleeding from the stomach is a gastric ulcer. Films of the highest quality should be obtained in an attempt to show a vessel which causes a round filling defect in the base of the ulcer. When varices are present, a careful search should be made for a gastric or duodenal ulcer which, if found, may be the cause of the haemorrhage.

Gastric erosions may cause haematemesis but only rarely can they be detected by a barium meal. They show as superficial ulcer craters 2 to 3 mm. in diameter surrounded by a circular filling defect due to oedema.

GAS IN THE STOMACH WALL

Streaks of gas may be present in the stomach wall after severe vomiting or retching, presumably from a mucosal tear with sub-mucosal spread.

POST-OPERATIVE APPEARANCES

Pyloroplasty

This is usually carried out in association with a vagotomy for a chronic duodenal ulcer. The pylorus is wide and the deformity of the duodenal bulb remains. Large niches are usually present due to 'dog ears' as a result of transverse suturing and these must not be mistaken for ulcer craters. The barium can usually be displaced from these 'dog ears' more readily than from an ulcer crater, but in some cases the differentiation is difficult or even impossible.

Occasionally the ulcer becomes reactivated, usually because of an incomplete vagotomy, and its demonstration depends upon persistence of barium in a sharply defined rigid crater.

Polya Gastrectomy

Following a high partial gastrectomy, reflux may occur into the oesophagus because of interference with the normal hiatal mechanism. A high partial gastrectomy also predisposes to excessive filling of the afferent loop, but normally without dilatation or stasis.

Billroth I Gastrectomy

Barium passes into the duodenum through the normal route.

Gastro-enterostomy

Following a gastro-enterostomy, an attempt should be made to distend the antrum—the prone position being the best. If the stoma functions well, some contraction of the antrum always occurs and exclusion of a carcinoma may thus be difficult.

A variable amount of barium—sometimes none—leaves the stomach through the pylorus. Normally most of it leaves through the stoma. The mucosal pattern of the jejunum is usually a little coarser than normal.

Some filling of the afferent loop commonly occurs, but there should be no dilatation or stasis.

Sometimes, for example, because of malabsorption the gastro-enterostomy has to be dismantled and a gastro-duodenostomy performed. In these cases there is usually some irregularity of the greater curvature aspect of the stomach at the site of the previous stoma, and sometimes 'dog ears' are present. Thus a carcinoma or ulcer should not be erroneously diagnosed.

Interposed Jejunal Loop

Following a Polya partial gastrectomy with a small gastric remnant, it may be necessary because of malabsorption or excessive filling of the afferent loop, to dismantle the gastro-jejunostomy and interpose a segment of jejunum between the gastric remnant and the first part of the duodenum. A vagotomy is usually performed, but in spite of this, severe jejunitis may occur in this segment with coarse, thickened mucosal folds which produce excessive mucus. If the vagotomy is incomplete, a peptic ulcer, sometimes very large, may occur in the interposed segment.

EARLY POST-OPERATIVE COMPLICATIONS

OBSTRUCTION

After an operation on the stomach or duodenum, a high intestinal obstruction may develop. Even although the majority of these settle down with conservative measures, radiological investigations are of great value in determining the site and cause. Plain erect and supine films of the abdomen to include the diaphragm are taken as a preliminary, but it is usually necessary to give a Gastrografin meal either through a naso-gastric tube or by mouth to identify the loops and to note the precise nature of the obstruction. In some instances—e.g. a suspected retrograde jejuno-gastric intussusception, barium is safe as it can be washed out afterwards and detail is clearer. Sometimes elevation of the head of the table and raising of the left side of the patient initiates emptying of the stomach after a Polya or Billroth I gastrectomy.

In some cases of efferent loop obstruction following a gastro-enterostomy, barium or Gastrografin leaves the stomach through the pylorus and re-enters it by way of the afferent loop.

Causes of Obstruction

1. *Oedema of the Stoma.* The swollen mucosal folds cause a polypoidal filling defect protruding into the stomach and simulating an intussusception. A variable degree of obstruction results. This is most frequently seen following a gastro-enterostomy, but only rarely after any other type of operation.

2. *Retrograde Jejuno-gastric Intussusception.* The intussuscepted loop of jejunum causes a whorled filling defect in the stomach. Care must be taken not to mistake overlapping coils of small bowel for an intussusception. Rotation of the patient usually clarifies the position. Sometimes the diagnosis is obvious even in one view, particularly if the intussuscepted loops displace a pool of Gastrografin in the stomach.

3. *Retraction of the Gastro-enterostomy Stoma through the Transverse Meso-colon.* This serious complication may follow a retro-colic gastro-enterostomy causing complete stomal and afferent loop obstruction. A Gastrografin meal gives a characteristic appearance, namely the medium leaves the stomach through the pylorus and none through the stoma. The afferent loop, particularly the duodenum, is dilated with vigorous but ineffective peristaltic waves due to a jejunal obstruction at the stoma. This is, of course, a serious complication and a second operation is necessary to relieve the obstruction.

4. *Compression of Efferent Loop by a Dilated Afferent Loop.* This usually follows a degree of obstruction at the beginning of the efferent loop. The increasing dilatation of the afferent loop aggravates the condition by causing a valve effect. Subsequently adhesions may occur between the two loops.

5. *Stammer's Hernia.* Following a Polya gastrectomy, loops of jejunum may pass behind the stoma to the right or left, and become obstructed or even strangulated. The patient, of course, is very ill—often complaining of severe back pain—except in a few rare instances when the hernia is intermittent. The diagnosis can sometimes be made on a plain

film by noting the distended loops of jejunum usually to the left of the anastomosis. The gastric remnant is distended and there is dilatation of the proximal colon due to compression of the transverse colon opposite the stoma. A Gastrografin meal shows stomal obstruction with displacement of the anastomosis forwards and sometimes to the right.

6. *Obstruction by an Inflammatory Mass.* A soft-tissue shadow is present indenting, displacing and narrowing the bowel in the neighbourhood of the stoma. Commonly, the mucosa of the bowel is seen to be swollen and oedematous when the lumen is outlined by contrast medium or gas.

PERFORATIONS (LEAKS)

Following any abdominal operation gas is obvious under both domes of the diaphragm—seen most clearly on a chest film. It gradually becomes less and by the tenth post-operative day has normally been completely absorbed. Following a post-operative leak an increased amount of sub-diaphragmatic gas may be noted. For confirmation, a Gastrografin meal is necessary and barium must not be given. The sinus can usually be outlined and in most cases it arises from the stomal region.

INFECTIONS

Infection may be generalised in the peritoneal cavity causing ileus of the small and large bowel. More commonly it is localised forming an abscess or inflammatory mass usually in the neighbourhood of the stoma. One loculation of gas or several bubbles may be present. In all cases there is delay in the absorption of sub-diaphragmatic gas.

A Gastrografin meal helps to identify individual bowel loops from local abscesses and usually demonstrates a degree of stomal obstruction.

PANCREATITIS

The radiological diagnosis of this complication is difficult in the immediate post-operative period. It cannot usually be differentiated from a local infection.

LATE POST-OPERATIVE COMPLICATIONS

A barium meal forms a necessary part of the investigation of these cases.

ULCERATION

Films of the highest quality are necessary, and the greatest error is to mistake barium in a mucosal fold for an ulcer.

A peptic ulcer may occur on the suture line or in the jejunum usually within two or three inches of the stoma. It may be seen in profile extending beyond the normal outline of the jejunum, or *en face*. The mucosal folds in the base of the ulcer are destroyed giving a smooth appearance and barium usually persists in the crater. Occasionally barium does not adhere to the base of the ulcer especially if it is acutely inflamed, but in such cases the periphery of the ulcer is depicted by a sharp line.

After either a partial gastrectomy or a gastro-enterostomy some mucosal swelling of the upper jejunum is usually seen. This is considerably more obvious, together with hypermotility when an ulcer is present.

On fluoroscopy a metallic clip or groups of clips at the suture line can be mistaken for an ulcer but the nature of the opacity is obvious on inspection of the films.

In rare cases, a gastro-colic fistula develops from perforation of a stomal or jejunal ulcer into the colon. In these cases, a barium enema may be necessary for diagnosis because sometimes such a fistula is not outlined by a barium meal.

In chronic ulceration or extensive superficial erosions near the stoma some rigidity is present and the stomach and jejunum may be separated from each other as by a collar. Neither superficial erosions, even when extensive, nor exposed unabsorbed suture material can be demonstrated by a barium meal.

OBSTRUCTIONS

Stomal obstruction usually results from ulceration and only in rare instances is it due to an inadequate stoma at the original operation. Less commonly it is due to distortion of the stoma from adhesions or a haematoma.

A common site of jejunal obstruction following either a gastro-enterostomy or Polya gastrectomy is two or three inches from the stoma on the efferent loop. This is usually due to the jejunum being drawn up and kinked by adhesions, but occasionally a jejunal ulcer is the cause. Adequate films, especially spot films of the narrowed area, are essential. When due to adhesions the mucous membrane pattern is intact. Dilatation of the jejunum opposite the stoma, sometimes to a marked degree, may occur. In the erect position the dilated jejunum can be mistaken for the lower part of the stomach, but the situation is obvious in the horizontal position. There is usually also dilatation with stasis in the afferent loop. If the obstruction is marked a disordered X-ray pattern with segmentation and flocculation is present in the small bowel due to intermittent passage of barium through the narrowed area.

Dilated Afferent Loop

It is quite normal for some filling of the afferent loop to occur, especially if a high gastrectomy has been carried out. Dilatation and stasis, however, especially if associated with hyperperistalsis and a fluid level, are definitely abnormal. The dilatation may be caused by obstruction of the efferent loop or the mechanics of the anastomosis causing food to enter the afferent loop in preference to the efferent loop. As the result of this, bile vomiting or malabsorption may occur.

Retrograde Jejuno-gastric Intussusception

Only rarely is a chronic obstruction due to this cause. The appearances are similar to those in the immediate post-operative period (p. 46).

GALL-STONES

The occurrence of gall-stones is becoming increasingly recognised following a partial gastrectomy or vagotomy. The dilatation and atony of the gall-bladder which commonly follow these operations is presumably the precipitating factor. Subsequently cholecystitis or even pancreatitis may develop.

BILE VOMITING

This distressing complication may follow either a Polya gastrectomy or a gastro-enterostomy. In some cases it is associated with excessive filling of the afferent loop and is relieved by surgical correction. In others, probably the majority, there is a normal stoma and efferent loop, and little or no barium enters the afferent loop. In a few of these cases there is probably some obstruction of the afferent loop near the stoma. Attempts have been made without success to demonstrate the afferent loop by late films following intravenous Biligrafin.

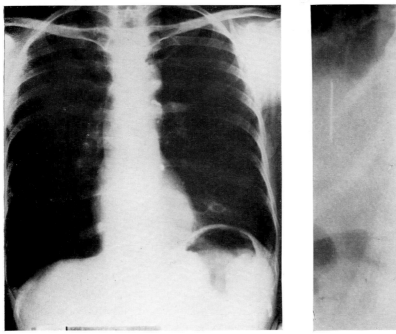

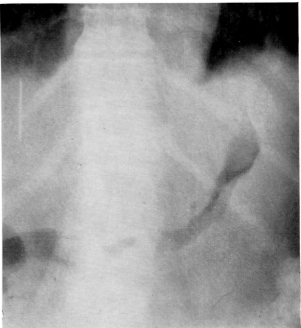

FIG. 101   FIG. 102

Fig. 101. Large fungating carcinoma encircling upper part of body of stomach detected on chest film.   The filling defect indents the gas-filled fundus.

Fig. 102. Gastric carcinoma detected on plain film of abdomen.   The gas in the stomach outlines clearly the diffusely contracted stomach.   Subsequently confirmed by barium meal.

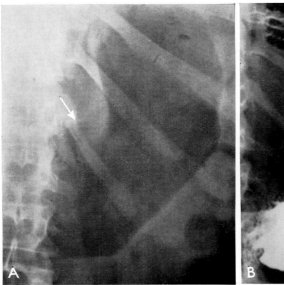

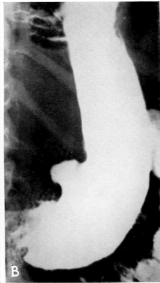

FIG. 103

Fig. 103. Gastric ulcer at incisura shown. A: On plain film of abdomen.   The ulcer crater (arrowed) is outlined by gas. B: By barium meal. Prone position. (Print reversed.)

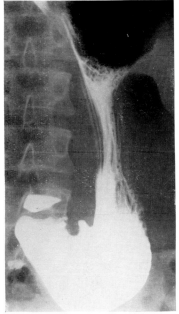

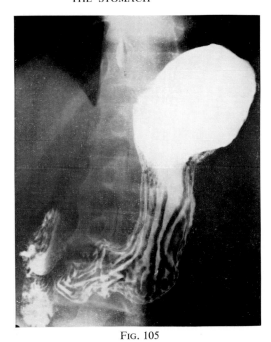

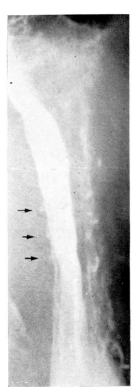

FIG. 104

FIG. 105

FIG. 106

Fig. 104. Two peristaltic waves near incisura simulating a gastric ulcer. A few seconds later the appearance was quite different. Erect position.

Fig. 105. 'Furrowing' of greater curvature of antrum simulating a greater curve ulcer. This appearance was due to two peristaltic waves and was transient.

Fig. 106. Mucosal folds of greater curvature (arrowed) appearing around lesser curvature of stomach simulating ulceration. Erect film.

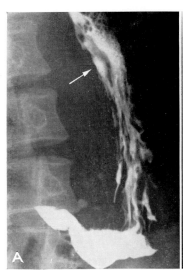

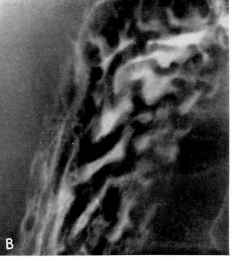

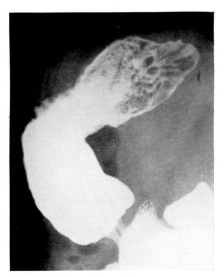

FIG. 107

FIG. 108

Fig. 107. Normal appearance high up on posterior wall of body of stomach. A: Erect. The mucosal folds (arrowed) simulate an ulcer. B: The folds are seen *en face* and are normal. This film is obtained by turning the patient from the supine position to the right lateral position and slightly elevating the head of the table.

Fig. 108. Two mucosal folds at gastro-oesophageal junction rather more prominent than usual but conforming to normal pattern. Thus they should not be confused with varices. Patient lying on right side with head of X-ray table slightly elevated to show the fundus.

D

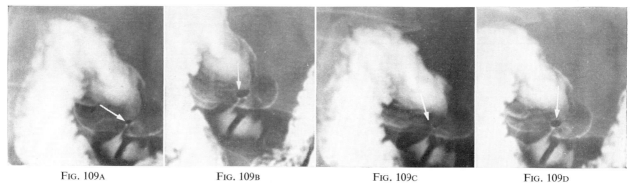

FIG. 109A　　　　FIG. 109B　　　　FIG. 109C　　　　FIG. 109D

Fig. 109. Normal pyloric canal (arrowed) seen in varying degrees of patency.　Supine views.

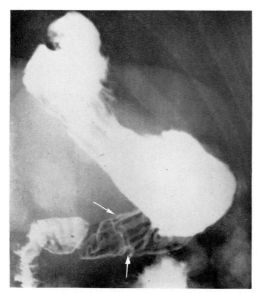

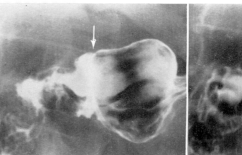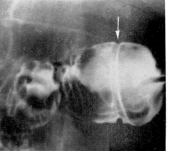

FIG. 111

Fig. 111. Two films (at an interval of a few seconds) showing transverse mucosal fold (arrowed) in antrum simulating an incomplete diaphragm.　The films show the progress of a peristaltic wave which has distended the antrum.　Operative confirmation of absence of diaphragm at the time of a cholecystectomy.

FIG. 110

Fig. 110. Mucosal fold (arrowed) causing tortuous ridge in prepyloric region. Such a fold is not uncommon and may resemble an incomplete congenital diaphragm.　Hiatus hernia also present. Supine film.

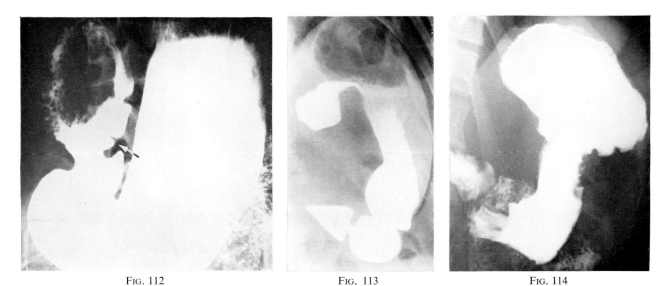

FIG. 112   FIG. 113   FIG. 114

Fig. 112. Thin shelf-like incomplete congenital diaphragm (arrowed) in antrum. Incidental finding.

Fig. 113. Cup and spill deformity (cascade stomach)—usually considered to be due to spasm of oblique muscle. The deformity had practically disappeared by the end of the examination. Note normal duodenal bulb and pylorus.

Fig. 114. 'Fringe effect' causing ulcer-like projection at upper end of lesser curvature. It is obviously due to the posterior aspect of the fundus crossing the body of the stomach. Supine view.

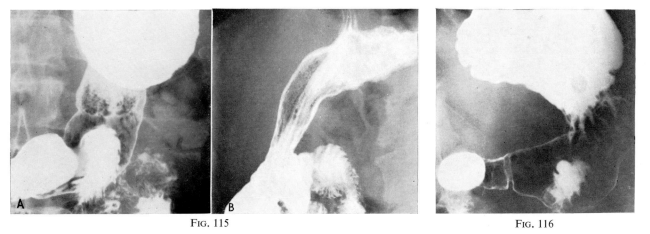

FIG. 115   FIG. 116

Fig. 115. Loaded transverse colon overlying the stomach and simulating a carcinoma. Case of pernicious anaemia with gross mucosal atrophy. A: Filling defect seen in P.A. view opposite middle of body of stomach. B: Lateral view showing clearly the smooth mucosal pattern (of pernicious anaemia) without evidence of a tumour. The loaded transverse colon is clear of the stomach.

Fig. 116. Congenital hymen-like diaphragm causing constant smooth rigid indentation in antrum. The indentation is deeper on one aspect—in this case the greater curvature. This helps to differentiate it from a transverse mucosal fold. Incidental finding.

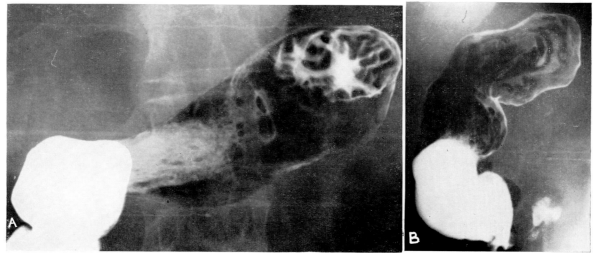

FIG. 117

Fig. 117. Funnelling of cardiac orifice simulating varices or a carcinoma. A: Supine view. B: Patient lying almost in the right lateral position and with the head of the table slightly raised. The fundus is clearly seen and is normal. This is an excellent position for demonstrating the region of the cardiac orifice.

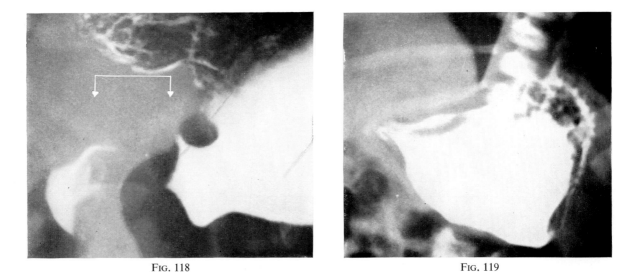

FIG. 118   FIG. 119

Fig. 118. Congenital hypertrophic pyloric stenosis. Characteristic smooth elongated filling defect (arrowed) continuous with the pylorus. Typical indentation of base of duodenal bulb. Baby between prone and right lateral position. (Print reversed.)

Fig. 119. Antral spasm causing typical conical narrowing without indentation of duodenal bulb. Baby aged 6 weeks with attacks of vomiting.

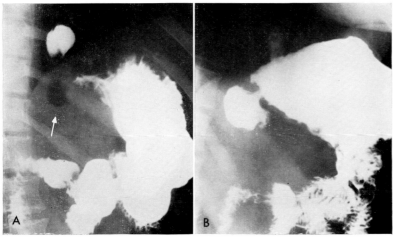

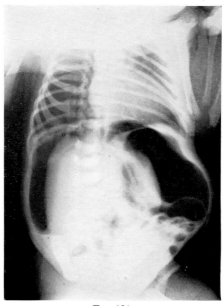

FIG. 120

Fig. 120. Gastric diverticulum arising from fundus posteriorly—the common site.

A: The diverticulum (arrowed) is outlined with gas. Note also normal phrenic ampulla.

B: The diverticulum is filled with barium showing clearly its characteristic smooth neck.

FIG. 121

Fig. 121. Perforation of stomach in a new-born infant due to congenital absence of muscle coat. Large amount of gas present in peritoneal cavity.

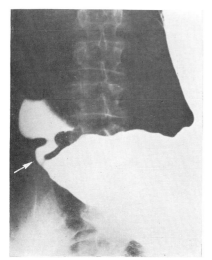

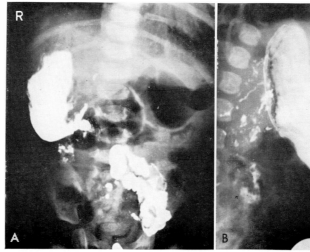

FIG. 122   FIG. 123

Fig. 122. Cholecyst-duodenal band (arrowed) indenting antrum and causing a degree of obstruction. Laparotomy performed as a carcinoma could not entirely be excluded. This band more commonly indents the duodenum.

Fig. 123. Malrotation of the foregut. Gross congenital heart disease also present. Small bowel and colon in normal position. Autopsy confirmation. A: Supine view. The stomach lies opposite the liver on the right side. B: Lateral view. The stomach is behind the liver.

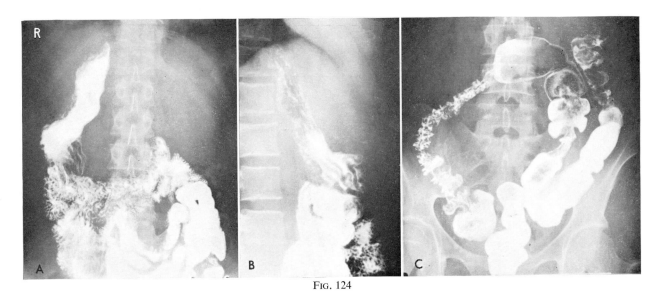

FIG. 124

Fig. 124. Malrotation of the foregut.   A: Supine view.   The stomach is on the right side opposite the liver.   The disposition of the small bowel loops is normal.   One hour follow-through film.   B: Lateral view.   The stomach is posterior to the liver. C: After evacuation film of barium enema showing the colon in its normal position.

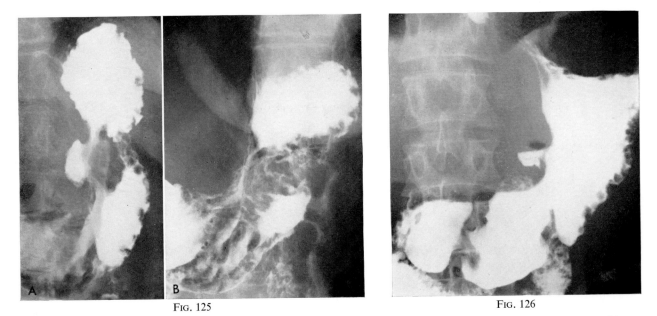

FIG. 125   FIG. 126

Fig. 125. A: Large gastric ulcer on lesser curvature with filling defect around its margins due to oedema.   Coarse hypertrophic gastric folds also present commonly seen in ulcers of this size.   The fine linear dark streaks in the antrum are due to mucus. B: Three months later.   The ulcer has healed.   Supine films.

Fig. 126. Large simple gastric ulcer with a fluid level on lesser curvature.   Erect film.

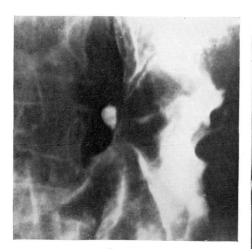

FIG. 127

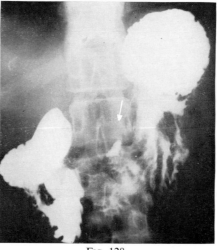

FIG. 128

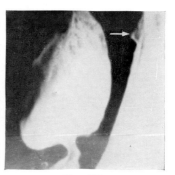

FIG. 129

Fig. 127. Chronic gastric ulcer with radiating folds situated near incisura. Supine film. In the erect position the ulcer could not be seen with certainty.

Fig. 128. Gastric ulcer at incisura (arrowed)—in a case of duodenal ileus (arterio-mesenteric occlusion). Dilated duodenum with a powerful peristaltic contraction in second part at the moment the film was taken. Characteristic obstruction in the third part. Supine view. The ulcer healed following treatment with mecothane.

Fig. 129. 'Spot' film of duodenal bulb which fortuitously showed shallow gastric ulcer (arrowed) on posterior wall of stomach—the only film on which it was demonstrated. Whenever possible this area should be included in a spot film. Normal duodenal bulb.

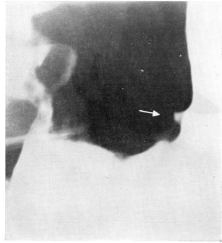

FIG. 130

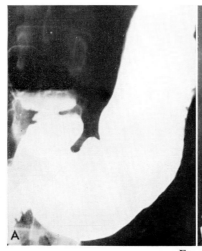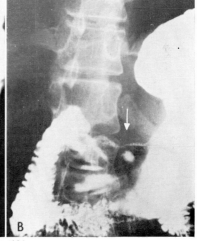

FIG. 131

Fig. 130. Gastric ulcer (arrowed) at incisura—seen only with compression when patient erect.

Fig. 131. Gastric ulcer on posterior wall of antrum seen only in supine position. A: Erect. Ulcer not seen even with compression. B: Supine and with right side slightly raised. Ulcer (arrowed) now clearly seen.

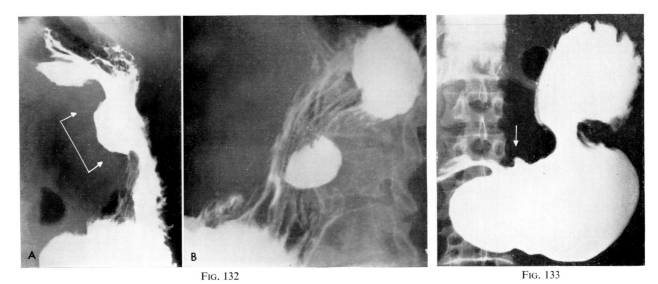

FIG. 132   FIG. 133

Fig. 132. Very large gastric ulcer high up on posterior wall. A: Ulcer (arrowed) shown in profile. Some irregularity with a filling defect around its margins, especially on its proximal aspect. Erect film. B: Ulcer shown *en face*. Normal mucosal pattern right up to edge of ulcer suggesting that it is simple. Supine film with left side raised. Laparotomy confirmation. The ulcer had burrowed into the pancreas.

Fig. 133. Chronic antral gastric ulcer (arrowed) with shortening of lesser curvature—the 'scrotal' or 'tea-pot' stomach. Prone view—(Print reversed).

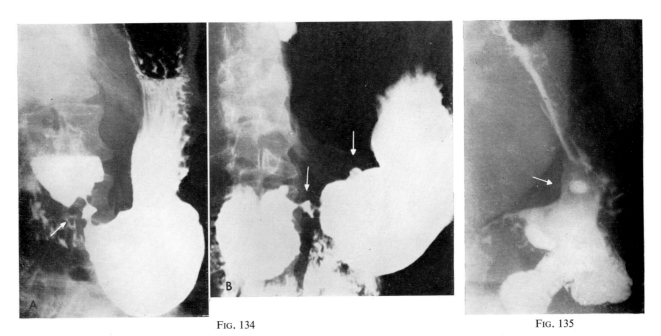

FIG. 134   FIG. 135

Fig. 134. Two gastric ulcers. A: Erect, The prepyloric ulcer (arrowed) is obvious and has caused stenosis but the ulcer near the incisura cannot be seen. B: Prone. (Print reversed.) Both ulcers (arrowed) are clearly seen.

Fig. 135. Gastric ulcer (arrowed) following well-functioning gastro-enterostomy—an unusual occurrence. The operation had been performed for a chronic duodenal ulcer.

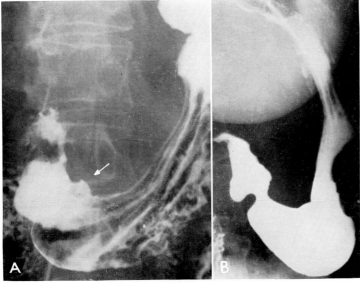

FIG. 136

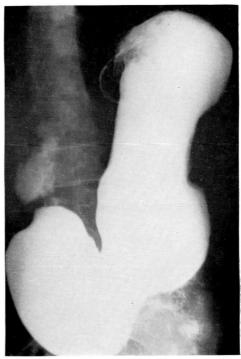

Fig. 136. Flattening of lesser curvature aspect of prepyloric region following healing of a gastric ulcer. A: Gastric ulcer (arrowed) on lesser curvature aspect—the usual site. Incisura on greater curvature opposite the ulcer. B: Eight months later, the ulcer has healed with flattening, causing an eccentric pylorus.

FIG. 137

Fig. 137. Gross stenosis proved at operation to be due to a healed prepyloric ulcer. Markedly dilated stomach with vigorous peristalsis and delay in barium entering duodenum.

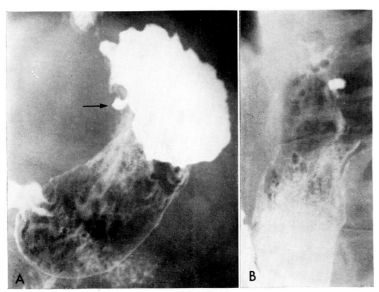

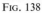

FIG. 138

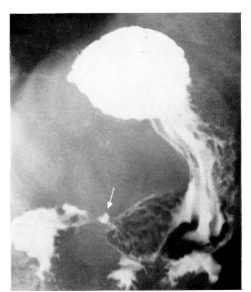

FIG. 139

Fig. 138. Gastric ulcer high up on posterior wall. A: Supine. Ulcer (arrowed) could readily be mistaken for a coarse mucosal fold. B: When the fundus is coated with barium and the gastric air bubble gives a double contrast, the ulcer is clearly seen *en face*. This view is achieved by turning the patient over on his right side and tilting the table slightly towards the vertical.

Fig. 139. Pyloric ulcer (arrowed). In this case there is singularly little stenosis. Some fibrosis has extended proximally into the prepyloric region and distally into the base of the bulb. Supine view.

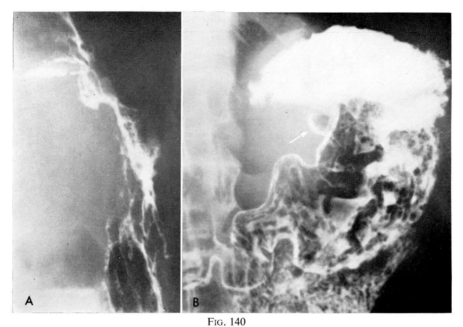

Fig. 140

Fig. 140. Gastric ulcer high up on posterior wall. A: Erect. Considerable irregularity with suggestion of a filling defect around the ulcer initially arousing suspicion of malignancy. B: Supine. Ulcer (arrowed). The gastric mucosal folds are coarse. Barium does not adhere satisfactorily to the mucosa due to an excess of mucus from an associated gastritis.

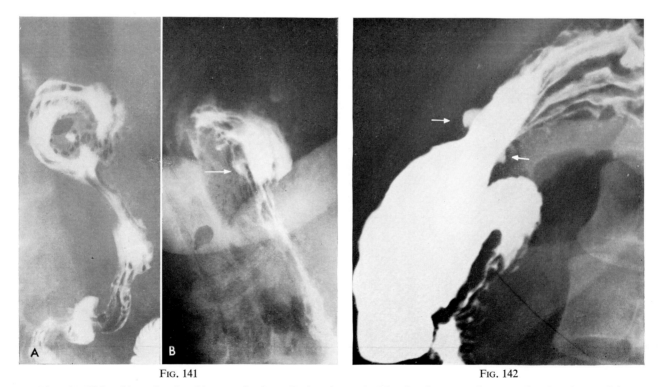

Fig. 141   Fig. 142

Fig. 141. Sliding hiatus hernia with a gastric ulcer. Supine views. A: The ulcer is seen *en face*. B: The ulcer (arrowed) is seen in profile.

Fig. 142. Two gastric ulcers (arrowed), one on anterior wall and one on posterior wall Film taken with patient lying on right side and head of table slightly raised. This is the best position for demonstrating lesions on the anterior wall of stomach.

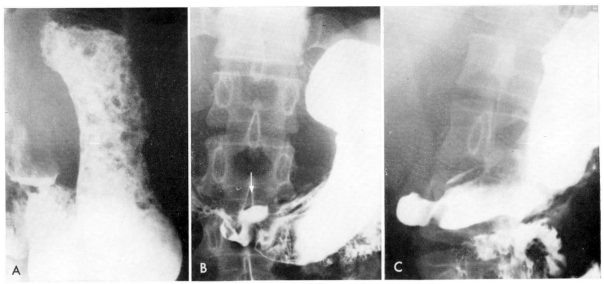

FIG. 143

Fig. 143. Gastric atony with a gastric ulcer. A: Large residue of sticky consistency containing food particles which simulated polypi and which masked the ulcer in all positions. B: Second barium meal following prolonged gastric lavage. Large gastric ulcer (arrowed) now clearly seen in the prepyloric region. C: Three months later. The ulcer has healed following simple gastro-enterostomy with adequate drainage. No gastric lavage was necessary on this occasion.

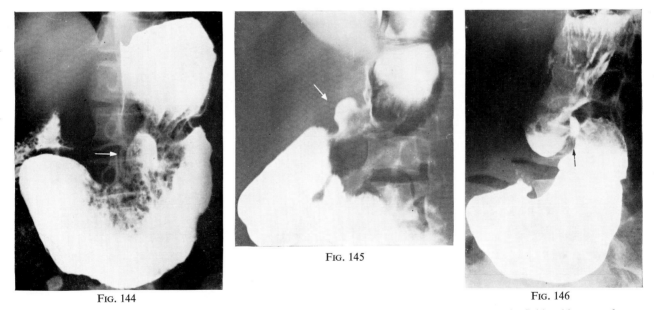

FIG. 145

FIG. 144   FIG. 146

Fig. 144. Large gastric ulcer (arrowed) on posterior wall above incisura in a case of gastric atony. The fluid residue was of a sticky consistency and contained food particles which simulated polypi. Only with the patient supine and the left side elevated could the ulcer be satisfactorily demonstrated.

Fig. 145. Large gastric ulcer (arrowed) high up on anterior wall of body of stomach. *En plateau* appearance simulating malignancy, found at operation to be due to oedema and inflammatory reaction around the ulcer. Patient lying on right side and head of X-ray table slightly elevated.

Fig. 146. Chronic gastric ulcer (arrowed) with hour glass deformity. Fluid residue in proximal part of stomach. It is now rare to see such gross deformity presumably due to earlier diagnosis and treatment.

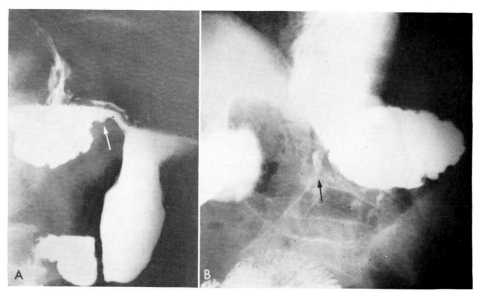

FIG. 147

Fig. 147. Cup and spill deformity with gastric ulcer (arrowed) high up on posterior wall. A: Erect. Ulcer crater seen in profile. B: Supine and with patient's left side raised. The ulcer is clearly seen *en face*.

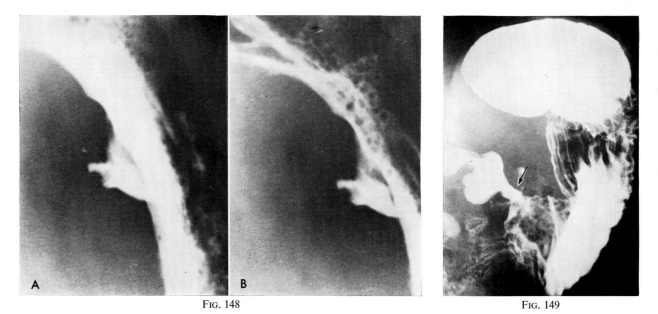

FIG. 148   FIG. 149

Fig. 148. Large irregular gastric ulcer high up on posterior wall. Indentation on the floor of the ulcer considered to be due to an artery but at gastroscopy was seen to be due to granulations. A: First profile view. B: Second profile view with approximately 7° of rotation so that A and B are a good stereoscopic pair.

Fig. 149. Gastric ulcer (arrowed) in prepyloric region. Radiologically, the ulcer was considered more likely to be simple than malignant. Gastroscopically the ulcer was not seen, but an irregular and oedematous antrum suggested the probability of malignancy. Gastric cytology—no malignant cells seen. At laparotomy macroscopically the ulcer was considered malignant but careful microscopy showed it to be simple. Congenital duodenal diverticula also present.

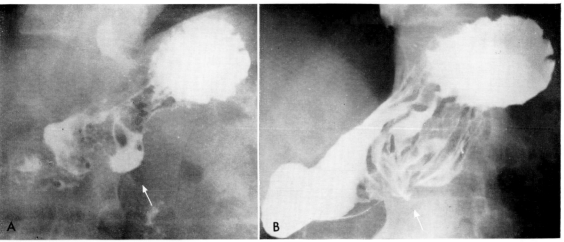

Fig. 150

Fig. 150. Simple gastric ulcer (arrowed) on greater curvature aspect of stomach—operative confirmation. Supine views. A: Because of its position and size it was considered likely to be malignant. B: After three weeks medical treatment the ulcer (arrowed) has almost healed with radiating folds suggesting that it is simple. A partial gastrectomy was performed because of recurrence of symptoms.

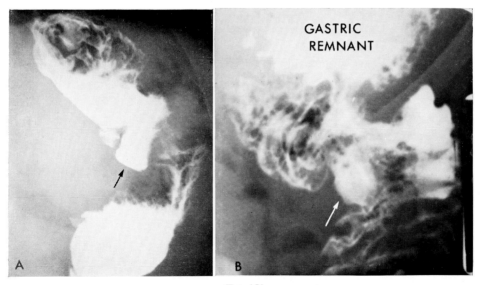

Fig. 151

Fig. 151. Large peptic ulcer (arrowed) in a segment of jejunum interposed between the gastric remnant and duodenum. Previously partial gastrectomy with small gastric remnant. Because of the development of dumping and malabsorption the normal route was reconstituted. A: Profile view of the ulcer. B: Spot film showing the ulcer *en face*.

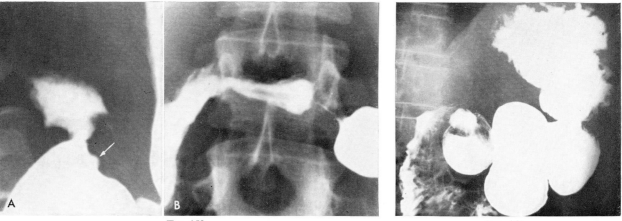

FIG. 152   FIG. 153

Fig. 152. Prepyloric ulcer causing elongation of pylorus on healing. A: Ulcer crater (arrowed) clearly seen on spot film. Indentation of base of duodenal bulb suggesting adult hypertrophic pyloric stenosis but in view of subsequent findings, presumably due to spasm of pyloric muscle. B: After medical treatment for one month. The ulcer has healed with some narrowing in the prepyloric region—the lumen being continuous with the pyloric canal. The indentation seen in A is not now evident.

Fig. 153. Vigorous hyperperistalsis in a patient with duodenal stenosis from a chronic duodenal ulcer. Three powerful peristaltic waves present and a fourth starting near the fundus.

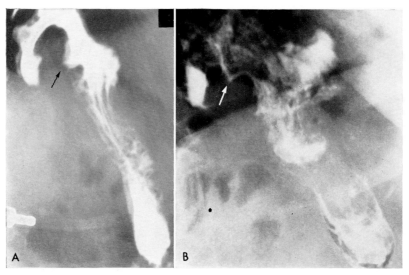

FIG. 154

Fig. 154. Gastric ulcer (arrowed) in a hiatus hernia causing massive haematemesis. Operative confirmation. Supine views with right side elevated. A: Ulcer seen in profile. B: Ten minutes later. Extensive fluffy filling defects due to blood from recurrence of haemorrhage during the course of the barium meal—a rare occurrence.
(By courtesy of the Editor of the *British Journal of Surgery*.)

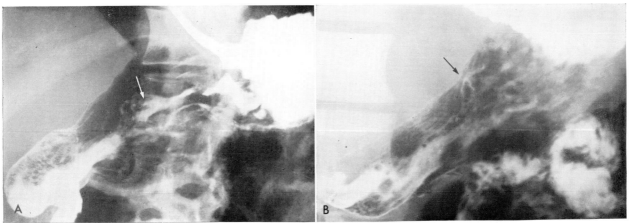

FIG. 155

Fig 155. Massive haematemesis from gastric ulcer on posterior wall of body of stomach. Operative confirmation. A: Organised clot causing irregular filling defect around ulcer (arrowed) and obscuring it. B: The blood clot fortuitously became displaced and the ulcer crater (arrowed) is now revealed.

No active attempt must be made to displace the clot because of the danger of provoking a further haemorrhage.
(By courtesy of the Editor of the *British Journal of Surgery*.)

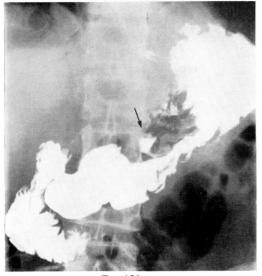

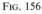

FIG. 156

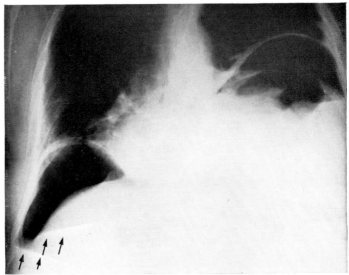

FIG. 157

Fig. 156. Gastric ulcer (arrowed) on lesser curvature of stomach causing massive haematemesis. Filling defect around the ulcer due to organised blood clot which had fortuitously formed around the bleeding lesion drawing attention to it at an early stage in the examination.

Fig. 157. Perforation of a gastric ulcer with a large amount of gas under both domes of the diaphragm. The two straight lines (arrowed) initially suggesting fluid levels under the right dome of diaphragm are due to the visceral and parietal layers of peritoneum coming together. One line is anterior and the other posterior. They obviously do not represent fluid levels, as they are not horizontal and parallel. Commonly only one such line is present.

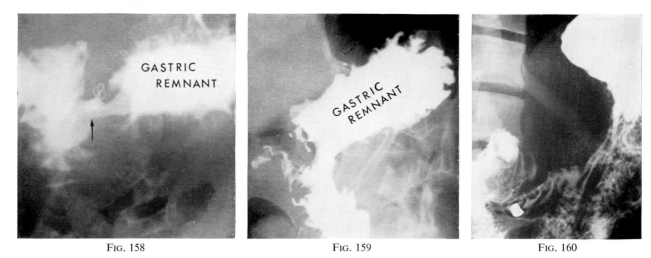

FIG. 158   FIG. 159   FIG. 160

Fig. 158. Stomal ulcer (arrowed) with characteristic separation of gastric remnant from jejunum by a collar of fibrosis. Metallic clips also present at suture line. Supine view with left side raised. Previous Polya gastrectomy.

Fig. 159. Polya gastrectomy with fibrosis from previous ulceration at the stoma causing a collar separating the gastric remnant from the jejunum. Multiple erosions were present around the anastomosis—seen gastroscopically but could not be detected by barium meal.

Fig. 160. Metallic foreign body in stomach. On fluoroscopy it looked remarkably like a prepyloric ulcer but its nature is obvious on the improved detail of the film. Malingerer.

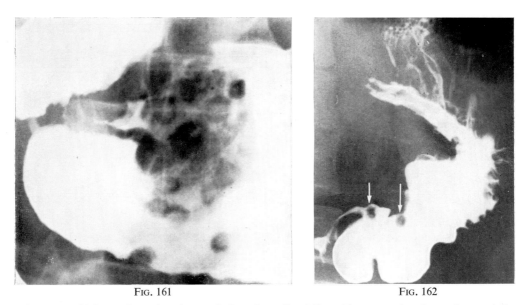

FIG. 161   FIG. 162

Fig. 161. Multiple gastric erosions in prepyloric region. 'Spot' film with compression shows characteristic shallow ulcers with surrounding translucency presumably due to oedema.

Fig. 162. Two round foreign bodies (arrowed) proved subsequently to be composed mainly of fat— diagnosed radiologically as polypi. Previous pyloroplasty for a chronic duodenal ulcer.

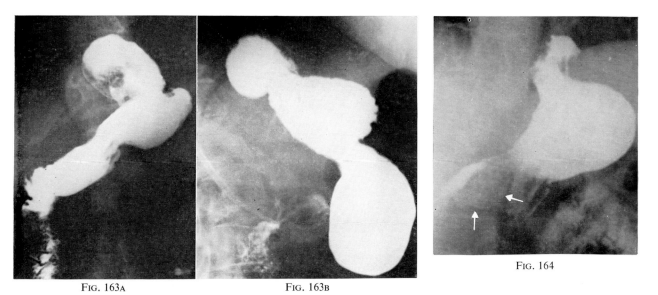

FIG. 163A   FIG. 163B   FIG. 164

Fig. 163. Food bolus simulating a carcinoma in a hiatus hernia. A: Sliding hiatus hernia with large filling defect. B: Three days later—filling defect is no longer seen.

Fig. 164. Bezoar (arrowed) in antrum causing smooth filling defect initially suggesting a simple tumour. It was easily displaced and at the end of the examination was in the hiatus hernia.

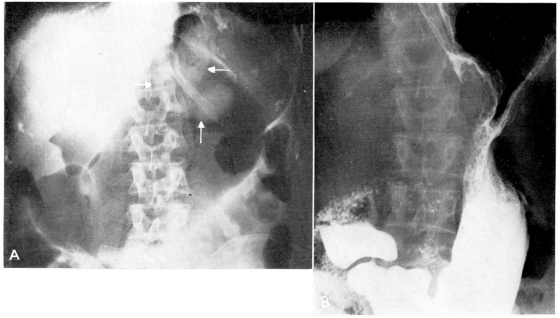

FIG. 165

Fig. 165. Villous papilloma of stomach. A: Plain film. The bulky tumour (arrowed) surrounded by gas is seen adjacent to the cardia. The distension of the stomach is presumably due to difficulty in belching. B: Barium meal. Smooth tumour coated with barium indistinguishable from a carcinoma. At laparotomy the tumour was so soft that it could not be palpated through the intact stomach.

E

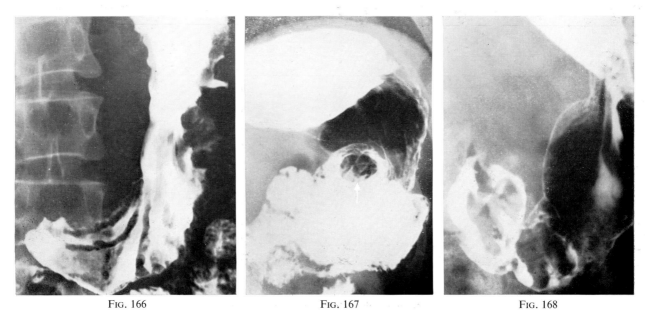

FIG. 166   FIG. 167   FIG. 168

Fig. 166. Multiple benign adenomata of stomach causing smooth filling defects particularly on crests of mucosal folds. Gastroscopic confirmation. Radiologically the appearances could not be differentiated from a mammillary gastritis.

Fig. 167. Large papilloma at stoma (arrowed) causing intermittent obstruction. Previous partial gastrectomy following which the patient was well for many years. Recent attacks of pain and vomiting.

Fig. 168. Large antral polyp which had partially prolapsed into the duodenal bulb. Operative confirmation. Supine film.

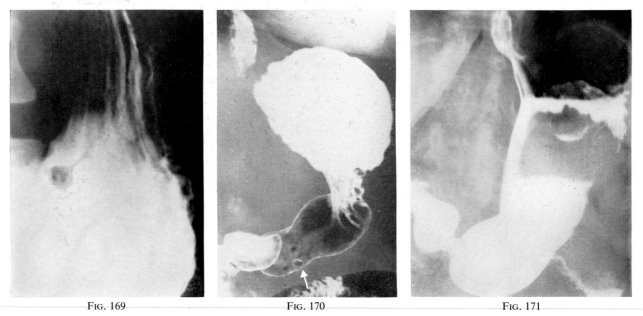

FIG. 169   FIG. 170   FIG. 171

Fig. 169. Round polyp on a stalk at incisura. Gastroscopic confirmation. The patient presented with anaemia.

Fig. 170. Small simple tumour (arrowed), ? pancreatic rest, ? fibromyoma, in pyloric antrum. It could only be shown satisfactorily in the supine position when coated with barium and surrounded by the normal gastric air bubble. Incidental finding.

Fig. 171. Leiomyoma of body of stomach causing large smooth filling defect projecting into gastric air bubble. Large ulcer crater present in middle of the tumour due to central necrosis—a common finding. Erect film showing a barium-fluid level in the ulcer crater.

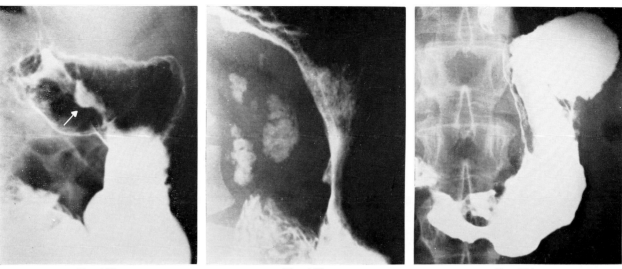

FIG. 172   FIG. 173   FIG. 174

Fig. 172. Malignant ulcer (arrowed) in fundus of stomach. At gastroscopy the ulcer was considered to be simple. Patient returned a year and a half later with a large tumour of the fundus of the stomach. Prone view. (Print reversed.)

Fig. 173. Malignant ulcer on lesser curvature of body of stomach. Radiologically considered to be simple because of extension beyond the normal outline of the stomach and its smooth margins. Large mass of calcified glands behind the stomach also present.

Fig. 174. Malignant ulcer of antrum showing the meniscus sign, i.e. translucency around the crater caused by the rolled margin. Supine film.

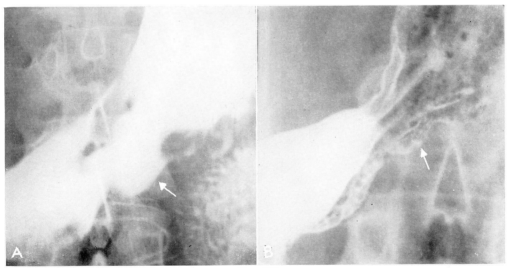

FIG. 175

Fig. 175. Malignant ulcer (arrowed) of greater curvature of stomach. A: Prone film. (Print reversed.) Irregular filling defect opposite base of ulcer suggesting malignancy. B: Supine film. The mucosal pattern around the ulcer looks reasonably normal. This is because the mucosa lining the wall opposite to lesion seen in A is now depicted. All ulcers on greater curvature and at the fundus must be considered malignant until proved otherwise.

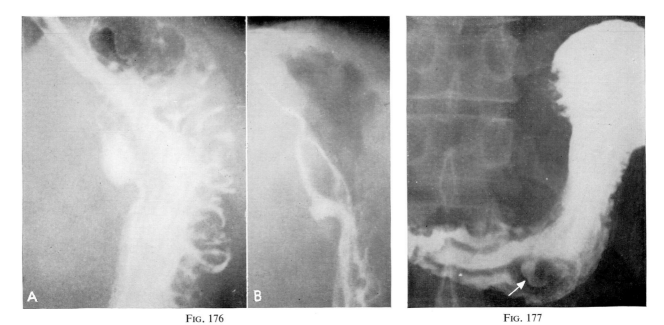

FIG. 176   FIG. 177

Fig. 176. Malignant ulcer high up on posterior wall of body of stomach. A: Irregular filling defect around its margin—the meniscus sign. B: One month later. No improvement. Irregularity even more marked, strongly suggesting malignancy. Laparotomy confirmed this ulcer to be malignant.

Seven years previously a barium meal elsewhere reported a gastric ulcer at this site. Thus, this is either a case of malignancy supervening on a simple gastric ulcer or a very slowly growing malignant ulcer.

Fig. 177. Malignant ulcer of stomach. Irregular 'comma' shaped ulcer (arrowed) with filling defect around its margins.

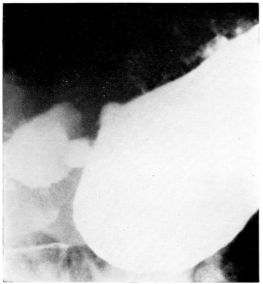

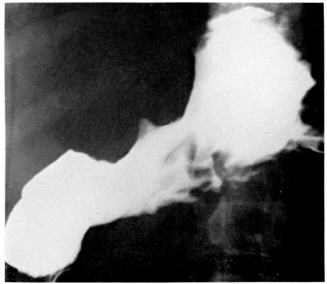

FIG. 178   FIG. 179

Fig. 178. Malignant ulcer in immediate prepyloric region. Radiologically and gastroscopically it was considered more likely to be simple than malignant. Gastric cytology was negative for malignant cells. Maximum acid output 29 mEq/hr. At laparotomy the lesion was proved to be a well differentiated adeno-carcinoma. This case illustrates the difficulty in some cases of making a precise pre-operative diagnosis.

Fig. 179. Large malignant ulcer *en plateau* on anterior wall of body of stomach demonstrated most clearly with patient lying on right side and head of table slightly elevated. The deepest part of the ulcer does not extend beyond what would have been the normal margin of the stomach. The mucosal folds on greater curvature aspect of stomach are rather coarse.

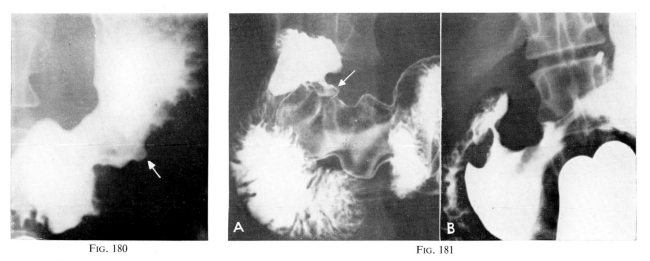

Fig. 180   Fig. 181

Fig. 180. Large irregular malignant ulcer (arrowed) on greater curvature aspect of stomach with some contraction opposite it.

Fig. 181. Gastric ulcer in prepyloric region with malignancy supervening. A : Initial film. Ulcer (arrowed). B : Three and a half years later. Large filling defect proved to be due to thickened muscle and inflammatory reaction. On microscopy early malignant change in floor of ulcer.

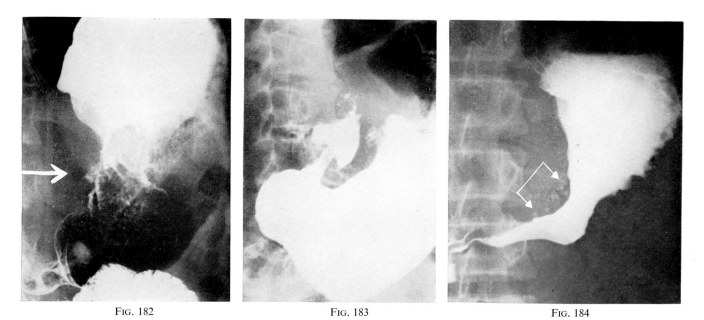

Fig. 182   Fig. 183   Fig. 184

Fig. 182. Massive haematemesis caused by irregular ulcer (arrowed) on lesser curvature aspect of stomach considered radiologically to be simple but subsequently proved to be malignant. Filling defect in the cavity of the ulcer and surrounding it due to organised blood clot which drew attention to the lesion at an early stage of the barium meal.

(By courtesy of the Editor of the *British Journal of Surgery*.)

Fig. 183. Localised scirrhous carcinoma of 'napkin-ring' type in prepyloric region resembling an adult hypertrophic pyloric stenosis. Some indentation also of base of duodenal bulb. In such cases the mucosal pattern of the abnormal area must be carefully examined for destruction suggesting malignancy.

Fig. 184. Diffuse scirrhous carcinoma of stomach with calcification (arrowed). Irregular contraction and mucosal destruction of body and antrum with rigidity on palpation.

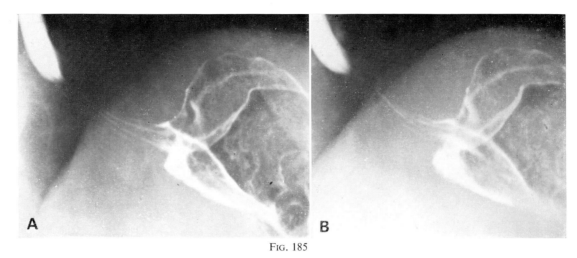

Fig. 185

Fig. 185. A and B: Carcinoma of fundus of stomach—only capable of demonstration by air contrast.   Persistence of abnormal rigid folds and complete destruction of normal mucosa.   Good stereoscopic pair.   Prone views.   (Prints reversed.)

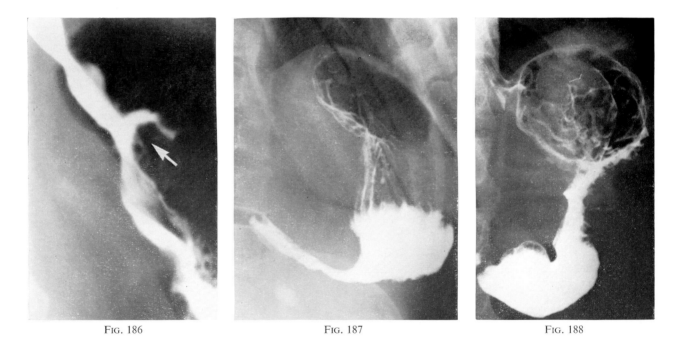

Fig. 186   Fig. 187   Fig. 188

Fig. 186. Carcinoma of fundus.   On swallowing the initial mouthful the stream of barium split at the fundus (arrowed).

Fig. 187. Diffuse scirrhous carcinoma of the antrum with gross contraction.   Well marked rigidity on fluoroscopy but the mucosal pattern in the affected area presented an almost normal appearance.   At operation the mucosa looked normal macroscopically, but on microscopic examination the tumour had infiltrated deeply into the wall.   The symptoms were typical of chronic duodenal ulceration.

Fig. 188. Large carcinoma of fundus of stomach—demonstrated clearly by double contrast.   The smooth outline and absence of oesophageal obstruction suggested a simple tumour, e.g. leiomyoma.   At laparotomy macroscopically the tumour appeared simple, but microscopically it was a carcinoma of low malignancy.

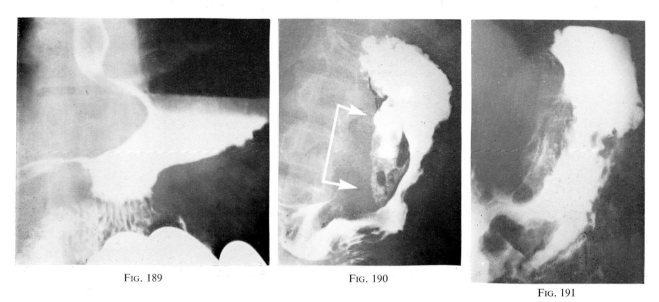

Fig. 189   Fig. 190

Fig. 191

Fig. 189. Diffuse scirrhous carcinoma involving the body and antrum with well marked rigidity and mucosal destruction. Gastro-enterostomy performed 20 years previously for a chronic duodenal ulcer. Normal jejunal folds clearly seen. Tumour restricted to stomach.

Fig. 190. Carcinoma of stomach. Large irregular filling defect with a huge ulcer (arrowed) on lesser curvature.

Fig. 191. Diffuse carcinoma of body and antrum with grossly thickened rigid folds which were persistent on palpation.

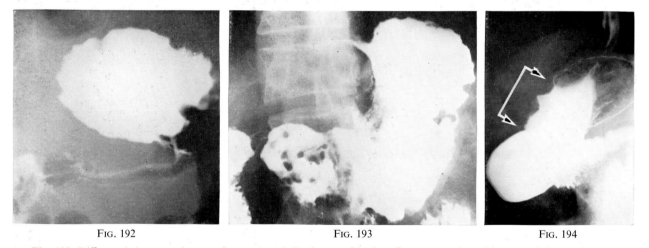

Fig. 192   Fig. 193   Fig. 194

Fig. 192. Diffuse scirrhous carcinoma of antrum and distal part of body. Gross narrowing with mucosal destruction and inability to distend even with appropriate positioning. The barium poured rapidly into the duodenum—a characteristic feature of a scirrhous carcinoma when the pylorus is affected.

Fig. 193. Large ulcerated fungating carcinoma of antrum causing an extremely irregular filling defect—occurring in an old standing case of Menétrier's disease. Barium meal 11 years previously showed extremely coarse hypertrophic mucosal folds. As a carcinoma at that time could not be excluded a laparotomy and biopsy were performed confirming Menétrier's disease.

Fig. 194. Carcinoma of anterior wall of stomach (arrowed) in a known case of pernicious anaemia. Large irregular filling defect only demonstrated by turning the patient to lie on his right side and slightly elevating the head of the table. Atrophic mucosal folds elsewhere—characteristic of pernicious anaemia.

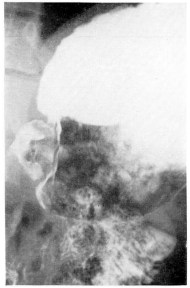
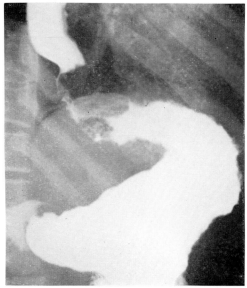
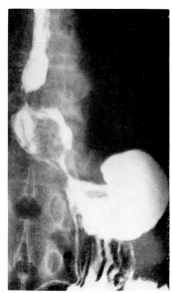

FIG. 195   FIG. 196   FIG. 197

Fig. 195. Carcinoma of antrum.   Large filling defect with a huge ulcer causing considerable stenosis.   Male aged 36.   Very high basal acid output.   Some of the clinical features suggested the Zollinger-Ellison syndrome.

Fig. 196. Carcinoma of fundus of stomach involving lower oesophagus with a characteristic filling defect.   Some dilatation also of the oesophagus proximal to the tumour.   Prone position.   (Print reversed.)

Fig. 197. Carcinoma of stomach in a case of hiatus hernia causing a filling defect in the herniated pouch and also in the stomach below the diaphragm.   Long history of regurgitation but with recent dysphagia and weight loss.

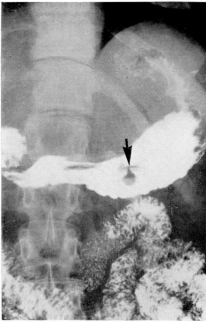
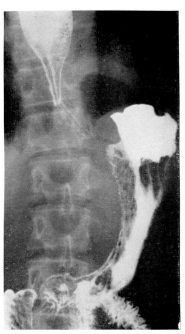
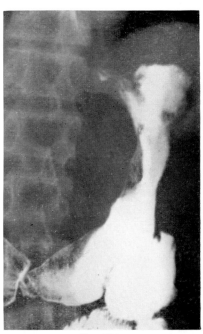

FIG. 198   FIG. 199   FIG. 200

Fig. 198. Malignant polyp (arrowed) opposite incisura causing filling defect readily detected on barium meal.   At operation the tumour could not be felt through the intact stomach nor was there any external evidence of malignancy.

Fig. 199. Diffuse scirrhous carcinoma of proximal half of stomach with marked rigidity, contraction and mucosal destruction. The tumour had spread to involve the lower oesophagus causing obstruction.   No increase in the distance between the lumen of the stomach and the base of the lung.

Fig. 200. Carcinoma of proximal half of stomach including fundus.   Diffuse contraction with filling defects, mucosal destruction, and greatly increased distance between fundus of stomach and base of lung due to thickening of fundal wall.

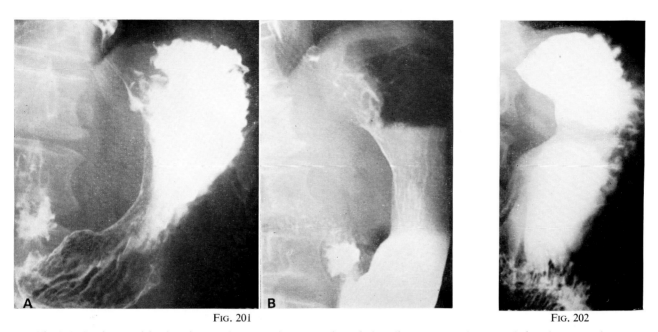

FIG. 201   FIG. 202

Fig. 201. Carcinoma of fundus of stomach. A: Supine. Some irregularity adjacent to oesophago-gastric junction suggesting a tumour but the appearances are not diagnostic. B: Erect film immediately following tilting the table from the supine position producing a double contrast of the fundus. The tumour is now coated with barium and clearly seen through the gastric air bubble. **Fig. 202.** Multifocal superficial carcinoma causing thickened mucosal folds but with absence of rigidity—similar to hypertrophic 'gastritis'. Body of the stomach mainly involved. History of loss of weight and indigestion with a high E.S.R. Total gastrectomy performed. Microscopic examination showed a diffuse carcinomatous infiltration involving the mucosa with some superficial ulceration.

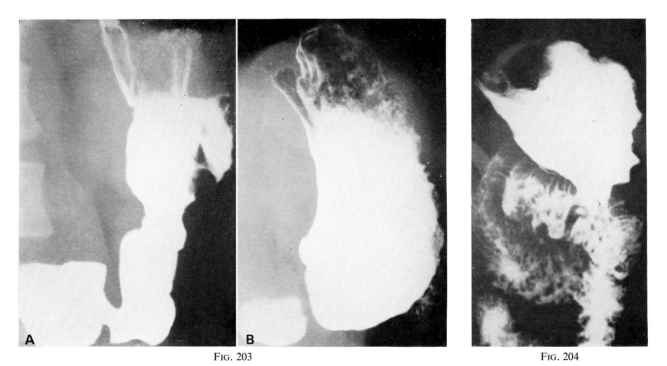

FIG. 203   FIG. 204

Fig. 203. Carcinoma of stomach treated by cytotoxic drugs. A: Large persistent irregular filling defect of body and antrum. The clinical, radiological and operative findings were all strongly suggestive of a carcinoma. Unfortunately at laparotomy no biopsy was taken as the surgeon was confident of the diagnosis. B: Five months later following treatment by cytotoxic drugs. The stomach presents an almost normal appearance. The patient had gained two stones in weight. Patient alive and well two years later. **Fig. 204.** Recurrence of carcinoma in gastric remnant causing rigidity, irregularity and mucosal destruction. Previous partial gastrectomy for malignant ulcer.

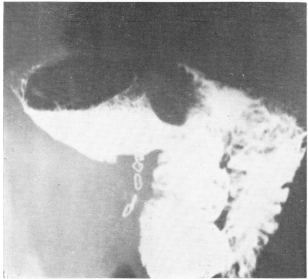

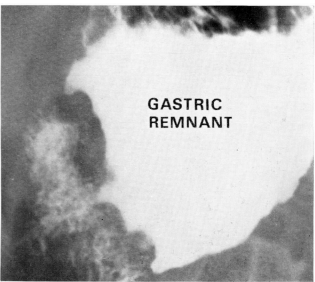

FIG. 205   FIG. 206

Fig. 205. Recurrence of carcinoma following partial gastrectomy causing collar-like filling defect at the stoma.   Metallic clips at suture line clearly seen.

Fig. 206. Recurrence of carcinoma of stomach at the suture line causing rigidity and irregularity with some stomal obstruction. Partial gastrectomy six years previously for a malignant ulcer in the antrum.   Supine view with left side raised.   Jejunum not involved.

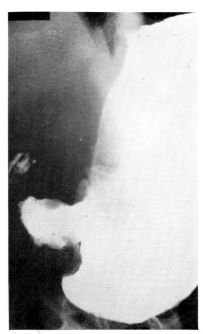

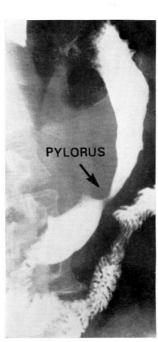

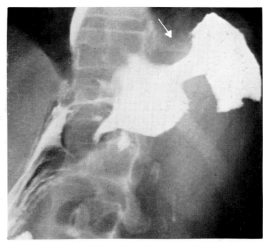

FIG. 209

FIG. 207   FIG. 208

Fig. 207. Lymphosarcoma of stomach.   Large bulky tumour in antrum with mucosal destruction—a characteristic appearance.   Supine position with left side slightly raised.

Fig. 208. Lymphosarcoma of stomach causing diffuse contraction and rigidity similar to a scirrhous carcinoma.   At laparotomy the stomach was opened and macroscopically looked and felt normal.   The first biopsy report was non-committal but subsequent study showed this to be a lymphosarcoma.

Fig. 209. Perforation of lymphosarcoma of fundus with fistula (arrowed) to sub-phrenic abscess on left side.   Note large tumour opposite cardiac orifice causing a filling defect.

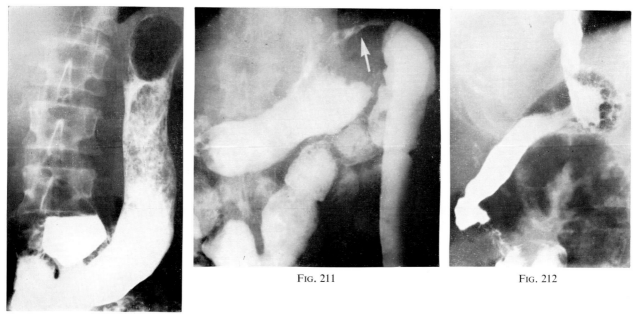

Fig. 210.   Fig. 211   Fig. 212

Fig. 210. Amyloidosis of stomach—radiologically indistinguishable from a diffuse scirrhous carcinoma. Some contraction with rigidity, mucosal atrophy and absence of peristalsis. The filling defects are due to food particles. **Fig. 211.** Gastro-colic fistula (arrowed) following perforation of lymphosarcoma of fundus of stomach into splenic flexure of colon. Note filling defect in the fundus due to the tumour. Film half an hour after barium meal showing colon extensively filled with barium. **Fig. 212.** Generalised contraction of stomach with mucosal atrophy in a case of anorexia nervosa. Normal motility and pliable walls differentiated it from a scirrhous carcinoma. Patient supine and turned almost on right side.

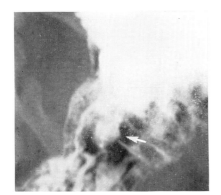

Fig. 213

Fig. 213. *Formation cavitaire d'origine dynamique de Moutier*—usually considered due to a circular area of spasm around an erosion. *En face* view. Characteristic ulcer-like appearance (arrowed) with surrounding translucency simulating a malignant ulcer. Half an hour later this area was normal. **Fig. 214.** *Formation*

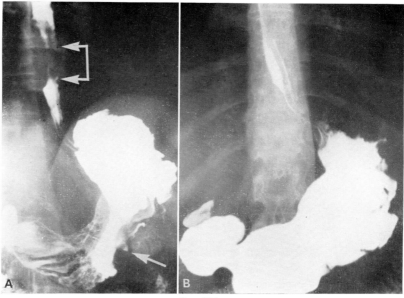

Fig. 214

cavitaire d'origine dynamique de Moutier. Incidental finding in a patient with a carcinoma in lower third of oesophagus. A: Initial film. Appearance suggests an irregular malig-nant ulcer *en plateau* (arrowed) on greater curvature. The filling defect and soft tissue shadow due to the oesophageal carcinoma are also arrowed. B: Two months later following radiotherapy to the oesophageal carcinoma. Normal greater curvature now present apart from a rather coarse mucosal pattern. Note excellent result in the oesophagus following treatment of the carcinoma.

In view of the previous suspicion of a gastric carcinoma a laparotomy was performed, but a tumour was excluded.

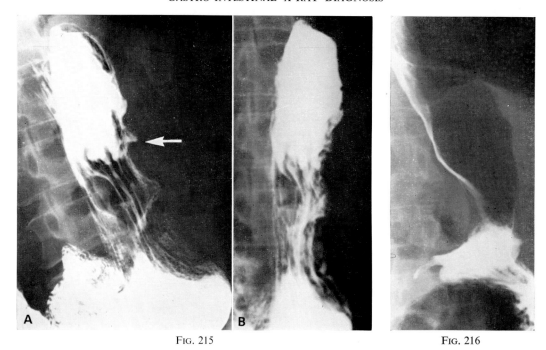

FIG. 215   FIG. 216

Fig. 215. *Formation cavitaire d'origine dynamique de Moutier.* A: The appearance (arrowed) suggests a malignant ulcer on greater curvature with a marginal filling defect. B: Half an hour later the greater curvature presents a normal appearance. (By courtesy of the Editor of the *British Journal of Surgery*.) **Fig. 216.** Syphilis of the stomach—a very rare condition. Complete mucosal atrophy, absence of peristalsis and with generalised contraction particularly affecting the antrum—indistinguishable from a scirrhous carcinoma. Gastro-enterostomy had been performed 20 years previously for an ulcerated filling defect in the antrum now known to have been a gumma but presumed at that time to be a carcinoma.

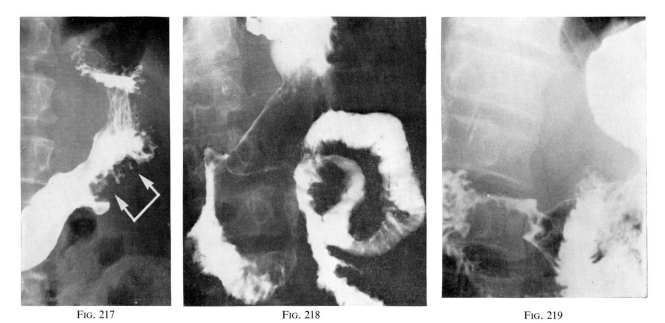

FIG. 217   FIG. 218   FIG. 219

Fig. 217. Menétrier's disease of greater curvature (arrowed). Gastroscopic confirmation. The coarse hypertrophic mucosal folds cause a localised bulky filling defect. Initially this looked like a carcinoma but on palpation the folds were pliable. Patient subsequently had resection of pelvic colon for a carcinoma and examination of stomach revealed no evidence of a tumour. **Fig. 218.** Plasmacytosis of stomach, duodenum and upper jejunum. Operative confirmation. Rigidity with some contraction of body and antrum with absence of normal mucosal pattern. Gross coarsening of mucosa of duodenum and upper jejunum due to oedematous mucosal folds. The barium in the bowel is also diluted by excess of fluid. No definite radiological diagnosis could be made. **Fig. 219.** Crohn's disease of stomach. Irregular filling defect with ulceration in immediate prepyloric region. Similar deformity in first and second parts of duodenum previously proved to be due to Crohn's disease. Diffuse Crohn's disease was also present in the ileum with a long normal intervening segment.

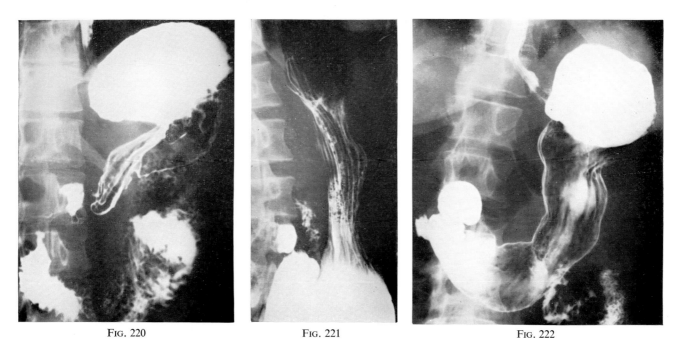

FIG. 220   FIG. 221   FIG. 222

Fig. 220. Crohn's disease of stomach. Diffuse rigidity of lower part of greater curvature and antrum with abnormal mucosal pattern—presumably due to oedema and inflammatory thickening. Gastroscopic confirmation. Crohn's disease present in upper part of second part of duodenum causing an irregularly narrowed segment. Diffuse Crohn's disease also present in ileum.

Fig. 221. Atrophic mucosal folds. Note fine parallel folds and smooth greater curvature and fundus. Low acid output. Long-standing hypochromic anaemia.

Fig. 222. Atrophic mucosal folds in a case of hypothyroidism. Smooth outline particularly obvious on greater curvature aspect and at fundus.

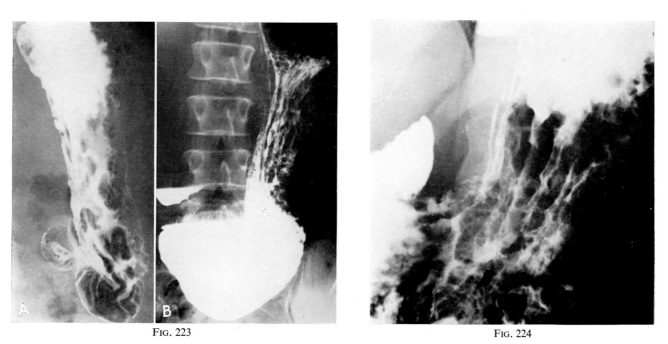

FIG. 223   FIG. 224

Fig. 223. A: Extremely coarse thickened folds, especially on greater curvature aspect—presumably representing a form of hypertrophic gastritis. No evidence of peptic ulceration. History of vague indigestion. B: Two months later. The folds are practically normal. Now clinically well.

Fig. 224. Coarse mucosal folds—confirmed gastroscopically. Chronic duodenal ulcer present.

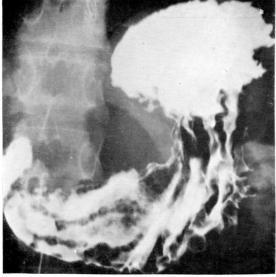

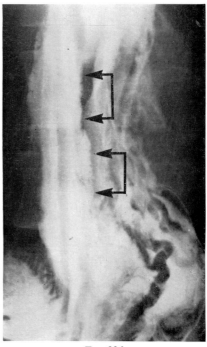

FIG. 225

Fig. 225. Mammillary gastritis causing multiple round filling defects on crests of mucosal folds especially in antrum. Chronic duodenal ulcer also present.

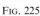

FIG. 226

Fig. 226. Streaks of mucus causing dark thread-like appearances in the lower part of body of stomach and also scalloped appearances (arrowed). Case of antral carcinoma with secondary gastritis in proximal part of stomach.

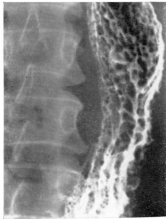
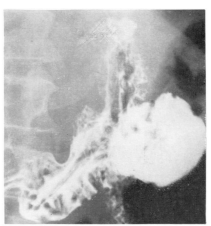
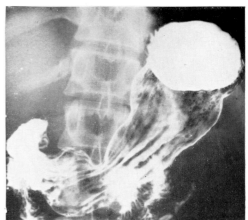

FIG. 227   FIG. 228   FIG. 229

Fig. 227. Mammillary gastritis causing multiple small filling defects on crests of mucosal folds—proved gastroscopically. Basal acid output 1·1 mEq/hr. Gastric biopsy showed excess of plasma cells in mucosa and sub-mucosa with some thickening of wall. History of nausea and vomiting for 2½ years with vague epigastric pain.

Fig. 228. Biliary gastritis following gastro-enterostomy. Coarse hypertrophic gastric mucosal folds without any specific characteristic radiological appearance. Adjacent jejunal loops are dilated and matted together by adhesions causing an obstruction which presumably encouraged reflux of bile into the stomach. Swollen oedematous folds with free reflux of bile into the stomach seen gastroscopically. History of vague indigestion. Very low acid output.

Fig. 229. Pernicious anaemia. Atrophic mucosal folds particularly affecting greater curvature and fundus. Normal peristalsis. On fluoroscopy with palpation the walls were pliable.

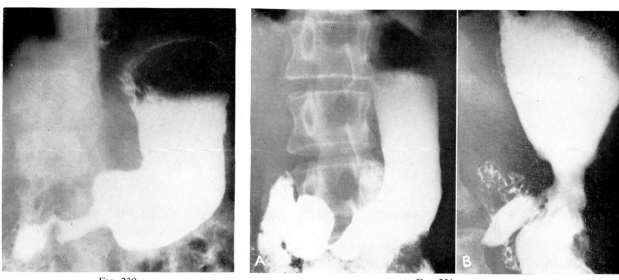

FIG. 230   FIG. 231

Fig. 230. Pseudo-malignancy in a case of pernicious anaemia. Persistent filling defect in antrum—considered radiologically to be due to a carcinoma. Note also atrophic mucosal pattern. At laparotomy the antrum initially appeared normal, but handling caused spasm producing the defect demonstrated on the film. A long myotomy was performed and biopsy showed no evidence of a carcinoma.

(By courtesy of Mr. A. A. Gunn and Dr. R. Saffley, Bangour Hospital.)

Fig. 231. Chronic form of gastritis simulating a scirrhous carcinoma in a case with pernicious anaemia. A: Gross mucosal atrophy, rigidity, absence of peristalsis and contraction of the stomach, particularly the antrum. Biopsy at laparotomy showed only a chronic inflammatory reaction. Gastro-enterostomy performed. B: Four years later. Gross contraction of antrum— more marked than commonly occurs after a gastro-enterostomy. The lower part of body is also affected and the appearances are now even more like a carcinoma. Gastric biopsy was non-committal but favoured a simple lesion. Careful follow up is being maintained. Patient still reasonably well two years later.

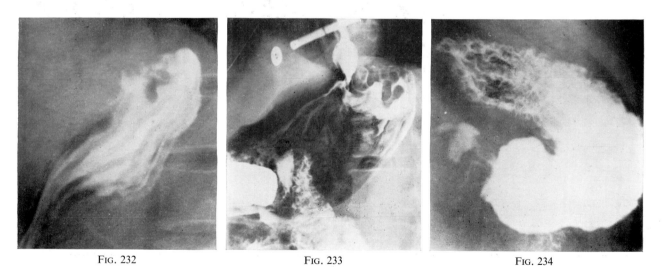

FIG. 232   FIG. 233   FIG. 234

Fig. 232. Varices of stomach causing filling defects in fundus adjacent to oesphago-gastric junction. These filling defects are obviously not in the line of mucosal folds and thus cannot represent hypertrophic mucosal folds. Case of cirrhosis of liver requiring porto-caval anastomosis. Oesophageal varices were also present. Supine film with left side raised.

Fig. 233. Gross fundal varices causing a rosette-like filling defect around oesophago-gastric junction. Oesophageal varices also present. Large gastric ulcer in the antrum difficult to see on this film, but clearly shown on others.

Fig. 234. Varices of fundus with characteristic sinuous filling defects and 'soap bubble' appearance. Gross oesophageal varices were also present. Scarring in antrum and duodenum with presence of an ulcer crater in duodenal bulb. This patient subsequently had a massive haematemesis which proved to be from the duodenal ulcer. Old case of viral hepatitis.

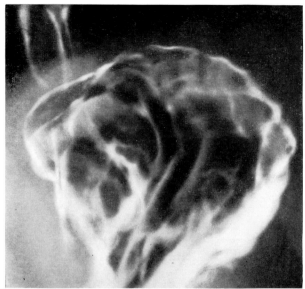
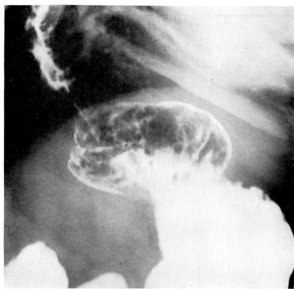

FIG. 235   FIG. 236

Fig. 235. Varices in fundus of stomach and lower oesophagus. Characteristic sinuous filling defects particularly around oesophago-gastric junction. Prone view. (Print reversed.)

Fig. 236. Varices of fundus causing polypoidal filling defects—at first sight suggesting a carcinoma. Obvious varices in lower oesophagus. Chronic alcoholic. Prone view. (Print reversed.)

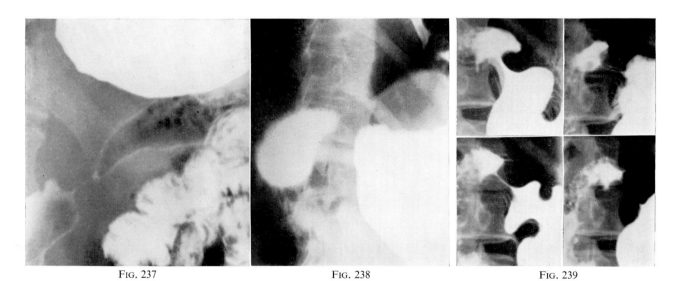

FIG. 237   FIG. 238   FIG. 239

Fig. 237. Adult hypertrophic pyloric stenosis in a patient with pernicious anaemia. The radiological appearances are far from typical and suggest a scirrhous carcinoma. Laparotomy performed and diagnosis of hypertrophic pyloric stenosis established.

Fig. 238. Adult hypertrophic pyloric stenosis. Smooth prepyloric filling defect with lumen same as pylorus. Barium meal five years previously with similar appearance—considered to represent a prepyloric carcinoma but operation at that time refused. Partial gastrectomy with operative confirmation of adult hypertrophic pyloric stenosis. Male aged 85.

Fig. 239. Adult hypertrophic pyloric stenosis. Four consecutive 'spot' films show smooth narrowing in prepyloric region with some variation in calibre but with normal mucosal pattern. Typical indentation of base of duodenal bulb. Patient treated conservatively since symptoms were relatively mild.

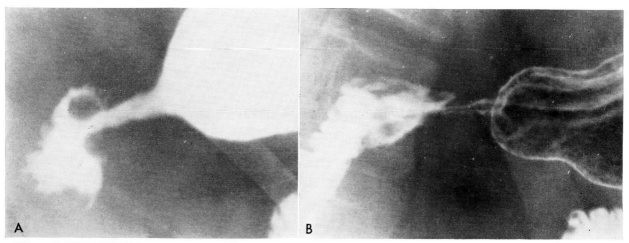

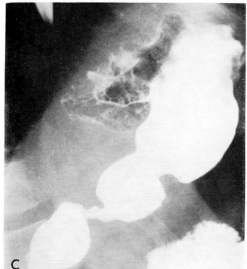

Fig. 240. Adult hypertrophic pyloric stenosis—operative confirmation. A: Prone film. (Print reversed.) Smooth narrowed prepyloric segment with lumen of approximately same calibre as true pylorus. Indentation of base of duodenal bulb by the muscular 'tumour'. Conical antrum proximal to hypertrophied muscle. B: Supine film. Normal mucosal pattern of antrum and narrowed prepyloric segment. C: Second prone film. (Print reversed.) Bend in middle of lumen of narrowed segment probably representing the change from the true pylorus to the hypertrophied muscle. This bend appeared in certain positions. Irregular filling defect of fundus of stomach confirmed to be due to a carcinoma.

F

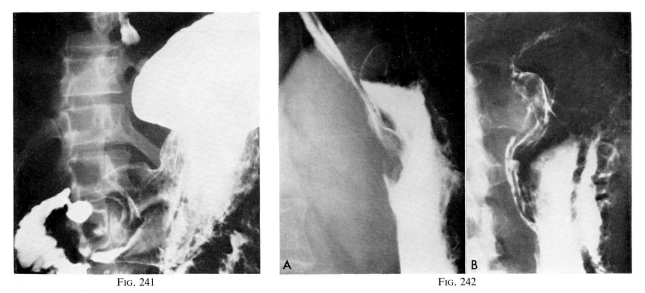

FIG. 241   FIG. 242

Fig. 241. Indentation of antrum by lumbar spine causing filling defect initially suggesting a carcinoma. On fluoroscopy with palpation the lumbar spine was obviously the cause of the deformity. Clinically a tumour had been suspected.

Fig. 242. Indentation of fundus of stomach by enlarged left lobe of liver. Operative confirmation. The filling defect near the cardiac orifice was considered most likely to be due to a carcinoma of the stomach, but the absence of oesophageal involvement cast some doubt upon this diagnosis. A: Conventional barium meal. Erect film. B: Double contrast barium meal. Prone view. (Print reversed.)

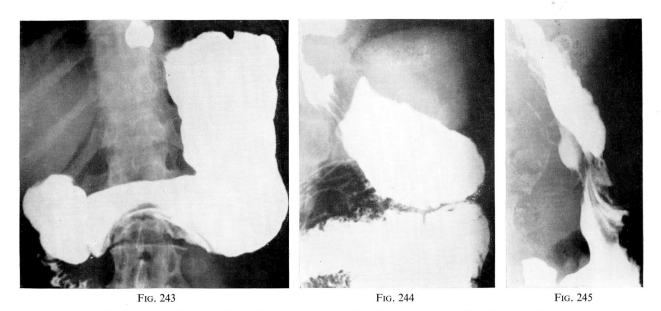

FIG. 243   FIG. 244   FIG. 245

Fig. 243. Displacement of stomach by kyphotic lumbar spine. Palpable mass present clinically suggesting a tumour.

Fig. 244. Displacement of fundus of stomach by a moderately enlarged spleen.

Fig. 245. Deformity with indentation of posterior wall of stomach caused by a grossly calcified dilated aorta. At first sight the appearances simulate a large malignant ulcer.

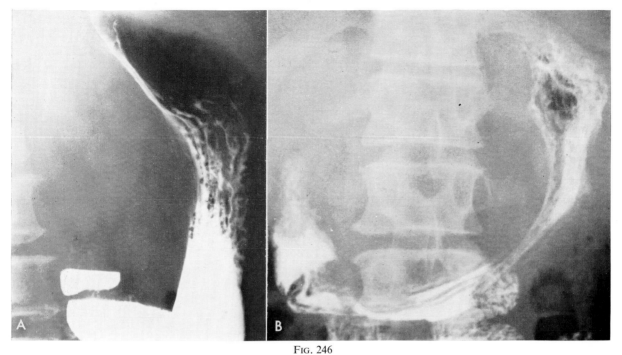

FIG. 246

Fig. 246. Displacement of stomach by large mass of glands (lymphosarcoma) adjacent to body of pancreas and causing appearances indistinguishable from a pancreatic tumour. A: Erect. The mass displaces the body of the stomach forwards. B: Supine. Downwards displacement with indentation of stomach.

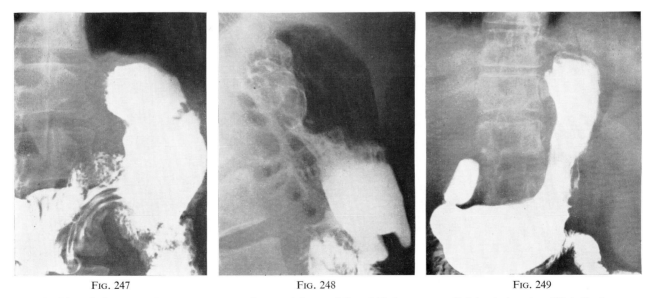

FIG. 247   FIG. 248   FIG. 249

Fig. 247. Displacement of greater curvature of stomach by partially calcified aneurysm of abdominal aorta. Clinically there was an abdominal mass of doubtful aetiology.

Fig. 248. Displacement of fundus of stomach by enlarged malignant glands. The filling defect is indistinguishable from an intrinsic gastric carcinoma. Double contrast film. Erect. Previous low partial gastrectomy.

Fig. 249. Displacement of stomach medially and downwards by grossly enlarged spleen. Some deformity of the greater curvature due to adhesions to the spleen.

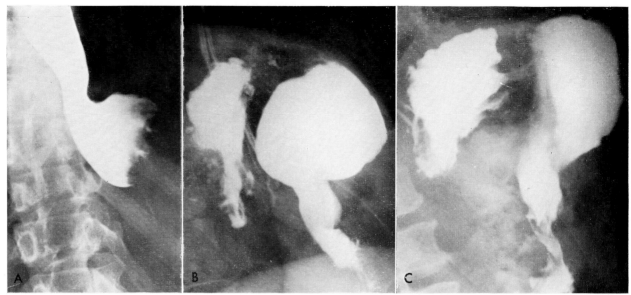

Fig. 250

Fig. 250. Volvulus of stomach on its transverse axis in a case of eventration of diaphragm. A: Irregular filling defect causing complete obstruction and suggesting a large carcinoma. B: Second barium meal three days later. Considerable clinical improvement. Only partial obstruction now present and obvious rotation of stomach on its transverse axis. C: A few minutes later. Further unfolding of the volvulus.

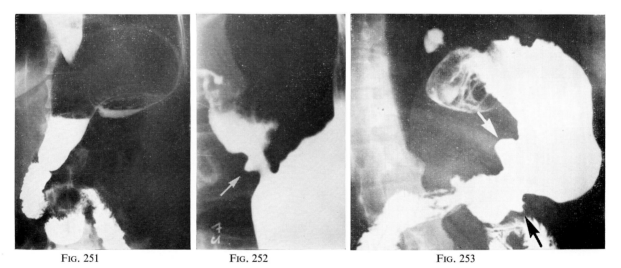

FIG. 251   FIG. 252   FIG. 253

Fig. 251. Intermittent volvulus of stomach on its cardio-pyloric axis. Considerable distension of stomach with gas probably due to inability to belch. Erect film almost true antero-posterior.

Six-year history of intermittent abdominal pain. Billroth I gastrectomy performed with excellent result.

Fig. 252. Previous pyloroplasty with the radiological appearances confirmed at subsequent operation. One of the 'dog ears' on the greater curvature aspect (arrowed) is clearly seen. The 'dog ear' was difficult to differentiate from an ulcer on the film but easy on fluoroscopy since barium could be readily expressed from it. Because of discomfort and pain in the right hypochondrium, laparotomy was performed. Considerable adhesions were present around the duodenum.

Fig. 253. Previous extensive pyloroplasty for adult hypertrophic pyloric stenosis causing large 'dog ears' (arrowed) resulting from transverse suturing. Because of megaloblastic anaemia and the uncertain nature of the deformity, a laparotomy was performed confirming that the 'dog ears' were in fact the result of the pyloroplasty and did not represent ulcer craters.

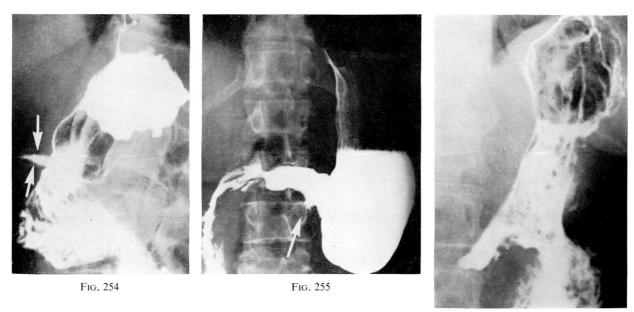

FIG. 254   FIG. 255

FIG. 256

Fig. 254. Antral contraction (arrowed) more gross than usual following well-functioning gastro-enterostomy. At laparotomy no evidence of a carcinoma.

Patient alive and well six years later.

Fig. 255. 'Dog ear' (arrowed) on greater curvature aspect of antrum due to dismantling of previous gastro-enterostomy at time of pyloroplasty. The 'dog ear' simulates an ulcer.

Fig. 256. Usual degree of antral narrowing following well-functioning gastro-enterostomy.

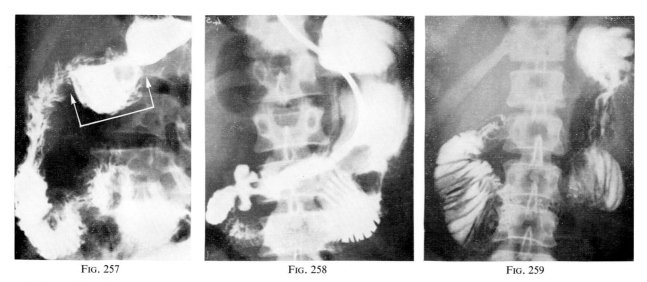

FIG. 257   FIG. 258   FIG. 259

Fig. 257. Jejunal segment (arrowed) interposed between small gastric remnant and duodenum. This operation was performed because of severe dumping following a Polya gastrectomy.

Fig. 258. Obstruction in immediate post-operative period due to retraction of gastro-enterostomy stoma through transverse meso-colon. Retro-colic anastomosis. On fluoroscopy no Gastrografin left the stomach through the stoma. Vigorous but ineffective peristaltic waves in duodenum. No Gastrografin entered the efferent loop. Obvious ulcer deformity of duodenal bulb. Loculated effusion below right dome of diaphragm containing a large amount of gas.

Fig. 259. Post-operative obstruction due to retraction of gastro-enterostomy stoma through transverse meso-colon. No Gastrografin left the stomach through the stoma. Dilatation of the duodenum with powerful but ineffective peristalsis. No Gastrografin entered the efferent loop either through the stoma or through the afferent loop.

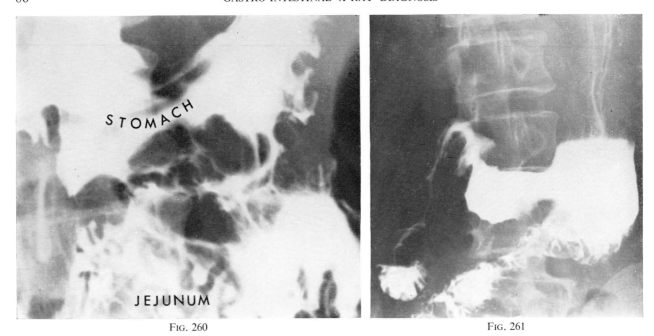

FIG. 260   FIG. 261

Fig. 260. Prolapse of oedematous mucosal folds through gastro-enterostomy stoma causing a polypoidal filling defect. Gastroscopic confirmation. History of abdominal pain and vomiting. **Fig. 261.** Stomal oedema following gastro-enterostomy causing a filling defect especially on antral side of anastomosis. Moderate fluid residue in the stomach.

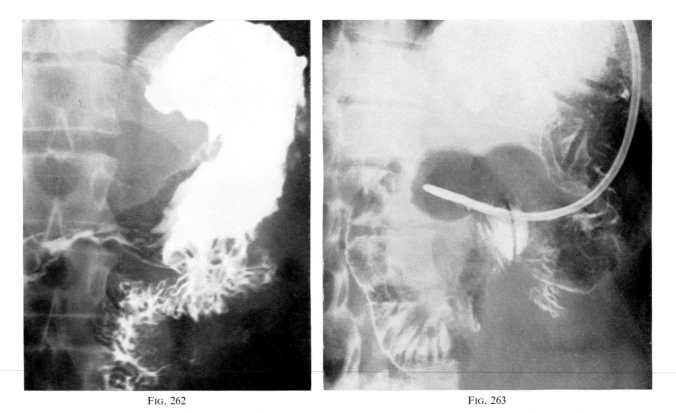

FIG. 262   FIG. 263

Fig. 262. Prolapse of swollen jejunal mucosal folds through gastro-jejunal anastomosis causing a polypoidal defect in stomach. Patient presented with bile vomiting. **Fig. 263.** Retraction of gastro-enterostomy stoma with adjacent jejunum through transverse meso-colon. History of vomiting and large aspirates in immediate post-operative period. Gastrografin meal. No Gastrografin left through the anastomosis. Dilatation and hyperperistalsis in duodenum with complete obstruction in stomal region. Operative confirmation.

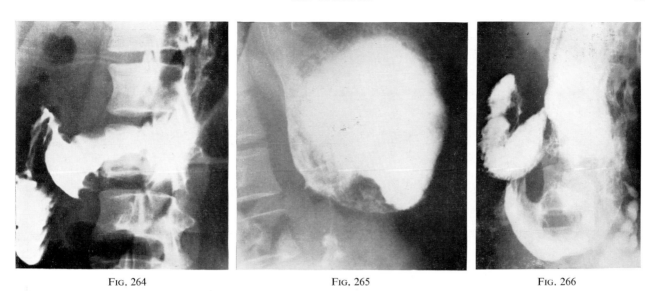

FIG. 264   FIG. 265   FIG. 266

Fig. 264. Prolapse of swollen oedematous jejunal mucosal folds into stomach causing a cauliflower like filling defect at gastro-jejunal anastomosis. Gastroscopic confirmation. Obstruction with vomiting seven days after gastro-enterostomy. Some Gastrografin left the stomach through the pylorus but none through the stoma.

Fig. 265. Stomal obstruction due to large inflammatory mass around stoma eight days after Polya partial gastrectomy. Dilatation of gastric remnant. Only a trace of Gastrografin left the stomach after considerable delay through an extremely narrowed stoma.

Fig. 266. Retrograde jejuno-gastric intussusception following gastro-enterostomy causing a large filling defect in stomach. This complication occurred in the immediate post-operative period. Gastrografin meal.

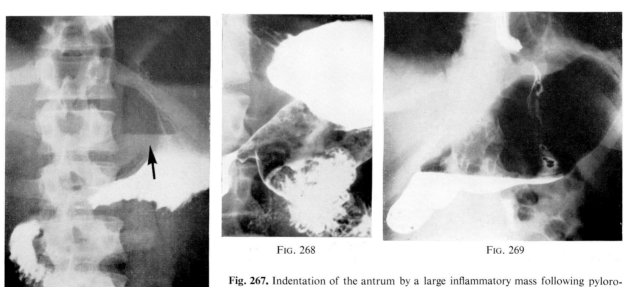

FIG. 268   FIG. 269

Fig. 267. Indentation of the antrum by a large inflammatory mass following pyloroplasty. Fluid level (arrowed) in an abscess cavity. Gastrografin meal ten days after operation. No fistula.

FIG. 267

Fig. 268. Gastro-enterostomy with chronic retrograde jejuno-gastric intussusception causing a filling defect in the stomach. Gastroscopic confirmation. No barium left through the stoma—the jejunum being filled through the duodenum. Some scarring in the prepyloric region from a prepyloric ulcer.

Fig. 269. Transient damage to vagi causing dilatation with atony of stomach following operation for hiatus hernia. Return to normal after two weeks. Erect film.

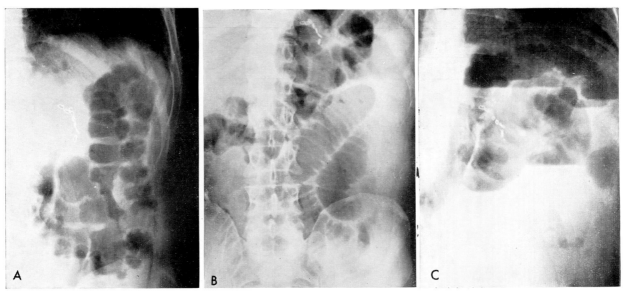

Fig. 270

Fig. 270. Stammer's hernia following Polya partial gastrectomy. A: No hernia present. Some post-operative distension. Note the position of the splenic flexure and the adjacent parts of the descending and transverse colon. Metallic clips on suture line easily identified. B: Supine. Two days later. Hernia now present. The patient developed severe abdominal and back pain. Distended loops of jejunum with typical cross-hatched appearance on the left side displacing the colon medially strongly suggesting a Stammer's hernia. C: Erect film at same time as B showing fluid levels in the distended loops of jejenum. Note difference from A. Operative confirmation.

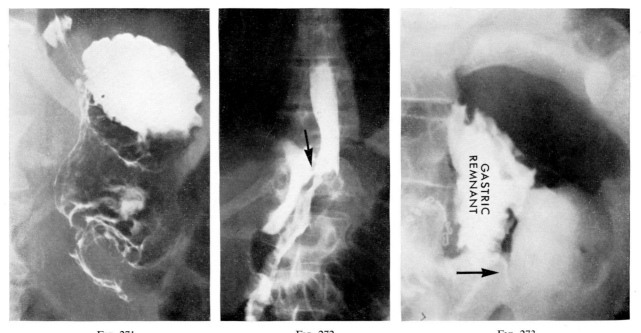

Fig. 271   Fig. 272   Fig. 273

Fig. 271. Stammer's type hernia following gastro-enterostomy. Operative confirmation. Displacement of stoma with stomal obstruction demonstrated by Gastrografin meal. Gas-distended jejunal loops on left side.

Fig. 272. Fistula (arrowed) arising from stomach. High partial gastrectomy eight days previously for large gastric ulcer. The abscess cavity lay between the liver and the gastric remnant. Gastrografin meal.

Fig. 273. Leak in immediate post-operative period following Polya partial gastrectomy. Fistula (arrowed) arising from the stomal region and extending into a cavity containing a large amount of gas. The gastric remnant is completely filled with Gastrografin. Note different appearance of the Gastrografin in the loculation where it is mixed with muco-pus.

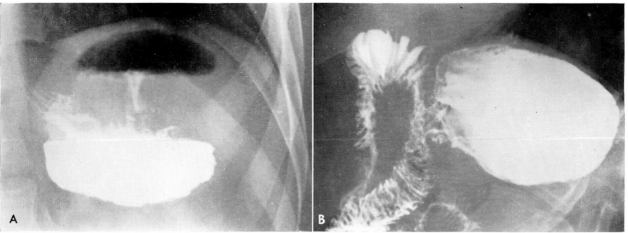

Fig. 274

Fig. 274. Stomal obstruction after Polya gastrectomy. A: Erect film. Large fluid residue seen in dilated gastric remnant. B: Supine film with left side raised and head of the table elevated—the best manoeuvre to cause emptying. Some narrowing of the jejunum at the stoma due to an inflammatory mass which settled down with conservative measures.

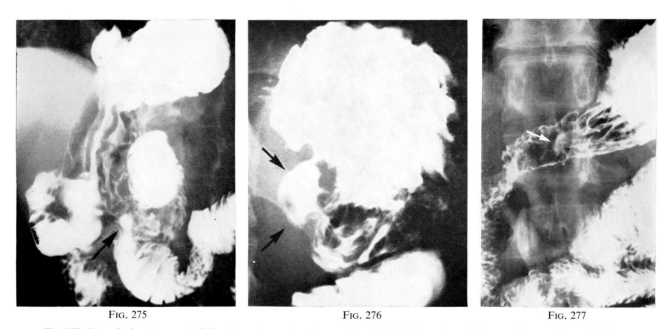

| Fig. 275 | Fig. 276 | Fig. 277 |

Fig. 275. Stomal ulcer (arrowed) following gastro-enterostomy. Considerable distortion of adjacent jejunum from adhesions. Supine film.

Fig. 276. Large stomal ulcer (arrowed) on the suture line with radiating folds following partial gastrectomy of Polya type. Gastroscopic confirmation.

Fig. 277. Stomal ulcer (arrowed) following Billroth I gastrectomy—an uncommon finding. Supine film showing large ulcer crater with radiating folds.

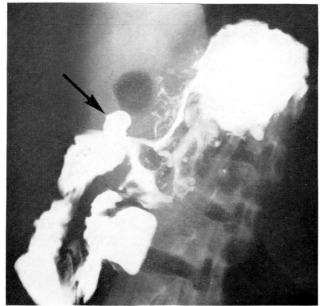

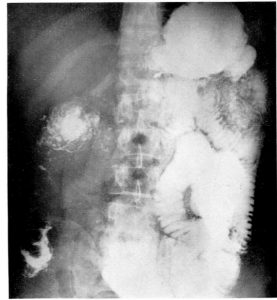

FIG. 278   FIG. 279

Fig. 278. Large stomal ulcer (arrowed) following Billroth I gastrectomy.   Recent perforation causing a localised abscess indicated by a pocket of gas adjacent to the ulcer.   Subsequent operative confirmation.   **Fig. 279.** Gastrocolic fistula following perforation of a jejunal ulcer into colon.   Polya gastrectomy several years previously.   Film half an hour after barium meal.   Note barium in proximal colon which fluoroscopically was seen to fill almost as soon as upper jejunum.

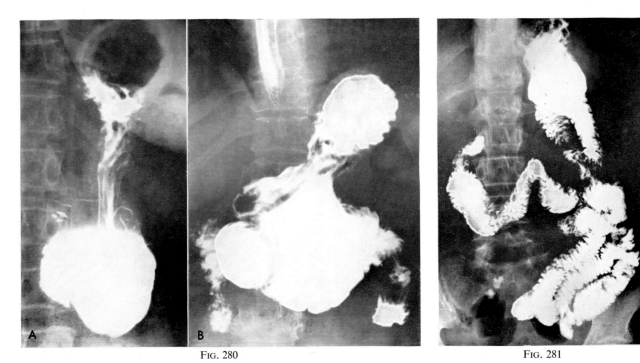

FIG. 280   FIG. 281

Fig. 280. Gastro-enterostomy with gross dilatation of jejunum opposite stoma—caused by adhesions which kinked and obstructed the efferent loop.   Complaint of heartburn, abdominal pain and bile vomiting.   A: Erect.   Initially the appearances suggested a dilated gastric remnant with a fluid level—the jejunum opposite the stoma being interpreted as the dependent part of the stomach. B: Supine.   Enormously dilated jejunal loop opposite the stoma.   Excessive filling also of the afferent loop.   **Fig. 281.** Bile vomiting following Polya gastrectomy.   Barium initially entered afferent loop presumably due to the mechanics of the stoma. Considerable stasis in afferent loop, including duodenum.   Treated by Roux-en-Y conversion with complete relief.

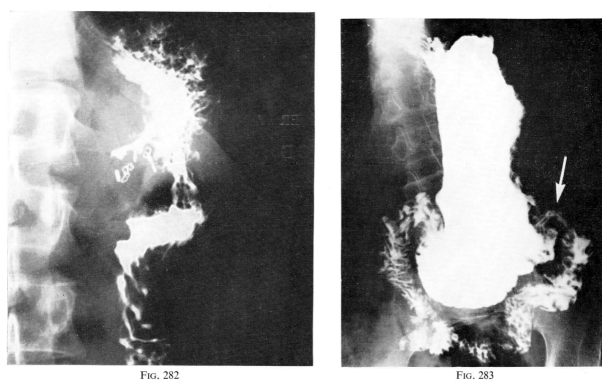

Fig. 282 Fig. 283

Fig. 282. Haematoma at stoma following Polya partial gastrectomy causing a large filling defect displacing gastric remnant upwards. Gastroscopic confirmation. Note metallic clips at suture line. **Fig. 283.** Bile vomiting following Polya partial gastrectomy. Wide stoma with distension of jejunum opposite anastomosis. Narrowing of efferent loop (arrowed) due to kinking by adhesions. Some filling of afferent loop.

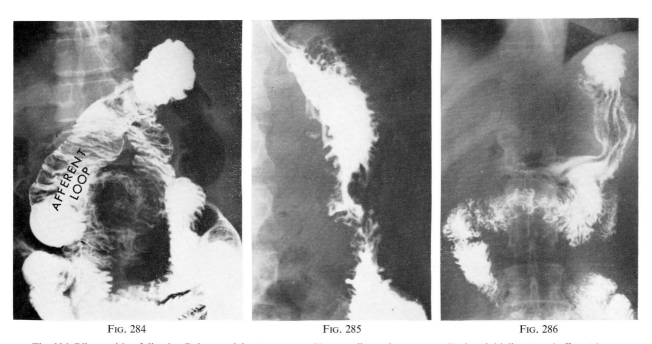

Fig. 284 Fig. 285 Fig. 286

Fig. 284. Bile vomiting following Polya partial gastrectomy. Very small gastric remnant. Barium initially entered afferent loop which was dilated and emptied slowly. Adhesions were divided and entero-anastomosis performed with clinical cure. **Fig. 285.** Bile vomiting following Polya gastrectomy. No abnormality detected on barium meal, the stoma functioning satisfactorily. No filling of afferent loop. This is quite a common finding in such cases. **Fig. 286.** Bile vomiting following iso-peristaltic gastro-enterostomy. The stoma functions satisfactorily and only a minimal amount of barium entered the afferent loop. The barium passed normally along the efferent loop. History of vague indigestion with heaviness building up over several days followed by an episode of bile vomiting.

CHAPTER IV

THE DUODENUM

RADIOLOGICAL METHODS OF EXAMINATION

Plain films are necessary in obstructions and in acute abdominal emergencies, particularly suspected perforations. They are important in the newborn for the diagnosis of lesions such as duodenal atresia.

A barium meal is the standard method for routine use and needs no further description. In selected cases barium is injected through a tube into the duodenum which has been rendered hypotonic (p. 4).

A Gastrografin meal is of value in investigating immediate post-operative complications, suspected perforations, and for the diagnosis or exclusion of acute cholecystitis and acute pancreatitis.

A cholecystogram and intravenous Biligrafin have been used in an attempt to outline the duodenum and afferent loop following partial gastrectomy and gastro-enterostomy but with little success.

CLINICAL RADIOLOGY

NORMAL APPEARANCES

The duodenal bulb is shaped like the ace of spades or an acorn and its walls are smooth and pliable. It empties usually with a strong contraction propelling barium distally. The mucosal folds tend to be parallel to the long axis but in the supine position they may be ironed out as in the pyloric antrum resulting in a smooth outline when the bulb is distended with air and coated with barium. Occasionally the folds are transverse. They may present a rosette appearance in the base of the bulb around the pylorus when it is seen partially *en face*.

At the apex of the bulb a small rest or niche of barium surrounded by a circular translucency causing a form of 'dot and ring' or 'target' appearance is a normal appearance and must not be mistaken for an ulcer or other abnormality. Because of its site it is unlikely to be due to the opening of the duct of Santorini as had at one time been thought.

The mucosa of the remainder of the duodenum is of the feathery type and barium is usually propelled rapidly onwards by peristaltic waves. The normal ampulla of Vater may be shown by air contrast.

In the third or fourth parts a transverse ridge due to indentation by the superior mesenteric vessels in the root of the mesentery is usually present.

In stout, thick-set individuals, the duodenal loop is large, particularly in the prone position.

CONGENITAL ANOMALIES

Duodenal atresia is particularly common in mongolism. On plain erect films the distended antrum and first part of the duodenum produce a 'double bubble' appearance. This anomaly is easily confirmed by a barium or Gastrografin meal.

Duodenal diverticula are common, may be single or multiple, and are usually situated on the concave border of the duodenal loop. Diverticula in the upper jejunum may also coexist and in the erect position show fluid levels simulating an obstruction. In the supine view on a barium follow-through they are readily recognised.

Food may be retained in a diverticulum causing a filling defect simulating a carcinoma. If there is doubt, the barium meal should be repeated after a few days when the filling defect, if due to food, will have disappeared. Rarely an ulcer may be present in a diverticulum and such an ulcer has a special tendency to bleed, sometimes profusely.

A diverticulum is common at the ampulla of Vater and sometimes the common bile duct and the pancreatic duct enter this diverticulum. Occasionally it is the site of chronic inflammation and may then cause obstruction of these ducts.

Intra-luminal diverticula, i.e. projecting into the lumen, are rare and cause a filling defect with smooth margins usually in the second part of the duodenum. If the diverticulum fills with barium its recognition is relatively easy. Otherwise it may be mistaken for a tumour.

Other minor anomalies, e.g. reversed duodenal loop, figure of eight duodenum, etc., need no further description. Congenital looping of the first part is common but is rarely of significance. In the erect position it forms a 'U'-shaped loop distal to the bulb.

In *situs inversus partialis commune mesenterium* the third part of the duodenum does not cross the midline but proceeds downwards to the right of the spine. The small bowel is mainly or entirely situated on the right side of the abdomen.

DUODENAL ULCERATION

A. In the Bulb

A duodenal ulcer at this site is by far the commonest lesion discovered during the course of a barium meal. In the early stages of the examination a fluid residue in the stomach with coarse gastric mucosal folds and a degree of pylorospasm suggests the possibility of a duodenal ulcer. However, a definite diagnosis can be made only with the demonstration of a crater usually *en face* but sometimes in profile. For this purpose the value of the supine view cannot be too strongly stressed. The ulcer *en face* is indicated by a persistent fleck of barium which is not displaced by pressure or palpation.

In the great majority of cases there is a typical butterfly deformity of the bulb due to the development of an incisura on each side opposite the ulcer. Occasionally the deformity is more complicated with additional incisurae. Sometimes a thickened ridge simulating a mucosal fold runs from the prepyloric region through the pylorus towards the duodenal ulcer. When the ulcer is recent the deformity is due to spasm and when healing occurs the bulb returns to normal. In some cases an ulcer is present in an otherwise normally shaped bulb. Likewise the ulcer may heal and the bulb return to normal.

In chronic cases the deformity of the bulb is permanent on account of fibrosis and with each exacerbation the fibrosis increases and eventually causes duodenal stenosis at the level of the ulcer.

When this happens, the fornices of the bulb distend producing the pre-stenotic diverticula of Åkerlund.

The development of duodenal stenosis is associated in the first instance with gastric hyperperistalsis, but later gives way to atony and dilatation of the stomach. When this occurs the pylorus dilates and ultimately becomes permanently patent. This condition of a dilated pylorus immediately proximal to duodenal stenosis from an ulcer is not sufficiently appreciated. True pyloric stenosis results only from an ulcer in the pyloric canal or immediately adjacent to it.

If an ulcer is adjacent to the pylorus on the superior aspect, it causes flattening of the fornix during the process of healing. This flattening may extend through the pylorus to the prepyloric region of the stomach.

Rarely an ulcer on the posterior wall extends backwards to involve the common bile duct. This may result in dilatation of the ducts with obstructive jaundice. In rare instances the ulcer perforates into the common bile duct allowing gas to appear in the biliary passages and barium following a barium meal.

A very large duodenal ulcer can be overlooked as it may mimic a normal bulb or a pre-stenotic diverticulum. However, its margins are sharp and rigid, it cannot be emptied readily by palpation, nor can its shape be altered as in the case of a normal bulb or pre-stenotic diverticulum.

Frequent barium meal examinations for progress of healing should be avoided because of the danger of excessive radiation. Furthermore, it is not always possible to demonstrate an actual ulcer crater in a grossly scarred bulb.

After gastro-enterostomy a duodenal ulcer usually heals satisfactorily and becomes reactivated only if stenosis of the stoma results. If an ulcer recurs following vagotomy and pyloroplasty, this usually means that the vagotomy has been incomplete.

In all cases of hiatus hernia with oesophagitis a careful search must be made for a duodenal ulcer as these two lesions not infrequently co-exist. Multiple peptic ulcers may occur, e.g. two in the bulb, one in the bulb and one post-bulbar, one duodenal ulcer and one gastric ulcer, etc.

DIFFERENTIAL DIAGNOSIS

The typical butterfly or clover-leaf deformity due to a duodenal ulcer can rarely be mistaken for anything else. Some deformity of the bulb can also be produced by the following:

1. *A cholecyst-duodenal band* may indent the superior aspect of the bulb producing a sharp incisura. More commonly it causes a vertical impression particularly obvious in the supine position. However, there is no evidence of a crater or of scarring and no disturbance of mucosal pattern.

2. *The common bile duct* may occasionally cause a similar impression but with a normal mucosal pattern.

3. *A congenital loop* of the first part of the duodenum may drag on the bulb and produce some deformity in the erect position. When supine the deformity disappears.

4. *The normal 'dot and ring' or 'target'* appearance at the apex of the bulb must not be mistaken for an ulcer.

Barium in a mucosal fold may sometimes be mistaken for an ulcer crater, but a careful study of the course of these folds—especially in the supine position—should prevent such an error.

B. Post-bulbar (including Ulcers of the Second Part)

Post-bulbar ulcers are common in India and Pakistan and comprise a small but definite proportion of duodenal ulcers in Britain. In the past there is no doubt that many were missed because the occurrence of an ulcer in this site was not sufficiently appreciated. Furthermore, many radiologists were not familiar with the technique of examination and the radiological appearances. At the site of the ulcer there is usually some narrowing of the duodenum due to spasm or fibrosis and sometimes more gross deformity when the ulcer burrows into the head of the pancreas. There is a variable degree of distension of the duodenal bulb and usually also some coarsening of the mucosa of the second part of the duodenum.

The ulcer may be seen either *en face* or in profile and is usually situated near the concave border, and only very rarely on the convex aspect. If it is very active, barium may not adhere to its base, but the margin is clearly depicted.

With careful radiological technique the diagnosis of an ulcer both in the bulb and distal to it should be made with a very high degree of accuracy. However, care must be taken not to mistake barium in a mucosal fold for an ulcer. When the condition is associated with a very high acid output, especially under basal conditions, the Zollinger-Ellison syndrome must be borne in mind.

Differential Diagnosis of Post-Bulbar Ulceration

Deformity with narrowing at the junction of the first and second parts of the duodenum can also be caused by the following conditions:

1. *Carcinoma of Head of Pancreas.* When the tumour is large enough to cause post-bulbar deformity jaundice is almost invariably present.

2. *Subacute Pancreatitis.* Deformity and indentation of the third and fourth parts of the duodenum are generally also present. However, as the mucosal folds are usually coarse there is added difficulty in differentiating from a second part ulcer.

3. *Pericholecystitis* may cause adhesions to the duodenum with some narrowing, but this is not so common as would be expected considering the proximity of the gall-bladder to the duodenum. Gall-stones may be present. Oral cholecystography and intravenous cholangiography are advised for confirmation.

4. *A carcinoma of gall-bladder* is a rare cause.

5. *Acute Cholecystitis.* The clinical features are most helpful. This will be discussed more fully in the section dealing with the biliary tract (p. 265).

6. *Infiltration by a Carcinoma of the Colon.* In these cases there is usually a large mass present. A barium enema provides the diagnosis.

7. *Right Renal Colic.* The swollen right kidney may cause spasm in the middle of the second part of the duodenum. An intravenous pyelogram is indicated when this diagnosis is suspected.

8. *Crohn's disease of the colon* may occasionally affect the second part of the duodenum by direct spread, especially from an ileo-colic anastomosis.

9. *Intrinsic Crohn's Disease of the Duodenum.* In these cases ulceration is usually present with deformity affecting a more extensive area than in the case of a post-bulbar peptic ulcer. Crohn's disease is always present elsewhere in the small bowel.

Haemorrhage

If a duodenal ulcer is seen the following are indications that it is the cause of the haemorrhage:

1. An artery in the base of the ulcer showing as a persistent round filling defect.

2. In the absence of stenosis, blood in the duodenum causing streaky filling defects in the column of barium with little blood in the stomach. The crater may initially be obscured by the blood clot.

3. In the presence of stenosis, blood in the stomach causing similar streaky filling defects, provided that no other lesion causing the haemorrhage is demonstrated in the oesophagus or stomach.

4. Impregnation with barium of stellate cracks in the blood clot in the ulcer crater.

Haemorrhage may occur from erosions. They can be demonstrated only rarely and present the same appearance as in the stomach, namely shallow ulcer craters 2 to 3 mm. in diameter surrounded by circular filling defects due to oedema.

Perforation of a Duodenal Ulcer

Following perforation, free gas is noted in a high proportion of cases, but in a significant minority none is apparent. Gas is usually seen on the right side below the diaphragm, and here it is more clearly and more frequently demonstrated on a chest film because of its radiographic quality. A chest film also helps to exclude pneumonia, heart disease, etc. If the gas is under the left dome of the diaphragm, the perforated viscus is more likely to be the stomach or the left half of the colon. It must be remembered, however, that adhesions on the right side from previous operations, etc., may prevent accumulation of gas under the right dome of diaphragm.

Streaks or bubbles of gas may occasionally be noted below the liver. Their exact situation often cannot be determined on plain radiography, particularly if adhesions are present from a previous operation. A Gastrografin meal is then of great value as it outlines the bowel lumen. If the gas is outside the bowel, a perforation is present except in rare conditions, e.g. infection of the gall-bladder or right kidney by gas-forming organisms. An ulcer crater may also be seen, and if the medium escapes into the peritoneal cavity, the diagnosis of a perforation is established beyond all doubt. Frequently however, even when a perforation is present, Gastrografin does not leak into the peritoneal cavity. In most cases there is a degree of adynamic ileus in the jejunum and ileum.

The detection of an extra-luminal bubble of gas may be difficult if it lies over the bulb. In such cases attention may be drawn to the gas as its translucency may cause the ulcer to be seen with unusual clarity. Fortunately the bubbles tend to be above the duodenal bulb and are thus more obvious.

Sometimes a loculated abscess or chronic inflammatory mass follows a perforation. This may deform the antrum, simulating a carcinoma. In such cases adhesions may also distort the distal part of the duodenum. A careful scrutiny of the soft-tissue shadow should be made for gas.

DISPLACEMENT OF THE DUODENAL LOOP
Causes

(a) *Carcinoma of the Head of Pancreas.* The earliest signs are narrowing at the junction of the first and second parts of the duodenum, local indentations of the concave border of the duodenal loop, or in rare cases, the reversed '3' sign of Frostberg. Ultimately the duodenal loop is enlarged. By the time any one of these signs is manifest, jaundice is usually present and the tumour inoperable.

(b) *Pseudo-cysts and diffuse lipomatosis of the pancreas* similarly cause enlargement of the duodenal loop, but jaundice is usually absent. In diffuse lipomatosis there is usually gross malabsorption with bony decalcification and Looser's zones.

(c) *Annular pancreas* causes narrowing of the second part of the duodenum and is a rare congenital anomaly.

(d) *In stout thick-set individuals* the duodenal loop is large particularly in the prone position. Thus before the diagnosis of a tumour of the head of the pancreas is made the build of the patient must be taken into consideration.

(e) *Tumours of the liver, kidney, colon or enlarged lymph nodes* occasionally indent the duodenum. A distended, loaded transverse colon may also cause some displacement but the gas and faecal content make its identification easy.

DILATATION OF THE DUODENUM
Causes

(a) *Duodenal Ileus (Arterio-mesenteric Occlusion).* This is usually considered to be due to compression of the third part of the duodenum by the superior mesenteric vessels in the root of the mesentery. However, when the patient is turned to the prone position, the obstruction is not always relieved as might be expected. Furthermore, at operation in some cases, the obstruction is not exactly at the point of crossing by the superior mesenteric vessels.

The proximal part of the duodenum shows dilatation, hyperperistalsis, and sometimes also retrograde movements. In all cases a careful search must be made for a gastric ulcer which may be present and is presumably caused by the stasis.

(b) *Carcinoid syndrome*, including cases of the Zollinger-Ellison syndrome when carcinoid features also exist. The ileus is of the adynamic type.

(c) *Diffuse Systemic Sclerosis (Scleroderma)*. The duodenum and proximal jejunum are sometimes affected, resulting in dilatation, stasis and atony. The valvulae conniventes are very obvious and clearly depicted owing to the diminished motility.

(d) *Administration of Anticholinergic Drugs*, e.g. *Atropine, Buscopan or Probanthine*. The appearances are almost identical with diffuse systemic sclerosis. The correct interpretation can be made only with the knowledge that one of these drugs has been given. The point of indentation by the superior mesenteric vessels is usually clearly seen.

(e) *Mechanical obstruction* from strictures, tumours, enlarged lymph nodes, etc., causes dilatation and hyperperistalsis. Rarely a retrograde jejuno-duodenal intussusception occurs following a duodeno-jejunostomy. It is easily recognised as it causes a whorled filling defect.

FISTULAE

Occasionally a cholecyst-duodenal fistula results from ulceration of a gall-stone or rupture of an empyema of the gall-bladder into the duodenum. In such cases gas is present in the biliary tract. Gas is also present following perforation of a posterior wall duodenal ulcer into the common bile duct. In rare instances a duodeno-colic fistula follows perforation into the duodenum of a carcinoma or Crohn's disease affecting the hepatic flexure of colon.

In all cases adequate clinical information must be available to the radiologist since gas (and barium following a barium meal) can be present in the biliary tract following cholecyst-duodenostomy, sphinctero-tomy, etc.

MISCELLANEOUS CONDITIONS

Coarse Duodenal Mucosal Folds

These are commonly seen in association with a duodenal ulcer, and their presence may make the demonstration of a crater difficult or even impossible. In doubtful cases, a second examination should be carried out following a short period of medical treatment. This usually results in diminution of the mucosal oedema which facilitates the detection of an ulcer. There is no doubt, however, that coarse mucosal folds can occur in association with a high acid output and a typical ulcer history but without an actual ulcer crater or scarring. In these cases there is sometimes a strong family history of duodenal ulceration.

Other causes of coarse duodenal mucosal folds are acute and subacute pancreatitis, the malabsorption syndromes, etc.

Hyperplasia of Brunner's Glands

These cause multiple round or slightly oval filling defects in the duodenal bulb. They may be associated with a vague form of dyspepsia.

Prolapse of Antral Mucosa

The mucosa of the antrum may prolapse through the pylorus into the base of the duodenal bulb. It is most common in cases of duodenal ulceration—presumably because of the associated hypertrophied gastric mucosal folds and the increased peristalsis. The prolapsed mucosa produces a mushroom-like filling defect in the base of the bulb. The diagnosis is easy, as the folds can be traced into the antrum and sometimes can be pressed back by palpation. The only condition likely to cause confusion is prolapse of an antral polyp. Only rarely do such prolapsed folds cause symptoms, e.g. of obstruction, or melaena due to superficial erosions.

Papillitis of Ampulla of Vater

This is sometimes present in cases of well-marked cholangitis and may occasionally cause spasm of the second part of the duodenum. The ampulla itself may be shown as a persistent niche of barium surrounded by a translucent zone due to oedema.

TUMOURS

Simple Tumours

Polypi cause round or lobulated filling defects with varying mobility depending on the length of the stalk. An antral polyp may prolapse into the bulb from the stomach and sometimes can be pushed back by palpation. A simple adenoma causes a smooth filling defect and usually cannot radiologically be differentiated from a pancreatic rest. Care must be taken not to mistake a normal 'target sign' at the apex of the bulb for a small tumour with a central ulcer.

Leiomyomata tend to be larger than other tumours and are usually situated in the second, third or fourth parts of the duodenum. They may recur following local excision.

Malignant Tumours

A carcinoma is the commonest type and causes mucosal destruction, ulceration or a localised filling defect. The commonest site is at the ampulla of Vater. In rare instances the duodenum is involved by direct spread from a carcinoma of the hepatic flexure of colon or the gall-bladder. In such cases a large mass is usually present.

G

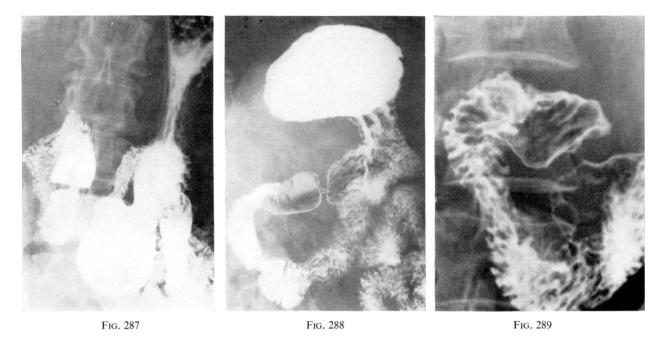

Fig. 287   Fig. 288   Fig. 289

Fig. 287. Normal duodenum. Bulb shaped like an acorn or ace of spades and feathery mucosal pattern distally. Erect film.

Fig. 288. Normal stomach and duodenum. Supine film. The duodenal bulb is coated with barium and distended with air. The mucosal folds of the bulb are ironed out causing a smooth appearance.

Fig. 289. Normal duodenum. Supine film. The duodenal bulb is distended with air giving excellent double contrast. In this case the folds of the bulb tend to be transverse. The feathery pattern of duodenum distal to the bulb is well demonstrated.

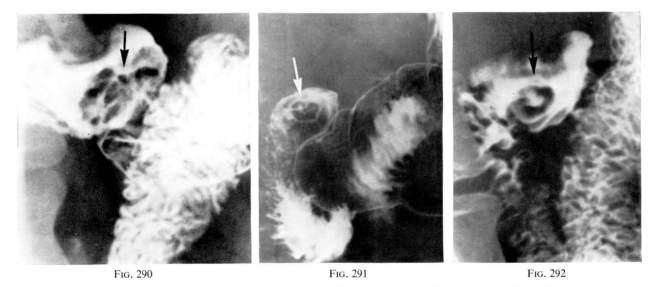

Fig. 290   Fig. 291   Fig. 292

Fig. 290. Normal bulb seen partially *en face*. The mucosal folds in the base of the bulb can be seen radiating from the pylorus (arrowed) shown as an oval translucency. The indentation of the superior aspect of the bulb is due to the lumbar spine.

Fig. 291. Normal circular mucosal fold (arrowed) at apex of bulb causing a 'target' appearance which must not be mistaken for a polyp or tiny ulcer with surrounding oedema. At operation for gall stones the duodenal bulb was carefully inspected and no abnormality was detected.

Fig. 292. Normal 'target' appearance (arrowed), i.e. persistent 'niche' of barium with surrounding translucency at the apex of the bulb. This is due to the disposition of the mucosal folds. No evidence clinically or radiologically of pancreatitis or duodenal ulceration.

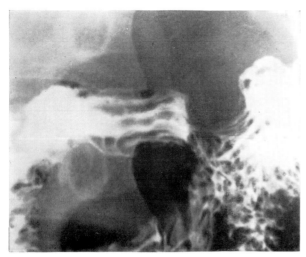

FIG. 293

Fig. 293. Normal duodenal bulb. The mucosal folds are disposed longitudinally. Supine film.

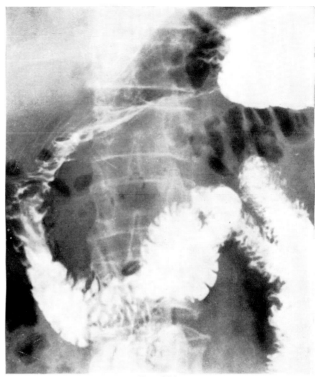

FIG. 294

Fig. 294. Enlargement of duodenal loop simulating a tumour of head of pancreas in a stout, thick set patient. The build of the individual must be taken into consideration before the diagnosis of a tumour of the head of the pancreas is made.

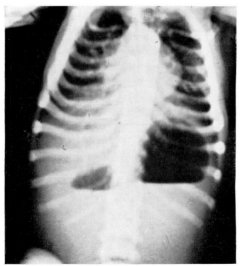

FIG. 295

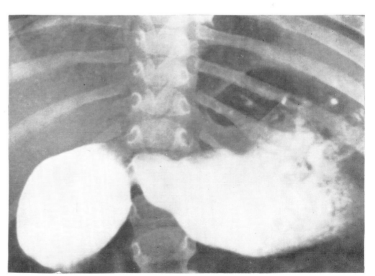

FIG. 296

Fig. 295. Duodenal atresia in the newborn. Erect film, showing 'double bubble' appearance. The fluid level on the patient's right side is in the dilated duodenal bulb and on his left side in the dilated stomach.

Fig. 296. Congenital stenosis of second part of duodenum causing gross distension of the bulb and to a lesser extent the stomach. Prone view. (Print reversed.)

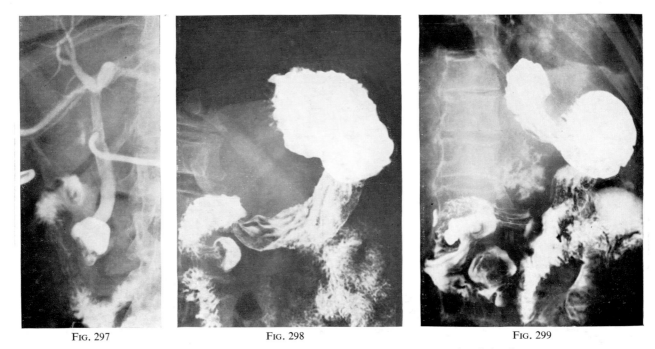

FIG. 297   FIG. 298   FIG. 299

Fig. 297. Common bile duct entering duodenal diverticulum. Post-operative cholangiogram.

Fig. 298. Duodenal diverticulum with redundant mucosa.

Fig. 299. Duodenal diverticula containing food causing mottled filling defects. Extensive calcification probably in body of pancreas. Hiatus hernia with oesophagitis at lower end of oesophagus. The patient presented with heartburn and oesophageal pain. The diverticula were symptomless.

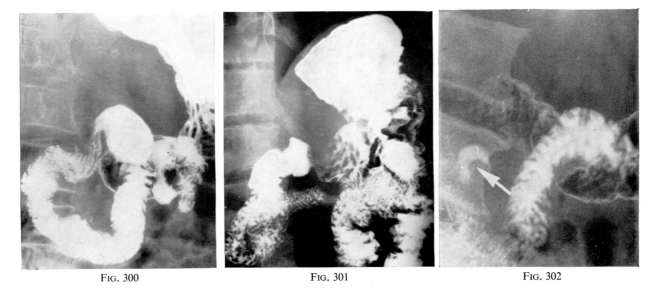

FIG. 300   FIG. 301   FIG. 302

Fig. 300. Congenital loop of first part of duodenum due to presence of a mesentery. Duodenum otherwise normal. Supine view. The diagnosis is easy when supine. When erect the loop dragged on the bulb causing deformity and distortion somewhat simulating ulcer deformity.

Fig. 301. Figure-of-eight duodenum—of no clinical significance.

Fig. 302. Duodenal diverticulum with persistent deformity (arrowed)—found at laparotomy to be due to chronic inflammation. The diverticulum had obstructed the lower end of the common bile duct causing deepening jaundice.

(By courtesy of the Editor of *Modern Trends in Gastroenterology*.)

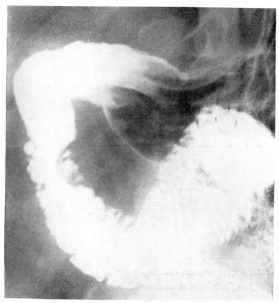
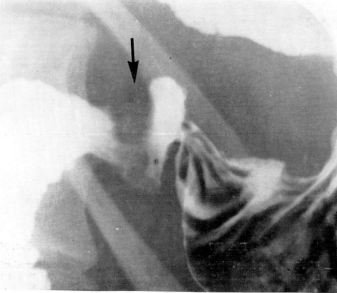

Fig. 303   Fig. 304

Fig. 303. Smooth filling defect in second part of duodenum probably due to an aberrant pancreatic nodule. Duodenal cytology negative. No operation performed because of the patient's cardiac condition. Normal E.S.R. Patient has remained free from gastro-intestinal symptoms on careful follow up.

Fig. 304. Cholecyst-duodenal band (arrowed) indenting the bulb—the common site. No evidence of ulcer crater or mucosal distortion from scarring. Supine view. Laparotomy confirmation at subsequent appendicectomy.

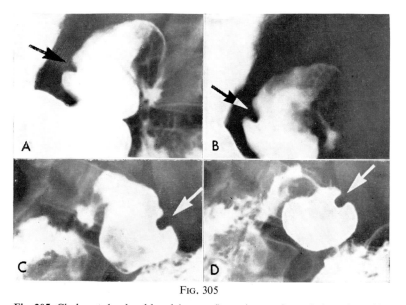
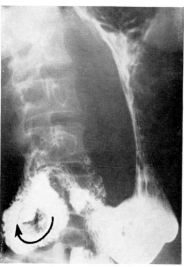

Fig. 305   Fig. 306

Fig. 305. Cholecyst-duodenal band (arrowed) causing persistent indentation of bulb on its superior aspect. Spot films A and B —prone. Spot films C and D—supine. No crater or scarring to suggest an ulcer. Incidental finding.

Fig. 306. Reversed duodenal loop the third part turning laterally. Incidental finding.

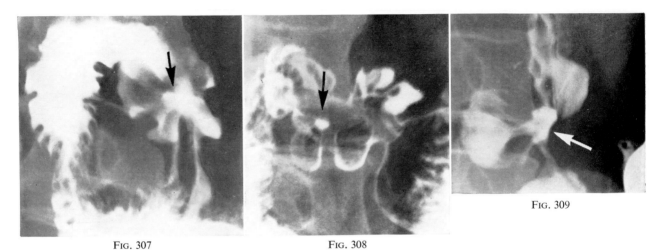

FIG. 307   FIG. 308   FIG. 309

Fig. 307. Duodenal ulcer (arrowed) with incisura on either side producing classical butterfly or clover-leaf deformity. Thickened mucosal fold extending through pyloric canal and pointing to the ulcer. This fold is occasionally seen in active duodenal ulceration.

Fig. 308. Duodenal ulcer (arrowed). Several incisurae producing a more complicated deformity—probably due to a second healed ulcer nearer the pylorus.

Fig. 309. Large duodenal ulcer (arrowed) adjacent to pylorus with typical persistent sharp rigid margins. Large pre-stenotic diverticulum present. Scarring extends from ulcer through pyloric canal causing apparent elongation of pylorus.

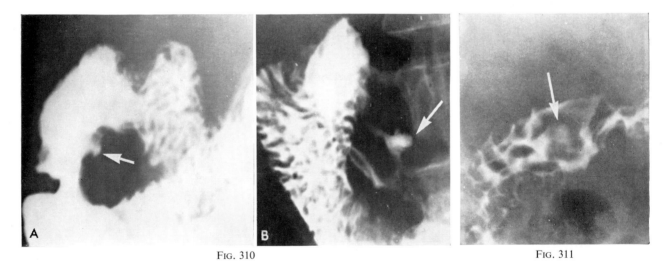

FIG. 310   FIG. 311

Fig. 310. Posterior wall duodenal ulcer in bulb demonstrated on two views. A: The ulcer (arrowed) is seen in profile. Note flattening extending across pylorus to immediate prepyloric region. B: The ulcer (arrowed) is seen *en face*.

Fig. 311. Shallow duodenal ulcer (arrowed) with a halo due to surrounding oedema. Ulcer only demonstrated in supine position. Coarse duodenal mucosal folds also present.

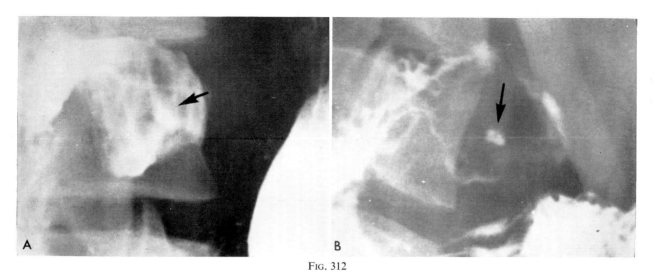

Fig. 312

Fig. 312. Duodenal ulcer without deformity. A: Erect. The ulcer (arrowed) is just visible. B: Supine. The ulcer crater (arrowed) is clearly seen when the bulb is distended with air and coated with barium.

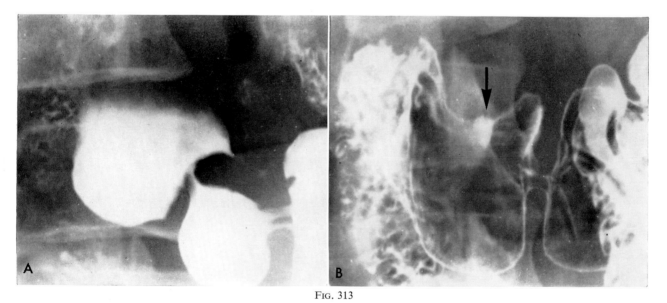

Fig. 313

Fig. 313. Duodenal ulcer—not demonstrated in erect position. A: Erect. No abnormality detected. The superior border of the bulb has not been outlined by barium due to pre-existing non-opaque fluid content. B: Supine. Duodenal ulcer (arrowed) is clearly seen.

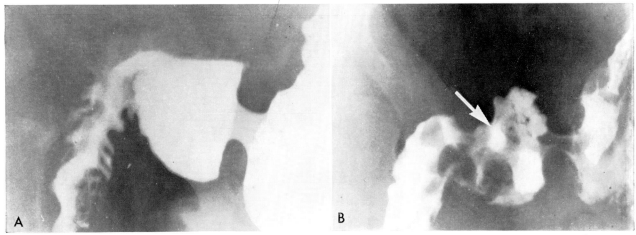

FIG. 314

Fig. 314. Duodenal ulcer not demonstrated in erect film, but clearly seen when supine. A: Erect. Ulcer obscured by barium in distended bulb. Even with palpation and firm compression the bulb could not adequately be emptied. B: Supine. The ulcer (arrowed) is now clearly seen. Typical radiating scars also present.

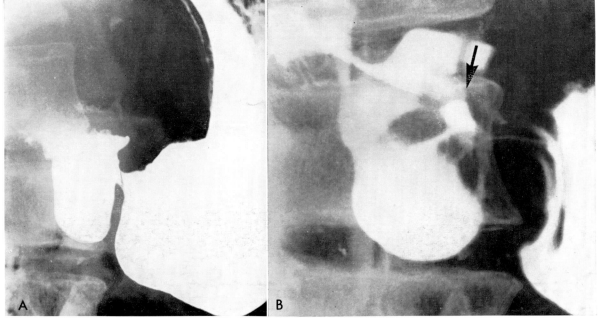

FIG. 315

Fig. 315. Large duodenal ulcer obscured in erect position but its presence suspected by flattening on the lesser curvature aspect of the prepyloric region of the stomach. A: Erect. Ulcer not seen. Prepyloric flattening. B: Supine. Large ulcer crater (arrowed) clearly seen adjacent to pylorus.

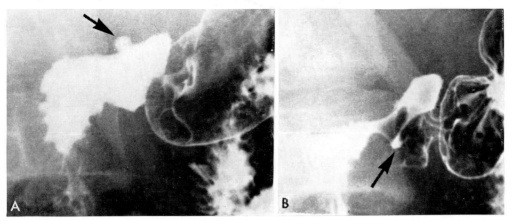

FIG. 316

Fig. 316. Two duodenal ulcers. Supine views. A: One ulcer crater (arrowed) demonstrated clearly in profile.
B: The second ulcer (arrowed) is seen *en face*—having been obscured in A by excessive barium.

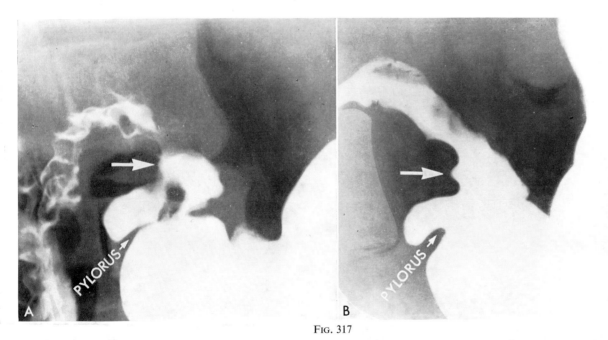

FIG. 317

Fig. 317. Development of widening of pylorus in a case of chronic duodenal ulceration. A: Pylorus of normal calibre. Chronic
duodenal ulcer (arrowed) in middle of bulb. Prominent mucosal fold extending through pylorus and pointing to the crater.
B: One year later. Marked widening of pylorus. This must not be mistaken for a narrowed area in the pyloric antrum. Duodenal
ulcer (arrowed) still obvious—seen on this occasion in profile.

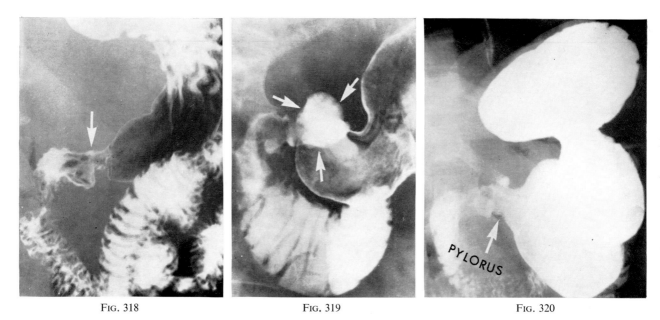

FIG. 318   FIG. 319   FIG. 320

Fig. 318. Duodenal ulcer (arrowed) on superior border adjacent to pylorus. Flattening of fornix—occasionally produced by ulcers at this site. The scarring extends across the pylorus to cause flattening of prepyloric region of stomach. Supine film. **Fig. 319.** Large duodenal ulcer (arrowed) which could be mistaken at first sight for the duodenal bulb. Recognition subsequently easy because of persistence of barium in the crater, inability to empty it by palpation, and its unaltered shape. **Fig. 320.** Wide pylorus in duodenal stenosis. Large duodenal ulcer on superior aspect with stenosis over a considerable length. The ulcer is further from the pylorus than would appear from this film since the first part of the duodenum points backwards. Dilated stomach with vigorous peristaltic waves.

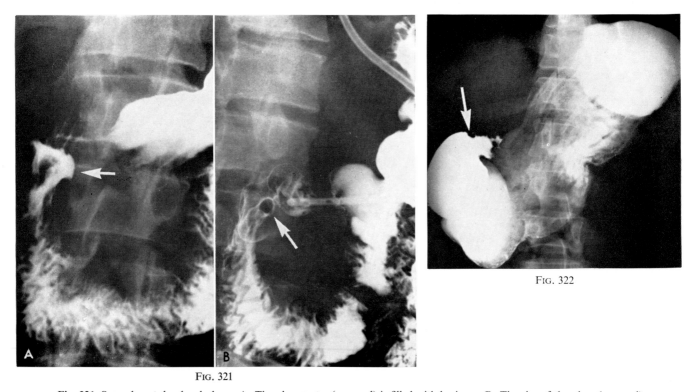

FIG. 321

FIG. 322

Fig. 321. Second part duodenal ulcer. A: The ulcer crater (arrowed) is filled with barium. B: The rim of the ulcer (arrowed) is outlined but barium has not persisted in the crater itself. This is presumably due to the marked activity of the ulcer. A little air has been insufflated through a duodenal tube to obtain better detail. Supine film. **Fig. 322.** Dilated pylorus (arrowed) following stenosis of duodenal bulb from a chronic duodenal ulcer. The stomach is also considerably dilated. Supine film with left side raised.

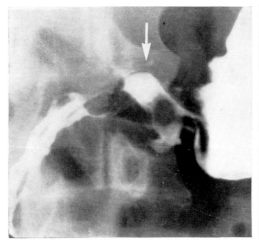

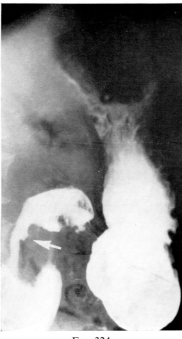

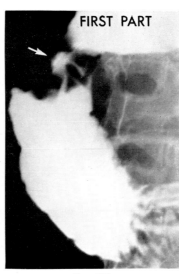

Fig. 323

Fig. 325

Fig. 324

Fig. 323. Recurrent duodenal ulcer (arrowed). Previous incomplete vagotomy. Before first operation maximal acid output 28·1 mEq/hr. After first operation 21 mEq/hr. At second operation further strands of vagus were discovered and divided.
Fig. 324. Second part duodenal ulcer (arrowed) with stenosis causing distension of duodenal bulb—the feature which on fluoroscopy initially drew attention to the probability of a second part ulcer. Operative confirmation. Prolapse of gastric mucosa into base of duodenal bulb. **Fig. 325.** Duodenal ulcer (arrowed) with some stenosis at upper extremity of second part of duodenum. Obvious radiating scars.

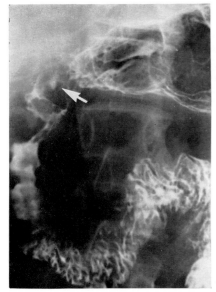

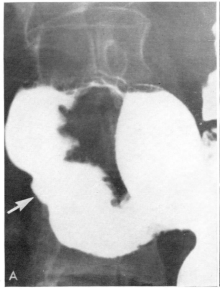

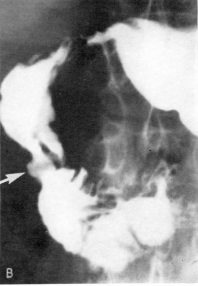

Fig. 326

Fig. 327

Fig. 326. Duodenal ulcer (arrowed) in bulb without deformity. Gross deformity with stenosis at junction of first and second parts of duodenum due to a post-bulbar ulcer. The mucosa in the second part of the duodenum is coarse—presumably due to the high acid output. **Fig. 327.** Second part duodenal ulcer arising from its convex border—an uncommon site. A: The ulcer (arrowed) is relatively large. B: One month later. The ulcer (arrowed) is smaller.

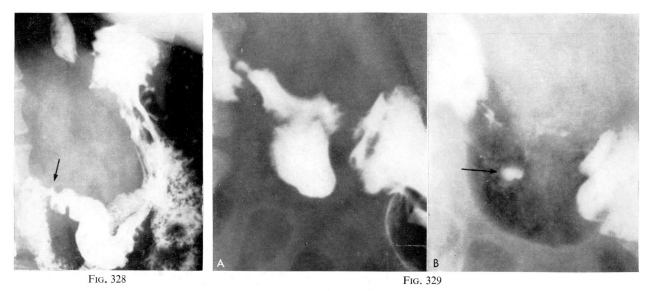

FIG. 328   FIG. 329

Fig. 328. Chronic duodenal ulcer (arrowed) with some stenosis causing massive haematemesis. Some streaky filling defects in proximal part of body of stomach due to blood clot.

Fig. 329. Duodenal ulcer causing massive haematemesis. A: Characteristic fluffy filling defects due to recent blood clot mixed with barium in duodenal bulb. Ulcer crater obscured by barium. B: After the barium and blood clot have been displaced the crater (arrowed) is revealed. There was very little blood clot in the stomach because of the absence of duodenal stenosis.

(By courtesy of the Editor of the *British Journal of Surgery*.)

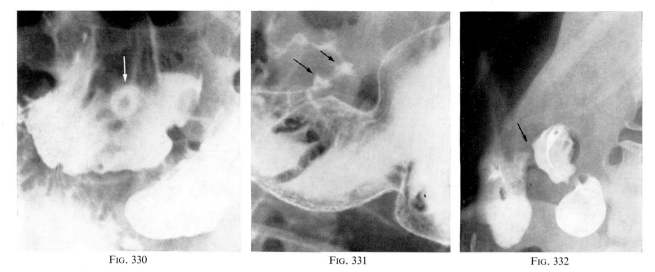

FIG. 330   FIG. 331   FIG. 332

Fig. 330. Duodenal ulcer (arrowed) with an artery in its base causing a round filling defect. Patient admitted with massive haematemesis which had settled down at the time of the barium meal. Subsequent operative confirmation.

(By courtesy of the Editor of the *British Journal of Surgery*.)

Fig. 331. Gross deformity of bulb with stenosis and the presence of two ulcer craters (arrowed). Case of massive haematemesis. No other lesion detected. Considerable blood clot was present in the stomach—not shown on this film.

Fig. 332. Perforation of a duodenal ulcer. Gastrografin meal shows leak (arrowed) from duodenal bulb. Large collection of gas also present below the diaphragm on right side. Patient supine with left side raised.

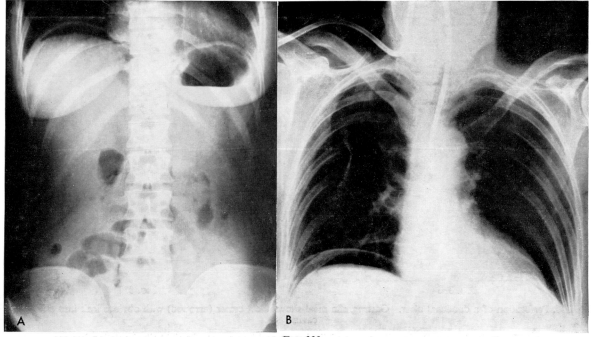

FIG. 333

Fig. 333. Perforation of a duodenal ulcer. A: Erect film of abdomen showing gas under right dome of diaphragm and only a trace under left dome of diaphragm. Degree of ileus of small bowel due to peritoneal irritation. B: Chest film. The gas under the diaphragm is even more obvious.

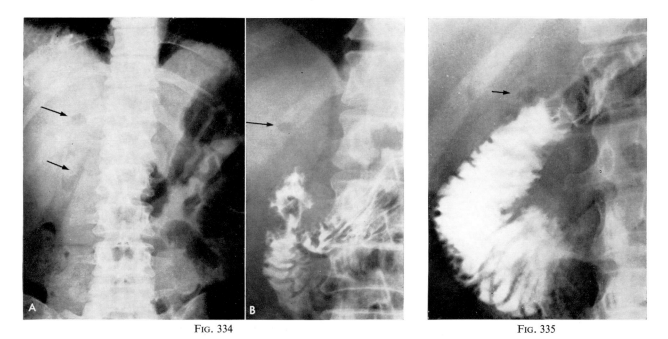

FIG. 334   FIG. 335

Fig. 334. Perforation of a duodenal ulcer. A: Plain film. Deformed duodenal bulb (lower arrow) outlined with gas. Bubble of gas (top arrow)—obviously not in the bowel and thus strongly suggesting a perforation. Coarse gastric mucosal folds—commonly present in cases of duodenal ulceration. B: Following Gastrografin, the bubble of gas (arrowed) is shown to be outside the lumen of the stomach and duodenum as was originally suspected. No leak of Gastrografin into the peritoneal cavity which in no way alters the diagnosis of a perforation.

Fig. 335. Perforation of a duodenal ulcer. Bubbles of gas (arrowed) present in right hypochondrium. Gastrografin meal shows these bubbles to be outside the lumen of the stomach and duodenum strongly suggesting a perforation. No actual leak of Gastrografin from the ulcer. Operative confirmation of a perforation.

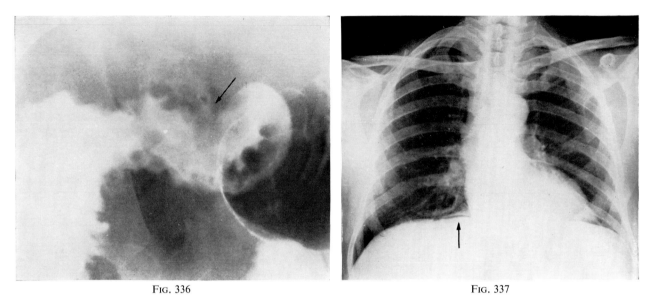

FIG. 336   FIG. 337

Fig. 336. Perforation of a duodenal ulcer. Gastrografin meal shows ulcer crater (arrowed) with obvious leak into peritoneal cavity.

Fig. 337. Overlap (arrowed) of medial aspect of diaphragm and lower part of a right rib simulating free gas.

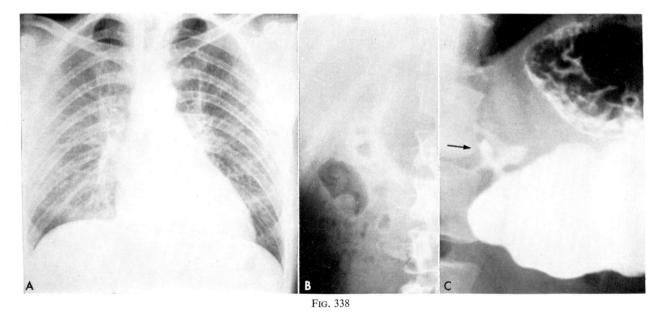

FIG. 338

Fig. 338. Perforation of a duodenal ulcer. A: No gas under diaphragm on plain film of chest. This never excludes a perforation. B: Possible bubbles of intra-peritoneal gas below the liver. C: Gastrografin meal shows deformity of the bulb with the presence of an ulcer crater (arrowed) shown with unusual clarity due to the overlying bubble of gas. No leak of Gastrografin into the peritoneal cavity. Operative confirmation of perforation.

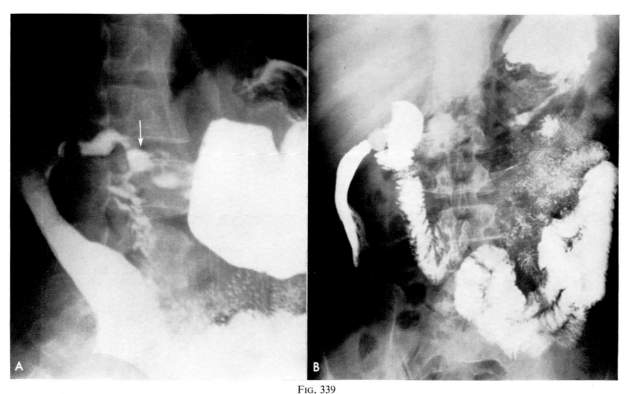

FIG. 339

Fig. 339. Old perforation of a duodenal ulcer with large abscess cavity. A: Ulcer crater (arrowed) with fistula leading into abscess on right side. B: Medial displacement of second part of duodenum by a large inflammatory mass around the abscess cavity.

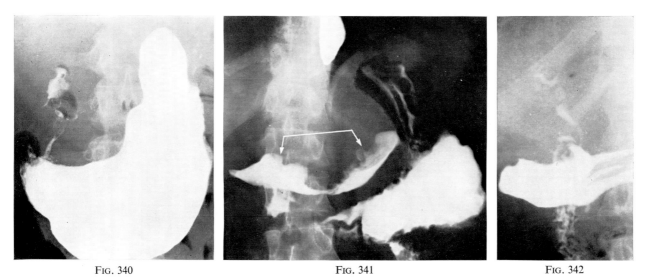

FIG. 340   FIG. 341   FIG. 342

Fig. 340. Old perforation of a duodenal ulcer with a local abscess and persistence of a fistula leading into the abscess cavity. These appearances initially simulated a carcinoma of the pyloric antrum.

Fig. 341. Perforation of a duodenal ulcer two weeks previously with formation of an abscess (arrowed) in the lesser sac and persistence of a fistula.

Fig. 342. Perforation of a duodenal ulcer into the common bile duct. Note barium and gas in the ducts. The patient presented with jaundice.

(By courtesy of Mr. A. A. Gunn and Dr. R. Saffley, Bangour Hospital.)

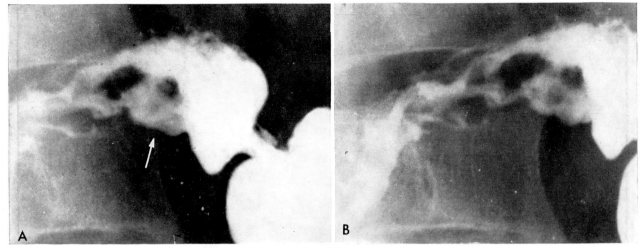

Fig. 343

Fig. 343. Crohn's disease of first and second parts of duodenum causing distortion, irregularity and ulceration. The patient had well marked Crohn's disease in the ileum. A: Linear ulcer (arrowed). B: Second spot film with 7° rotation. Good stereoscopic pair.

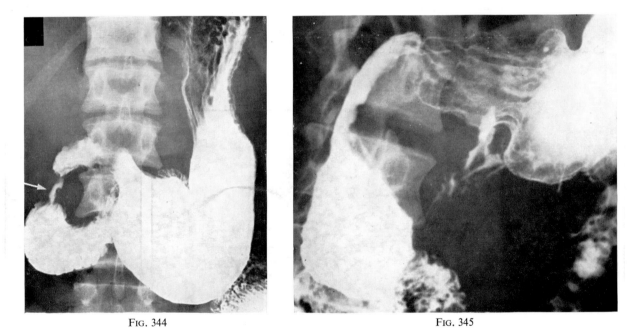

Fig. 344   Fig. 345

Fig. 344. Crohn's disease of second part of duodenum with linear ulcer (arrowed) and narrowing over approximately 2 cm. in length—more extensive than usually seen in post-bulbar peptic ulceration. Operative confirmation. Extensive Crohn's disease also present in the ileum.

Fig. 345. Crohn's disease of duodenum. Dilatation of junction of second and third parts with narrowing and mucosal destruction proximally and distally. Extensive Crohn's disease also present in jejunum and ileum.

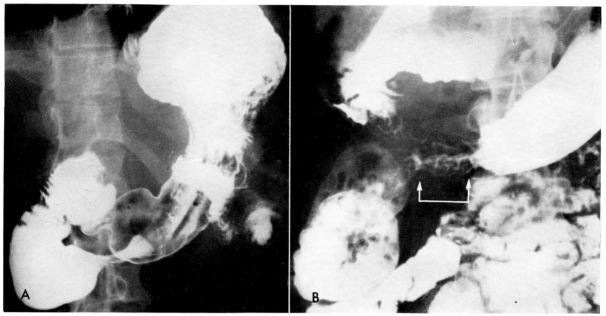

Fig. 346

Fig. 346. Crohn's disease of third part of duodenum due to extension from an adjacent ileo-colic anastomosis. A: Barium meal shows stenosis of third and fourth parts of duodenum. B: Follow-through of barium meal shows irregularity with narrowing and mucosal destruction indicating local recurrence of the disease at the ileo-colic anastomosis (arrowed). This is obviously adjacent to the area of involvement in the duodenum. The transverse colon distal to the stoma is smooth and shows lack of haustrations due to Crohn's disease.

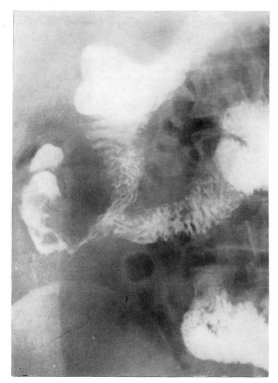

Fig. 347

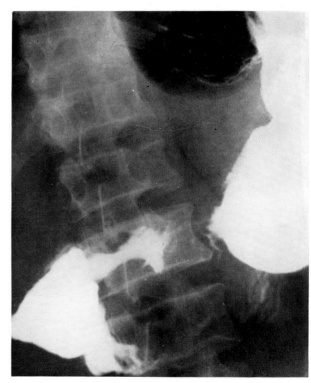

Fig. 348

Fig. 347. Crohn's disease of colon with fistula to second part of duodenum. Barium meal. No evidence of extension of Crohn's disease to the duodenum which is rather unusual in the presence of a fistula. In spite of the fistula and extensive Crohn's disease throughout the bowel the patient was in fact over-weight. **Fig. 348.** Crohn's disease of duodenum with irregularity, localised narrowing and mucosal destruction. Dilatation of second part due to marked obstruction in third part. The pyloric antrum is also affected with Crohn's disease by direct spread.

H

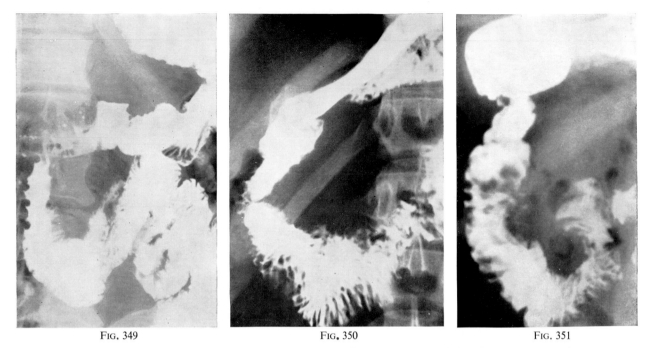

Fig. 349   Fig. 350   Fig. 351

Fig. 349. Displacement and distortion of first and second parts of duodenum. This followed a severe back injury which presumably caused a haematoma with subsequent fibrosis. **Fig. 350.** Deformity with localised narrowing in middle of second part of duodenum. This was considered radiologically to represent an annular pancreas but was found at laparotomy to be due to an adhesion probably congenital to the gall-bladder. Gall-bladder otherwise normal. Adhesion divided with subsequent complete recovery. Girl aged 14 with complaint of attacks of abdominal pain. **Fig. 351.** Displacement and indentation of second part of duodenum by a loaded transverse colon. On fluoroscopy the cause of the displacement and translucencies was uncertain. This illustrates the value of a film as opposed to prolonged fluoroscopy.

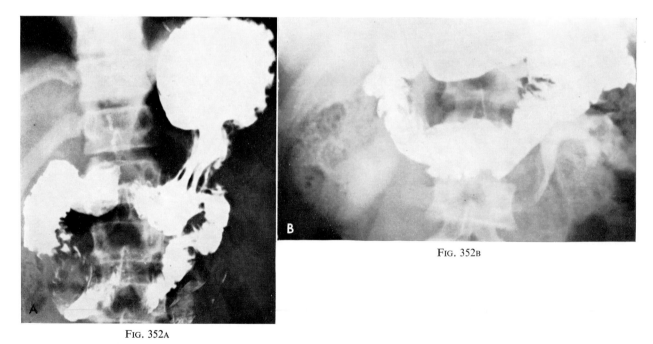

Fig. 352b

Fig. 352a

Fig. 352. Spasm of second part of duodenum due to a tender swollen right kidney from right renal colic. A: Barium meal—requested since the diagnosis was in doubt—showing narrowing of second part of duodenum due to spasm. B: Intravenous pyelogram showing characteristic appearances of renal colic, viz. delayed excretion, swelling of the kidney, a good but delayed nephrogram. The left side is normal. When this film was taken the pain had passed off and the duodenum presented a normal appearance.

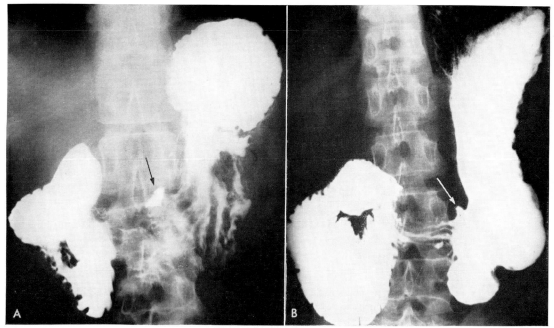

Fig. 353

Fig. 353. Duodenal ileus (arterio-mesenteric occlusion). A: Supine view. Dilatation of duodenum due to obstruction of third part. The narrowing in the second part in caused by a vigorous peristaltic wave. At the incisura there is a gastric ulcer (arrowed) which subsequently healed on mecothane. B: Prone view. (Print reversed.) Obstruction in third part still obvious with dilatation of proximal duodenum. The gastric ulcer (arrowed) is also clearly seen in this view.

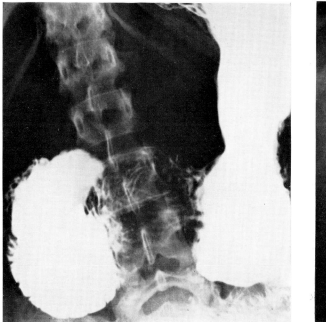

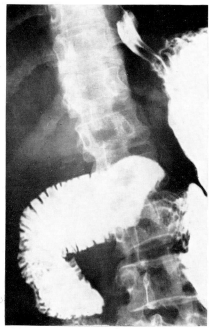

Fig. 354   Fig. 355

Fig. 354. Duodenal ileus with considerable dilatation of proximal duodenum. Prone view. (Print reversed.) Dilatation also present when the patient was supine. At operation the dilatation extended to a point beyond the crossing by the superior mesenteric vessels indicating that they were not the cause of the obstruction. Some adhesions were present and these were divided. History of recurrent attacks of abdominal pain and vomiting. **Fig. 355.** Diffuse systemic sclerosis (scleroderma) with marked dilatation and atony of duodenum. The third part of the duodenum runs up behind the second part—a minor congenital anomaly and of no significance. Hiatus hernia also present with reflux oesophagitis. Typical changes of scleroderma were also present in the oesophagus and jejunum. Raynaud's phenomenon and rheumatoid arthritis also present.

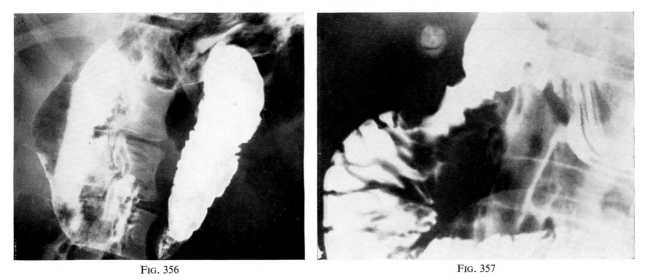

FIG. 356   FIG. 357

Fig. 356. Dilatation with marked atony of duodenum with smooth mucosal pattern due to Probanthine (given for intestinal hypermotility). The point of indentation by the superior mesenteric vessels in the third part is clearly seen. Unless the radiologist is informed when an anticholinergic drug has been given, an erroneous diagnosis e.g. of diffuse systemic sclerosis (scleroderma) might be made.

Fig. 357. Narrowing of junction of first and second parts of duodenum caused by adhesions from the gall-bladder. Case of chronic cholecystitis. Calcified gall-stone present in the gall-bladder.

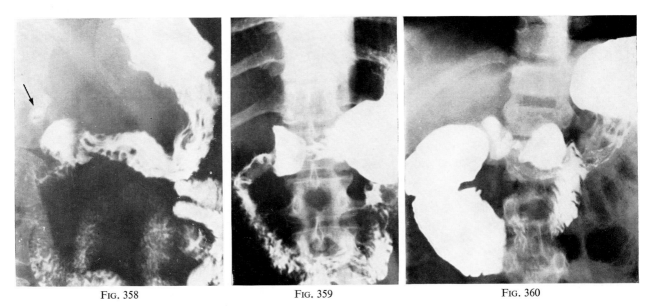

FIG. 358   FIG. 359   FIG. 360

Fig. 358. Narrowing of duodenum at apex of bulb due to adhesions from a chronically inflammed gall-bladder. Gall-stone (arrowed) present in the neck of the gall-bladder.

Fig. 359. Obstruction of first part of duodenum by adhesions following cholecystectomy. Complaint of vomiting since the operation. Prone film. (Print reversed.)

Fig. 360. Obstruction of third part of duodenum by a mass of tuberculous glands. Distension of proximal duodenum with vigorous peristaltic waves. Boy aged 14 with history of vomiting for a number of years.

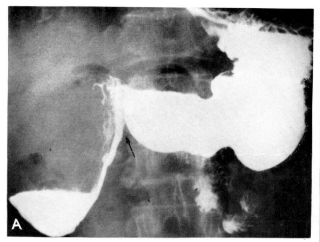

FIG. 361A

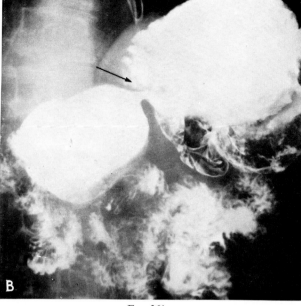

FIG. 361B

Fig. 361. Obstruction at junction of first and second parts of duodenum by adhesions with gross dilatation of bulb following cholecystectomy. A: Erect. Barium entering grossly distended first part of duodenum. Pylorus (arrowed). B: Supine. The dilated first part is more clearly seen. Pylorus (arrowed).

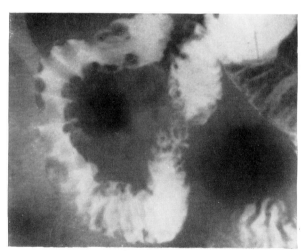

FIG. 362

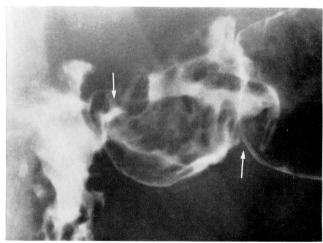

FIG. 363

Fig. 362. Coarse mucosal folds involving the whole of the first and second parts of duodenum. Maximal acid output 70 mEq/hr. Strong family history of duodenal ulceration. At operation no ulcer found.

(By courtesy of Dr. G. M. Fraser *et al.*, and Editor of *The Lancet*).

Fig. 363. Coarse mucosal folds involving both first and second parts of duodenum. Duodenal ulcer (top arrow pointing downwards) with some scarring at the apex of the bulb. Pylorus indicated (lower arrow pointing upwards.) Maximal acid output 81 mEq/hr.

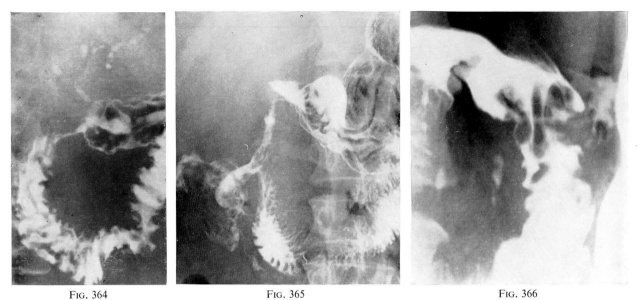

FIG. 364   FIG. 365   FIG. 366

Fig. 364. Coarse duodenal mucosa with high acid output and presence of a first part duodenal ulcer with stenosis. Thorotrast in para-aortic glands from a previous cerebral angiogram.

Fig. 365. Duodeno-colic fistula from a carcinoma of hepatic flexure of the colon—outlined by a barium meal. The fistula in such cases can usually only be demonstrated by barium enema.

Fig. 366. Prolapse of gastric mucosa through pylorus into base of duodenal bulb. The folds can be traced from prepyloric region into duodenal bulb. Incidental finding.

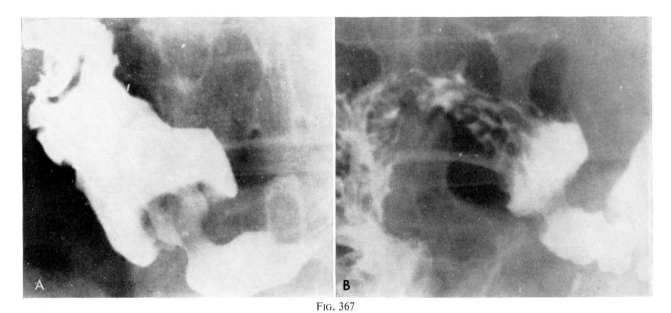

FIG. 367

Fig. 367. Prolapse of gastric mucosa through pylorus into base of duodenal bulb. Incidental finding. A: The folds can be clearly noted passing through the pylorus. B: The folds have been pushed back into the antrum.

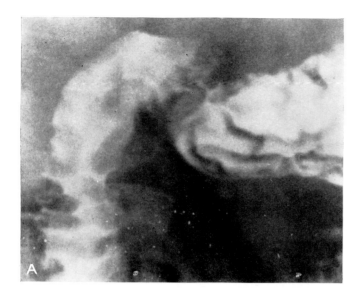

Fig. 368. Coarse mucosal folds initially obscuring a small duodenal ulcer. A: No ulcer seen. B and C: Stereoscopic pair. Second barium meal after three weeks medical treatment. Small but definite post-bulbar ulcer (arrowed) now seen since the folds are more normal. Basal acid output 21 mEq/hr. Maximal acid output 69 mEq/hr.

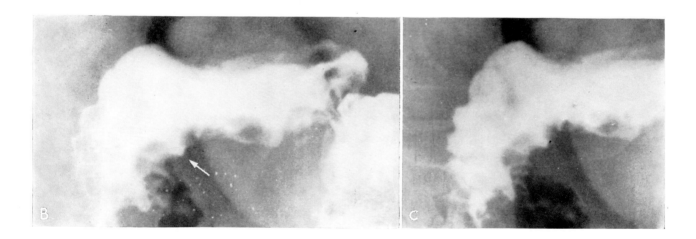

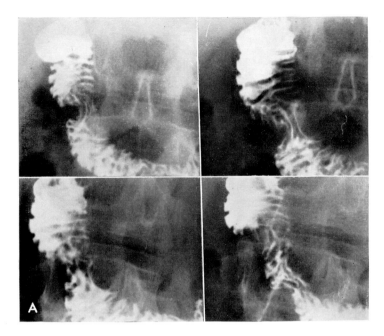

Fig. 369. Subacute inflammation of ampulla of Vater associated with a well marked cholangitis. Operative confirmation. A: Four spot films showing irritability and spasticity of second part of duodenum. B: Enlargement of one of spot films showing more clearly ampulla (arrowed) and circular translucent zone due to oedema. C: A few seconds later. More marked spasm causing increased deformity. Calcified gall-stone in the gall-bladder.

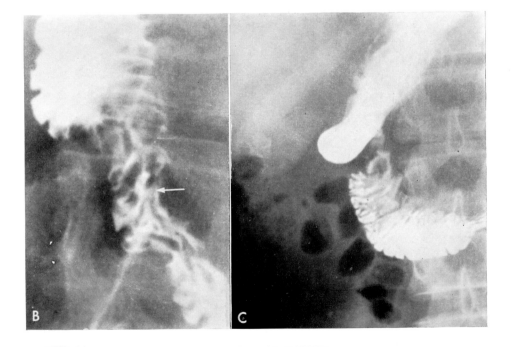

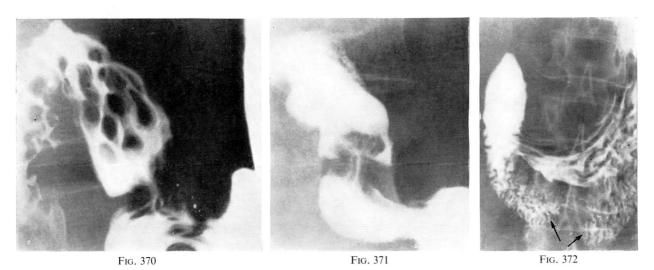

FIG. 370   FIG. 371   FIG. 372

Fig. 370. Multiple filling defects in duodenal bulb and second part of duodenum probably due to hyperplasia of Brunner's glands. History of vague dyspepsia.

Fig. 371. Prolapse of lobulated antral polyp through pylorus into duodenum producing a characteristic filling defect. The patient presented with attacks of pain and vomiting.

Fig. 372. Leiomyoma (arrowed) of third part of duodenum producing a persistent filling defect on greater curvature aspect. The tumour was removed and was considered to be simple but it subsequently recurred locally.

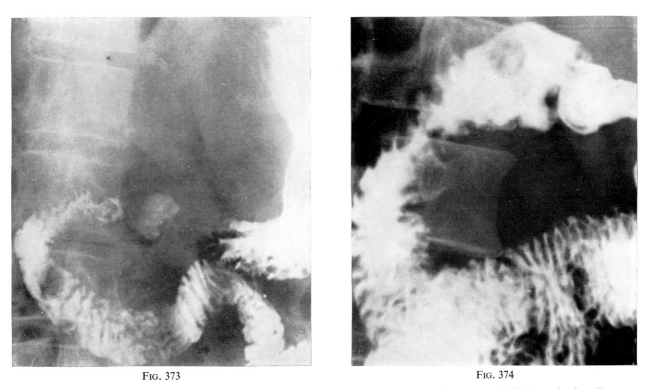

FIG. 373   FIG. 374

Fig. 373. Malignant papilloma of ampulla of Vater causing a persistent filling defect. Patient presented with deepening jaundice.

Fig. 374. Polyp in duodenal bulb causing a smooth round filling defect—incidental finding. The patient insisted upon its excision as he was going abroad.

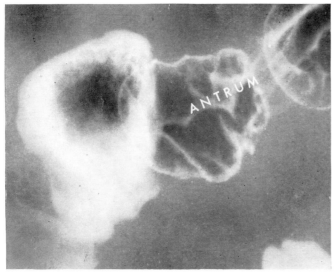

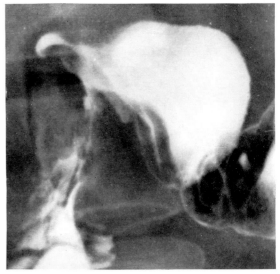

FIG. 375

FIG. 376

Fig. 375. Carcinoma of first part of duodenum causing a large irregular filling defect in the duodenal bulb.

Fig. 376. Carcinoma of hepatic flexure of colon which had infiltrated the duodenum and caused obstruction at junction of first and second parts.   Large mass present suggesting that an intrinsic tumour of the duodenum was unlikely.

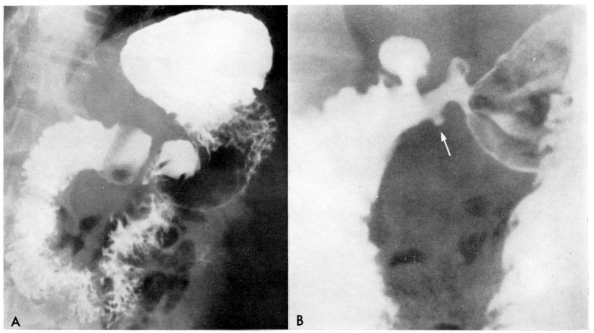

FIG. 377

Fig. 377. Pancreatic adenomata with change in nature of the pharmacologically active secretion causing different abnormalities. A: Dilatation with atony of duodenum. No ulcer seen. At this stage the patient presented with clinical features suggesting a carcinoid tumour and with elevation of the kinin levels. Basal acid output 1·3 mEq/hr. Maximal acid output 31 mEq/hr. At laparotomy the distal portion of the pancreas was removed and it contained a number of islet cell tumours. A similar tumour was enucleated from the head of the pancreas. Complete clinical recovery for approximately one year. B: One and a half years later. Severe duodenal ulcer symptoms. Basal acid output 7·6 mEq/hr. Maximal acid output 46 mEq/hr. Now gross deformity of the duodenal bulb with the presence of an ulcer crater (arrowed).

CHAPTER V

THE SMALL INTESTINE

RADIOLOGICAL METHODS OF INVESTIGATION

Plain or scout films are necessary in acute abdominal emergencies but are also of value in the diagnosis or exclusion of other abnormalities, e.g. stones in the biliary or renal tract, gas in the urinary bladder indicating a fistula, soft-tissue shadows suggesting tumours, etc. Erect and supine films are essential. The supine view (fortunately the easier to take) is of greater importance in determining the disposition of gas-filled loops and indicating the site and possible nature of an obstruction. If the patient cannot sit, a lateral decubitus view may be taken. It is not advisable to waste time taking complicated views of a seriously ill patient.

A follow-through of a barium meal is the standard method of investigation and in all cases the same type of non-flocculable barium (Micropaque is most satisfactory) should be used. Normally it follows examination of oesophagus, stomach and duodenum at the end of which the upper jejunum should be viewed fluoroscopically and films taken in the optimum position to show the loops. It is helpful to take these with compression and with the patient supine and his left side slightly raised. The patient may need to wait in his changing cubicle for 10 to 15 minutes to allow the barium to progress further down the jejunum before further films are taken. Following this, the remainder of the barium should be given and at least 10 oz. are required. Further films are taken usually at hourly intervals, preferably in the prone position, until the barium is in the ascending colon. These films must be inspected carefully. At any stage fluoroscopy, especially with compression, may be necessary to separate overlapping loops of bowel and to permit additional films to be taken of any abnormality or suspected lesion. Important information is also obtained about the relationship of a palpable mass to the small bowel.

Special attention must always be paid to the terminal ileum and the examination must be continued until there is positive evidence of barium in the colon.

This method has the great advantage of being simple and it has fewer variables than other more complicated procedures. The main disadvantage is that it is time-consuming and requires careful scrutiny of the films and personal attention by the radiologist.

Barium Enema. In most cases barium refluxes into the terminal ileum. Using the water contrast barium enema technique the ileum can be seen easily through the coated loops of pelvic colon but the detail is not so clear as on a follow-through. Unfortunately barium in the ileum is commonly mixed with faeces causing a mottled appearance. This not merely obscures detail but may give an erroneous impression of disease especially as there may also be a smooth or featureless mucosal pattern. Gross disease or a large ulcer however can usually be diagnosed with confidence. In doubtful cases it is desirable to confirm or exclude disease by a follow-through.

A follow-through using Gastrografin helps in emergencies and post-operative cases to identify individual gas-filled loops seen on plain film, to detect leaks, and to differentiate loculated abscess cavities from gas in the bowel. It is sometimes used to demonstrate the site of an obstruction. Usually 40 to 50 ml. are required.

Intestinal Intubation. When barium is instilled through an intestinal tube into the distal duodenum or upper jejunum a clearer view may be obtained of individual loops. Because of the difficulties of intubation and discomfort to the patient this has not proved to be a practical method for routine use.

Aortography and selective superior mesenteric angiography are valuable especially in the investigation of suspected vascular disease.

CLINICAL RADIOLOGY

NORMAL APPEARANCES

Plain Films. Normally little or no gas is present in the small bowel except in babies and young children. Small traces scattered throughout the jejunum and ileum however are of no significance, particularly in the aged and if the patient has been lying in bed. In air-swallowers there is a large amount of gas in the small bowel. This is distinguished from an obstruction or adynamic ileus as the loops are of normal calibre. The stomach of course is also distended with air.

Barium Follow-through. The mucosal pattern of the jejunum is fine and feathery while in the ileum it is a little coarser but the outline is smoother. On fluoroscopy the jejunum is in a state of restless activity while the peristaltic waves in the ileum are slow and regular. At the point of contraction the mucosal pattern is longitudinal. Except at the head and tail of the meal the barium forms an unbroken column. The transit time through the normal small intestine is variable but the ileo-caecal valve is reached in approximately two to two and a half hours. Thus, the three-hour film is most important as at that time the ileum is usually well filled and some barium is in the ascending colon.

In normal cases if the transit is unusually slow the bowel is a little dilated and the indentations in the jejunum by the valvulae conniventes are sharp because of the diminished motility. The ileum appears smooth, featureless, and relatively inert on fluoroscopy simulating the moulage sign of malabsorption.

In the presence of a high incomplete obstruction, e.g. from a duodenal ulcer or from kinking of the efferent loop following partial gastrectomy or gastroenterostomy, the barium passes intermittently into the jejunum. This results in segmentation and coarse flocculation in the small bowel simulating malabsorption. When the obstruction is less marked, initially the barium leaves the stomach at a reasonable speed but subsequently more slowly. Thus the column of barium at the head of the meal presents a normal appearance while in the middle and at the tail it is broken up and segmented.

Sometimes unabsorbed particles of food cause small filling defects in the column of barium. These should not be mistaken for polypi as their position is inconstant.

CONGENITAL ANOMALIES

In the newborn it is usually not possible radiologically to diagnose the precise cause of obstruction, e.g. *intestinal atresia, various forms of malrotation, etc.* In all cases plain erect and supine films should be taken and these will show dilated loops. A barium meal is usually contra-indicated but a Gastrografin meal or enema is helpful since it may be difficult to differentiate between a small bowel and colonic obstruction on the plain films.

In *congenital fibrocystic disease of the pancreas* with meconium ileus the small bowel is dilated and occasionally fine calcification is seen in the peritoneal cavity.

Enterogenous cysts are usually associated with multiple congenital anomalies of the spine and ribs. The cysts are frequently in the thorax and are seen as large opacities on a chest film.

Congenital diverticula are common. In the erect position they cause fluid levels which must not be mistaken for an obstruction. On rare occasions a calculus may form in a diverticulum.

The diverticula are readily detected on barium follow-through and they are usually more numerous than would appear at first sight as some are obscured by overlying loops of bowel. For this reason the majority of Meckel's diverticula escape detection even with careful fluoroscopy and palpation. After the meal has passed, residual barium mixed with food in a diverticulum may present a mottled or granular appearance somewhat resembling a calcified lymph node. Thus, a Meckel's diverticulum may be overlooked as it usually lies in the lower right quadrant of the abdomen—the common site for calcified nodes.

The various forms of malrotation, e.g. situs inversus, etc., have already been described (p. 93).

Congenital lymphangiectasia is a rare condition and is usually associated with malabsorption. The loops of small bowel are moderately dilated, but the indentations by the valvulae conniventes are sharp and thus the bowel margin has a regular saw-tooth appearance. A lymphogram may show lymph node hypoplasia.

INFLAMMATORY CONDITIONS

Acute Enteritis

Radiological investigation is rarely required unless symptoms persist or the diagnosis is uncertain.

Plain films show gas in the small bowel, especially the ileum and in the colon, but without significant distension. Fluid levels are present in the erect position. They are relatively small in the colonic haustrations which must not erroneously be identified as jejunal or ileal loops in an abnormal position.

A barium follow-through shows non-specific appearances of segmentation, flocculation, coarse mucosal pattern, with intestinal hurry. In infection by organisms of the salmonella group localised irregular narrowed areas with mucosal destruction may be noted in the terminal ileum.

In severe cases with profuse watery diarrhoea there is an almost complete absence of gas in the small and large bowel. Thus a plain film of the abdomen presents a ground-glass appearance. A barium meal is of course contra-indicated.

Transient or Non-sclerosing Ileitis

This condition is allied to 'the irritable small bowel'. In fact, it may be a form of that condition when it mainly affects the terminal ileum. The radiological appearances simulate Crohn's disease, namely hypermotility, spasticity and narrowing of the terminal ileum but without actual ulceration. An unfilled segment may be present on any one film simulating the 'skip' lesion of Crohn's disease. Intermittent fluoroscopy is recommended until this area is seen filled and films are then taken. The radiological appearances usually return to normal in a few weeks.

Mesenteric Adenitis

In the acute stage plain films may show dilatation of the terminal ileum similar to the findings in acute appendicitis from which it cannot be differentiated radiologically.

In the subacute stage a barium follow-through may be indicated if the diagnosis is in doubt. The appearances of the terminal ileum are similar to those found in transient ileitis. Sometimes when the terminal ileum is distended with barium indentation by enlarged lymph nodes may be noted.

Acute Meckel's Diverticulitis

A Meckel's diverticulum may become acutely inflamed and the clinical and radiological diagnosis of acute appendicitis is usually made (p. 186). There are gas-filled loops of ileum present but a careful scrutiny of the supine film sometimes reveals the diverticulum distended with gas which supports the diagnosis.

Post-operative Enteritis

Plain films show dilated loops of small and large bowel containing gas. The jejunum is particularly affected and its mucosal folds are coarse and thickened from oedema.

In the more severe form of necrotising enteritis—fortunately now rare—the appearances are more pronounced. In the late stages gas may be present in the portal circulation due to infection by gas-forming organisms derived from the bowel—a grave sign. In these cases the gas extends far out to the periphery of the liver.

Tuberculosis

As tuberculosis commonly affects both the small and large bowel it will be discussed fully in this section.

The disease was common in the past and sporadic cases still occur. The great danger is that it is mistaken for Crohn's disease which it closely resembles radiologically.

A follow-through of a barium meal is the best method of examination but in many instances a barium enema gives further information.

In acute tuberculous enteritis the whole of the small bowel shows non-specific appearances with coarsening and irregularity of the mucosal pattern and with segmentation and flocculation. The diagnosis fortunately is relatively easy on clinical and bacteriological grounds provided that it is borne in mind.

Chronic tuberculosis mainly affects the terminal ileum, caecum and ascending colon and only rarely is the bowel elsewhere involved. Radiologically there is irregularity, narrowing, distortion and ulceration. Shortening occurs particularly in the caecum and ascending colon so that the terminal ileum leads directly into the colon without the usual angle at the ileo-caecal valve.

A film of the chest should always be taken but this may show no evidence of active infection and, in fact, is often clear. An absence of calcified abdominal lymph nodes is also common.

Crohn's Disease

For convenience Crohn's disease will be fully discussed in this section.

PLAIN FILMS

The most common appearance is dilatation of loops of small bowel due to a variable degree of obstruction. Occasionally rigid segments filled with gas may be seen. Gas may be noted in the urinary bladder indicating the presence of a fistula. The spine and sacro-iliac joints should also be scrutinised for the presence of ankylosing spondylitis which is relatively more common in both Crohn's disease and ulcerative colitis.

During an acute exacerbation the clinical and radiological features sometimes resemble an acute appendicitis. Plain films thus show dilated atonic loops of ileum in the right lower quadrant of the abdomen with fluid levels in the erect position.

FOLLOW-THROUGH OF BARIUM MEAL

Early Stage. One or two short segments of bowel, in particular the terminal ileum, are usually affected with hypermotility, spasticity and mucosal irregularity. There may also be absence of filling of a segment—the 'skip' lesion. It cannot be too strongly stressed however that these appearances at one examination are in no way specific to Crohn's disease but can be caused by tuberculosis, transient (non-sclerosing) ileitis, idiopathic non-specific enteropathy, intestinal hurry, etc. The diagnosis is supported if these appearances persist on a second barium follow-through in three to four weeks' time. This is particularly so if ulceration and stricture formation have then occurred.

When the bowel is acutely inflamed there is stasis proximal to the affected segment due to local ileus. Barium subsequently passes through the acutely diseased areas of the small and large bowel with great rapidity producing extensive 'skip' lesions. Sometimes this erroneously arouses the suspicion of an entero-colic fistula.

Established Disease. As the disease progresses, increasing lengths of bowel including sometimes the colon but rarely the duodenum or stomach are affected, and fistulae, areas of stenosis, inflammatory masses, etc., may develop. Long tubular segments with a smooth outline due to diffuse mucosal destruction—the string sign—are common. Sacculations, though not so pronounced as those in vascular disorders or diffuse systemic sclerosis, may also occur both in the small and large bowel. The disease is frequently more widespread than would be suspected from the radiological appearances.

Sometimes the bowel is displaced by and may be adherent to an inflammatory mass, and mucosal swelling of the adjacent loops due to oedema may be noted. Following resection or by-pass procedures the disease tends to recur at the anastomosis and in the bowel proximal to the stoma. Thus special attention must be paid to these areas.

When obstruction is a prominent feature the bowel is dilated proximally and on fluoroscopy vigorous peristaltic waves are obvious. Segmentation and flocculation of the barium are also present and these may be exaggerated by co-existing malabsorption. On the other hand, if the patient has been careful to eat a low residue diet there may be no dilatation proximally in spite of an obvious area of stenosis.

BARIUM ENEMA

During a barium enema it may not be possible to fill the ileum because of spasm or obstruction at the ileo-caecal valve and if caecal spasm is present, the suspicion of Crohn's disease is increased. In other cases barium may flood into the ileum when the ileo-caecal valve is rigid and patent. A barium follow-through should always be carried out for confirmation and to estimate the extent of the small bowel disease. If the extreme terminal ileum is normal reflux should occur in the usual way and an affected segment proximally may be observed.

Crohn's Disease predominantly or solely affecting the Colon

In many cases both the small and large bowel are affected. Sometimes the colon is the more extensively involved and occasionally the disease is restricted to it.

Plain Films. These may show dilated loops of small and large bowel. Rarely the colon becomes grossly distended—the so-called toxic dilatation. In these cases pseudo-polypi may be present so that ulcerative colitis is suspected. An increase in the soft-tissue thickness between the gas in the stomach and the dilated transverse colon, however, suggests Crohn's disease. It must be remembered that thickened oedematous greater omentum wrapped around the transverse colon in ulcerative colitis gives a similar appearance.

Barium Enema. As in the radiological investigation of other colonic diseases a barium enema is the method of choice. Sometimes the colon contains faecal residues which may be difficult or even impossible to clear satisfactorily. In this respect it is no different from classical ulcerative colitis. It should be noted that contraction of the caecum cannot be diagnosed with certainty by a barium follow-through.

The right half of the colon is most frequently involved and as the disease extends distally the distribution tends to be segmental with normal intervening segments. The affected areas are narrowed, commonly with variation in degree, and ultimately stenosis may occur. The strictures may be either concentric or eccentric, usually the latter, and some general shortening usually results. Deep fissure-like ulcers causing a spikey or rose-thorn appearance, or long linear ulcers are common and fistulae may develop to other loops of bowel, the urinary bladder, etc. Large inflammatory masses may also be present. The bowel lumen commonly presents a cobble-stone appearance due to ulcers and granulations.

Frequently the diagnosis of Crohn's disease of the colon can be made with confidence but from time to time the differentiation between Crohn's disease and ulcerative colitis is impossible on radiological, clinical or even pathological grounds. Only a subsequent follow-up after a number of years may reveal the true nature of the disease. Tuberculosis also can mimic Crohn's disease.

Some of the features of Crohn's disease and ulcerative colitis are similar.

THE FOLLOWING FEATURES AND COMPLICATIONS ARE MORE COMMONLY SEEN IN CROHN'S DISEASE THAN IN ULCERATIVE COLITIS:

1. Disease starting in the proximal colon and extending distally in a patchy manner with intervening normal areas.
2. Deep fissure-like ulcers.
3. Inflammatory masses.
4. Long 'skip' lesions similar to those in the small bowel.
5. Fistulae.

THE FOLLOWING FEATURES AND COMPLICATIONS ARE MORE COMMONLY SEEN IN ULCERATIVE COLITIS THAN IN CROHN'S DISEASE:

1. Disease starting distally in the pelvic colon and rectum, and extending proximally in a continuous manner.
2. Collar-stud type of ulcers.
3. Smooth shortened hose-pipe type of colon with lack of haustrations and mucosal destruction.
4. Toxic dilatation.
5. Pseudo polypi.
6. Adenomatous polypi and malignant tumours.

Complications of Crohn's Disease of Small Bowel and Colon

1. Fistulae commonly occur between loops of bowel or to the skin surface or to the urinary bladder which may contain gas. There may be extensive ramifications which require to be carefully outlined with an opaque medium (Gastrografin is most suitable) before an operation is contemplated.
2. Inflammatory masses or even abscesses also occur causing displacement or obstruction. Sometimes a ureter, especially on the right side, is involved causing hydronephrosis or, in other instances, the bladder, causing chronic cystitis.
3. Recurrence of the disease tends to take place at an anastomosis.
4. Acute obstruction may occur at a stricture from a fruit stone, etc.
5. Associated lesions, e.g. ankylosing spondylitis may be present.

Crohn's Disease affecting the Duodenum and Stomach

In most instances the disease is widespread elsewhere in the bowel. In the duodenum the junction of the first and second parts is usually affected extending over a distance of two to three inches with mucosal destruction, narrowing and ulceration. In other cases it is even more extensive and may affect the entire duodenal loop. Occasionally the disease occurs by direct spread from the colon especially the neighbourhood of an anastomosis.

The stomach is only rarely affected with local rigidity and sometimes narrowing, but actual ulceration is uncommon.

Post X-irradiation Enteritis

Changes may occur in the bowel after radiotherapy. This is most commonly seen following treatment to the female pelvic organs. In the early stages the lumen is narrowed by mucosal swelling and barium passes through the affected area with great rapidity. In some cases there is complete recovery and the bowel returns to normal, but in others the condition progresses to mucosal atrophy with rigidity and diminution in calibre of the bowel lumen over a considerable length. Fistulae may subsequently develop.

Enlargement of the Ileo-caecal Valve

In some cases the lips of the valve are swollen causing a smooth filling defect seen best on a barium enema. This is rarely of significance.

Sarcoidosis

This rarely affects the small intestine. A barium follow-through may show segmentation, flocculation, etc.

Terminal Ileitis following Partial Gastrectomy

In some cases following partial gastrectomy severe malabsorption supervenes. In these cases the terminal ileum shows hypermotility, spasticity and sometimes even temporary absence of filling of a segment simulating a 'skip' lesion of Crohn's disease. This is particularly so if a blind or stagnation loop is present. Following treatment these appearances resolve.

JEJUNAL ULCERATION
See section on the stomach (p. 47)

INTESTINAL WORMS

Ascaris lumbricoides is the worm most commonly seen and it causes a smooth filling defect approximately 10 inches long. Occasionally the surface of the worm may be coated by the barium while on a 24-hour film barium may be noted in its alimentary canal. Infestation by certain parasites, e.g. *Giardia lamblia* or hookworm, causes segmentation and flocculation on a barium follow-through.

THE CARCINOID SYNDROME

The duodenum may be dilated. There is increased motility with hurry, often to a marked degree, in the jejunum and ileum and this may predispose to an intussusception. Only rarely can the filling defect or mucosal destruction caused by the tumour be demonstrated. Hepatomegaly may be present due to metastatic deposits.

COLLAGEN DISEASES

Diffuse Systemic Sclerosis

The most striking feature in this disease is atonic dilatation of the affected segments, especially the duodenum and jejunum, with marked stasis. The mucosal indentations, however, are sharp. Strictures may occur sometimes accompanied by sacculations. Segmentation and flocculation of the barium may be seen in the lower jejunum and in the ileum.

Dermatomyositis

The bowel is only rarely affected. Coarsening and irregularity of the mucosal folds with some variation in calibre of the bowel are sometimes present.

Disseminated Lupus Erythematosus

In the early stages the non-specific appearances of flocculation and segmentation may be noted on follow-through of a barium meal. In the late stage when the bowel wall is oedematous and a gross ascites is present the abdomen on a plain film presents a ground-glass featureless appearance with only a few loops of bowel outlined by gas.

Polyarteritis Nodosa

The bowel is only rarely affected and the appearances are similar to those in disseminated lupus erythematosus.

VASCULAR DISEASE

Henoch-Schönlein Purpura

Blood in the lumen produces streaky filling defects in the column of barium. In addition changes may occur in the bowel wall due to haematomata, viz. a spikey or picket-fence appearance, blurring and distortion of mucosal folds sometimes with local indentations. When the haematomata are diffuse there is extensive narrowing of the lumen. Sometimes enlarged glands in the mesentery cause local indentations of the bowel wall. When the bowel is diffusely involved segmentation and flocculation of the barium occur.

These appearances can also be caused by haematomata in the bowel wall and blood in the lumen from trauma or from the use of anticoagulants. The history in these cases is of course helpful.

Haemangiomata

These can rarely be diagnosed even following selective superior mesenteric angiography. Sometimes their presence may be suspected by clusters of phleboliths adjacent to the bowel wall.

Vascular Occlusion

The appearances depend upon the degree, duration and extent of interference with the blood supply.

Early or Mild Cases. Some dilatation of loops containing gas may be noted. If a barium meal is carried out there is irregularity with some narrowing and distortion of the affected areas with dilated loops proximally. The segments distended with gas are, in fact, the normal or less affected segments.

Aortography is of value in some cases demonstrating narrowing of the superior mesenteric artery or its branches. It should be remembered that stenoses are sometimes noted during the course of an aortogram for other reasons and in the absence of clinical or other evidence of vascular insufficiency of the small bowel.

Severe Cases. When gangrene is present, in the initial stages there is little or no gas in the affected segment as it is filled with fluid. Thus, if an extensive area of bowel is involved the abdomen presents on a plain film a ground-glass appearance. Some gaseous distension of the stomach and proximal unaffected bowel is of course present. Gas subsequently develops in the affected parts due to putrefaction

and it may subsequently be noted in the portal circulation in the liver—a grave sign.

INTESTINAL HURRY (INCLUDING THE IRRITABLE SMALL BOWEL)

Radiological changes may be caused by numerous widely differing conditions and diseases such as diabetic enteropathy, hyperthyroidism, and the persistence of diarrhoea, following gastro-enteritis. In a proportion of cases no cause can be found and it is then presumed to be a normal variant.

Radiological Appearances on a Barium Follow-through. In all cases barium reaches the ileo-caecal valve sooner than usual sometimes in an hour or less.

The following appearances may be noted:

(*a*) Vigorous peristaltic waves resulting in flocculation and segmentation. Sometimes a fuzzy outline of the bowel is seen. A transient break in the column of barium may also be noted and this may initially raise the suspicion of Crohn's disease.

(*b*) A fine saw-tooth margin due to excessive contractions of the muscularis mucosae. This produces sharp projections which are quite distinct and evenly spaced and thus should not be mistaken for ulceration.

(*c*) The column of barium is unbroken but the lumen is markedly narrowed. In some cases multiple regularly spaced localised areas of spasm are seen.

Disaccharidase Deficiency

Diarrhoea may result when there is a disaccharidase deficiency in the gut. With ordinary barium (Micropaque) the follow-through is normal. When the appropriate disaccharide (sucrose or maltose, etc.) is added marked dilution of the barium and sometimes fine flocculation occurs with intestinal hurry.

MECHANICAL OBSTRUCTION

The erect film shows distended loops with fluid levels. However, the supine film of the abdomen is the more valuable as the disposition of the gas-filled loops and therefore the site and possible cause of the obstruction are more obvious. The stomach is dilated unless the patient has vomited beforehand. Sometimes the loops of bowel, in particular the ileum, contain fluid alone and may not then be immediately obvious. The plain film of the abdomen then shows a ground-glass appearance. When the jejunum is distended with gas it shows a characteristic cross-hatched or coiled spring appearance while the outline of the ileum is smooth, somewhat resembling the colon. When the obstruction is in the jejunum there are relatively few distended loops and these are in the upper and mainly left side of the abdomen. When the obstruction is in the lower ileum there are a large number of dilated loops.

Acute Obstruction

Plain films are required but only rarely does a Gastrografin follow-through give further information. In many cases the acute obstruction is superimposed upon a chronic condition, e.g. Crohn's disease, tuberculosis, strictures, bands, adhesions from previous operations, etc.

THE FOLLOWING CAUSES ARE OF SUFFICIENT INTEREST TO WARRANT FURTHER DESCRIPTION

1. In the newborn an acute small bowel obstruction can be caused by a variety of congenital anomalies, e.g. stricture, atresia, anomaly of rotation particularly with a volvulus, etc. Radiology is of value in determining the site of the obstruction but usually not its nature.

2. In the immediate post-operative period a loop of small bowel adherent to an abdominal scar may cause an acute obstruction. The site of the obstruction is usually in the jejunum and it is generally obvious on a supine film. Occasionally a Gastrografin meal is of help in determining the site.

3. A calcified enterolith impacted at a stricture. The enterolith usually originates in the dilated segment proximal to the stricture.

4. Gall-stone ileus. A gall-stone may ulcerate into the duodenum or jejunum but it rarely causes an obstruction until the ileum is reached. In all cases gas is present in the biliary tract. A search should be made for the gall-stone but it usually cannot be detected with certainty. It must be remembered that in rare instances gas may be forced into the biliary tract through the ampulla of Vater in high intestinal obstructions from any cause. In all cases of intestinal obstruction associated with gas in the biliary tract a careful history should be taken in case there is a simple explanation for the presence of gas, e.g. previous sphincterotomy, choledocho-

duodenostomy, cholecyst-jejunostomy, etc. The gas in the hepatic ducts is always more clearly seen on the erect film.

Care must be taken not to confuse gas in the biliary tract with gas in the portal circulation. In the former it is usually confined to the main ducts near the porta hepatis while in the latter it extends almost to the periphery of the liver.

5. Intussusception caused by a polyp or tumour. In such cases other tumours or polypi may be shown as smooth filling defects in gas-filled loops.

6. Crohn's disease of distal small bowel. Sometimes a diseased gas-filled loop proximal to be obstruction shows persistent rigidity with tubular narrowing.

Acute Obstruction with Strangulation

In this serious condition the affected segment is dilated and filled with fluid producing a soft-tissue shadow which may be large and sometimes bean-shaped. In the erect position a tiny fluid level may sometimes be seen.

Subacute and Chronic Obstruction

A barium follow-through shows segmentation and clumping of the barium due to vigorous peristalsis. These changes adversely affect detail and occur in the absence of generalised small bowel disease. Thus, it may not be possible to make a precise diagnosis. If the obstruction has been present for a few days relative atony—especially obvious on fluoroscopy—may occur and give rise to extremely slow transit of the barium. In some cases of obstruction of longer duration affecting the distal ileum or colon atony supervenes with gross dilatation of the small bowel and barium remains uniformly dispersed throughout the small bowel for days or even weeks.

THE FOLLOWING CAUSES MERIT FURTHER DESCRIPTION

Intussusception. The diagnosis is usually easy on barium follow-through as the intussusception causes a characteristic whorled filling defect in a slightly dilated segment. A tumour or polyp may also be obvious as a smooth round filling defect at the apex of the entering loop. Sometimes it occurs following an operation, e.g. a retrograde jejuno-duodenal intussusception or intussusception of a Roux-en-Y loop into the jejunum. In the lower ileum a Meckel's diverticulum may also be a predisposing factor.

Adhesions. These cause varying degrees of distortion and stenosis with dilatation proximally. Sometimes a semi-erect view is helpful by showing kinking with angulation of an affected loop. In other cases fluoroscopy is of great value since on palpation the loops cannot be separated or displaced.

ADYNAMIC ILEUS

(a) Localised

An ileus may be localised to the neighbourhood of an inflammatory condition, e.g. an abscess or acutely inflamed appendix. Only rarely is it necessary or desirable to give Gastrografin for a more precise diagnosis.

A degree of adynamic ileus may develop if anticholinergic drugs, e.g. Probanthine or Buscopan, are used for therapeutic purposes. In such cases loops of bowel containing gas may be noted on a plain film and if the upper jejunum is involved the sentinal loop of an acute pancreatitis may be erroneously suspected.

(b) Generalised

There are many causes of this type, e.g. peritonitis, vascular occlusion, hypokalaemia, recent abdominal operations, retro-peritoneal haemorrhage and infections, severe generalised virus infection, herpes zoster, etc. The typical radiological features on plain films are dilatation of the small intestine with a striking absence of movement of the gas-filled bowel on fluoroscopy. The colon is usually dilated to a similar degree. Following operations on the appendix or the small bowel the dilatation usually involves the jejunum and ileum proximal to the lesion with the colon affected minimally or not at all. Fluid levels are seen in the erect position. If an ascites is present the loops are separated by fluid and there is bulging of the flanks. In reflex ileus associated with abdominal pain or injury, the degree of dilatation is usually only moderate.

Some dilatation and stasis not amounting to actual atony may occur following colectomy for ulcerative colitis and in a shortened small bowel following a resection.

POST-OPERATIVE ABSCESS

Following an abdominal operation an abscess may develop especially in the neighbourhood of an anastomosis. On the plain erect film a soft-tissue shadow with a fluid level may be detected. In other cases multiple small bubbles of gas are present. There is usually local adynamic ileus with mucosal swelling of the neighbouring loops. The dilatation, especially proximally, may be increased by a variable degree of mechanical obstruction.

IDIOPATHIC (NON-SPECIFIC) ENTEROPATHY

This is an unsatisfactory term applied to a clinical and radiological condition, the final outcome of which at the moment has not been precisely determined.

Acute Stage

This is characterised by attacks of abdominal pain, vomiting and diarrhoea. Macroscopically the bowel is heavy, swollen and oedematous with superficial mucosal ulceration. Petechial haemorrhages and enlarged glands are present in the mesentery.

Radiological Appearances. Plain films show dilatation of the small bowel with fluid levels, but the radiological appearances generally are unhelpful. When the very acute stage has passed so that a barium meal can safely be given, the jejunum presents a smooth featureless appearance with absence of mucosal pattern and greatly diminished peristalsis.

Subacute and Chronic Stage

Mucosal atrophy subsequently develops with cellular infiltration. This is accompanied by intermittent but gross steatorrhoea and other evidence of malabsorption. Osteomalacia commonly develops with the presence of Looser's zones.

Radiological Appearances. There are diffuse changes present with dilatation, flocculation, coarse mucosal pattern and sometimes 'skip' lesions. Crohn's disease may thus be suspected. Subsequently the moulage appearance may occur, sometimes with sacculations. An excess of mucus is present in the colon causing long worm-like filling defects which are seen on a barium enema. A string of mucus may also be coated by barium on a follow-through.

Remissions occur, especially following treatment with steroids and as expected the radiological appearances may then return virtually to normal.

OEDEMA OF MUCOSA AND SUBMUCOSA

The radiological changes due to oedema depend upon its degree and duration.

Acute Oedema (e.g. from a local inflammatory mass, acute intestinal allergy, post-operative enteritis, etc.)

Plain films show gaseous distension of bowel with swollen thickened folds. In the acute phase a barium meal is usually contra-indicated but in the stage of recovery a follow-through of a barium meal is sometimes carried out when the diagnosis is uncertain. In general this is not particularly helpful merely showing non-specific changes of flocculation and segmentation with coarse mucosal folds.

In other cases there is marked atony and the oedema irons out the folds so that the barium filled loops present a smooth featureless appearance.

Chronic Oedema (e.g. from portal hypertension, lymphatic obstruction from malignant glands, myxoedema, chronic intestinal allergy, plasma-cytosis, etc.)

A follow-through of a barium meal shows the mucosal folds to be obviously swollen and thickened, with some dilatation particularly in the jejunum. Flocculation and segmentation may also occur.

RADIOLOGY IN MALABSORPTION

Plain Films. These show dilated gas-filled loops of small and large bowel irregularly distributed throughout the abdomen sometimes with a mottled appearance, due to abnormal intestinal content.

Follow-through of Barium Meal. The main purpose is to detect any organic or structural cause, e.g. Crohn's disease, strictures, diverticula, blind loops, etc. This examination is of particular value following previous operations on the gut and provides information concerning the size of the gastric remnant, excessive filling with stasis of an afferent loop, size of small bowel remnant, etc.

In primary nodular hyperplasia multiple small filling defects due to lymphoid hyperplasia may be seen in the jejunum and ileum. In addition to the steatorrhoea and diarrhoea a chest infection is common and thus a film of the chest should also be taken.

The Disordered X-ray Pattern

This is present in the great majority of cases with malabsorption, but it must be remembered that idiopathic steatorrhoea with jejunal atrophy can occur with a normal pattern on barium follow-through. The pattern may also be normal in malabsorption from diverticulosis of the small bowel and following resections and by-pass procedures.

In all cases a non-flocculable type of barium should be used and Micropaque is most satisfactory. In the initial stages the radiological features are dilatation, segmentation, flocculation and a coarse mucosal pattern. On fluoroscopy the movements are abnormal and the transit time is usually prolonged. The radiological changes usually tend to become more obvious at the later stages of the follow-through examination. They are also most pronounced in gluten-sensitive enteropathy and reticulosis and less obvious in steatorrhoea of pancreatic origin. After cure the pattern returns to normal.

The disordered X-ray pattern has many other causes, including mechanical obstruction, hypo-proteinaemia, hypovitaminosis, purpura, amyloidosis, disseminated lupus erythematosus, motility disorders, infestation with certain parasites, non-specific entero-pathy, etc. It can be simulated by intermittent passage of barium from a duodenal or high intestinal obstruction. Cases with a high acid output, especially the Zollinger-Ellison syndrome, cause similar appearances, particularly the coarse mucosal pattern in the jejunum and duodenum. In Whipple's disease flocculation and segmentation are usually pronounced but there are no specific diagnostic radiological features. In this condition, following treatment with appropriate antibiotics the appearances return to normal.

As the disease progresses with increasing mucosal atrophy and muscular atony the moulage or plaster cast appearance is seen, i.e. the bowel is a little dilated, its outline is smooth and featureless but at the point of a peristaltic wave the normal mucosal pattern is distinguishable. There is no separation of loops unless there is co-existing ascites. It must be remembered that the moulage sign may be present in atony or delay in transit from any cause.

In cases that do not respond to treatment and especially if associated with a high E.S.R., leucocytosis and fever, an underlying reticulosis has seriously to be considered.

TUMOURS OF THE SMALL BOWEL

Simple Tumours, including Polypi

These cause smooth round filling defects in the column of barium and are difficult to detect. Films taken with compression in order to separate the loops (a foam-rubber pad between patient and fluorescent screen) in association with fluoroscopy are usually necessary. A polyp may cause an intussusception or an obstruction.

Neurofibromatosis occasionally affects the small bowel. It causes localised areas of irregularity, narrowing and distortion and may closely resemble Crohn's disease.

Endometriosis only rarely involves the small bowel causing a localised tumour in the ileum. By the time the bowel is affected the diagnosis has usually been established.

Localised Malignant Tumours (e.g. carcinoma, lymphosarcoma, leiomyosarcoma)

These cause irregular filling defects with mucosal destruction and sometimes ulceration with or without stenosis. Lymphosarcomata, especially following radiotherapy and leiomyosarcomata are particularly liable to ulcerate and perforate.

Diffuse Malignant Tumours, especially Reticulosis (including plasmacytosis, Hodgkin's disease, lymphosarcoma)

Malabsorption may precede the development of frank malignancy of this type by years. Flocculation, segmentation, etc., are well marked. In some cases the moulage sign occurs and on palpation the bowel is usually stiff and some loops may have straight borders with rigid, sharply defined angles. Radiotherapy may cause the bowel to return to normal but in other instances precipitates a perforation.

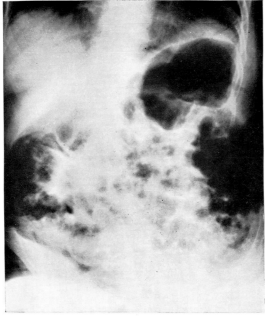

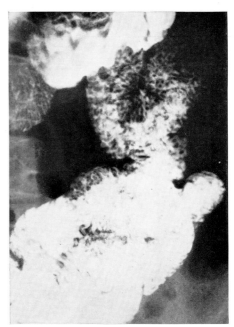

FIG. 378   FIG. 379

Fig. 378. Noisy air swallower without organic disease. Plain film of abdomen shows considerable amount of gas in stomach, small bowel and colon. The loops of small bowel are of normal calibre. **Fig. 379.** Normal jejunum. Follow-through film showing fine feathery pattern. Compare with smooth outline of ileum (Fig. 382).

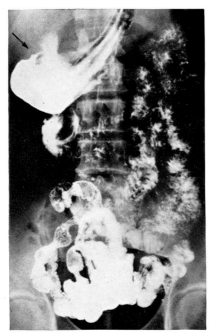

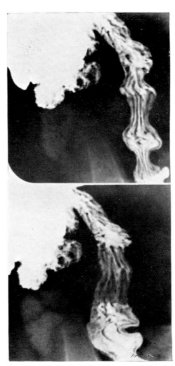

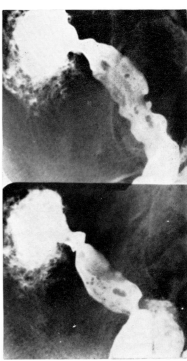

FIG. 380

FIG. 381   FIG. 382

Fig. 380. Normal jejunum and ileum. Case of obstruction of pyloric antrum by a large carcinoma (arrowed). The barium initially left the stomach at the normal rate, hence normal appearance of ileum and unbroken column at head of meal. The coarse floccular pattern in the jejunum is due to subsequent slow emptying rate of the stomach. **Fig. 381.** Normal terminal ileum on barium follow-through. Mucosal pattern showing parallel folds at the point of a peristaltic wave. The pattern is not so feathery as in the duodenum and jejunum and the peristaltic waves are at longer intervals. **Fig. 382.** Normal terminal ileum with a smooth outline, but which is within normal limits. There are several translucent filling defects due to unabsorbed food. They have obviously changed their position in the two films.

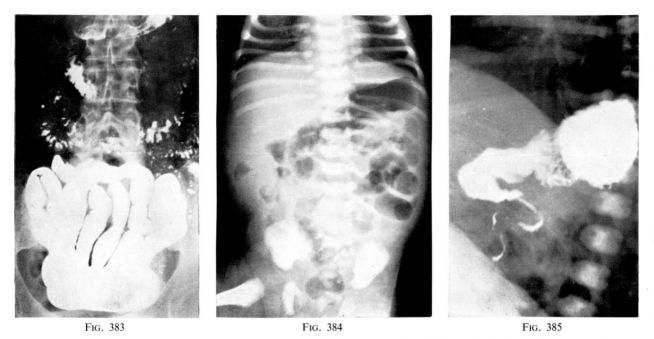

FIG. 383   FIG. 384   FIG. 385

Fig. 383. Normal small bowel showing a pseudo-moulage sign, i.e. smooth outline, diminished peristalsis—due merely to slow transit. No clinical evidence of small bowel disease. Five-hour barium follow-through film.

Fig. 384. Duplication of small bowel with obstruction. Distended loops of small bowel with little gas in the colon. The exact diagnosis could be made only at laparotomy.

Fig. 385. Congenital jejuna l stenosis. Long narrowed segment in upper jejunum but with some gas dista to the obstruction indicating that it is incomplete. Baby 7 days old.

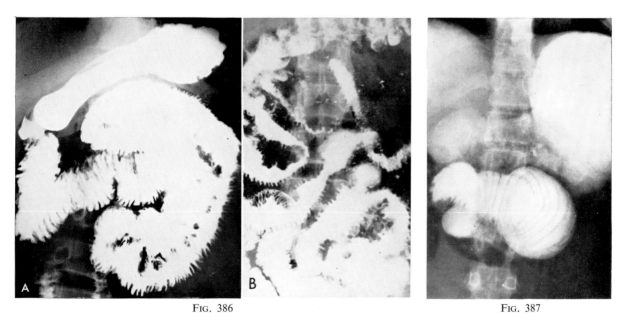

FIG. 386   FIG. 387

Fig. 386. Congenital lymphangiectasia. Marked prominence of mucosal folds with a regular saw-tooth appearance. A: Half-hour film. B: Two-hour film. History of gross steatorrhoea with protein loss resulting in severe hypoproteinaemia. Jejunal biopsy showed grossly dilated lymph sacs. Lymphogram had previously demonstrated generalised lymph node hypoplasia.

Fig. 387. Gross gastric and duodenal dilatation from a congenital anomaly of upper jejunum which caused intermittent obstruction. The barium meal was performed during such an attack. On fluoroscopy vigorous but ineffective peristaltic waves in the duodenum. Previous barium meal when symptomless was normal. Girl aged 18, markedly underdeveloped because of malnutrition. At laparotomy the upper jejunum was found to pass through a foramen in the root of the mesentery of the small bowel.

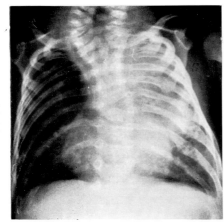

Fig. 388

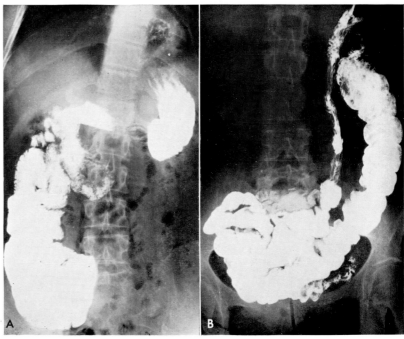

Fig. 388. Enterogenous cyst causing opacity of left upper zone. Operative confirmation. Gross spinal and rib anomalies present—a common association.

Fig. 389

Fig. 389. Situs inversus partialis commune mesenterium. The third part of the duodenum does not cross the midline but turns to the right. The small bowel is almost entirely on the right side of the abdomen and in the pelvis. The ascending colon is to the left of the spine and the descending colon still further to the left. A: One-hour follow-through film. Hiatus hernia also present. B: Five-hour follow-through film showing colon on left side of abdomen.

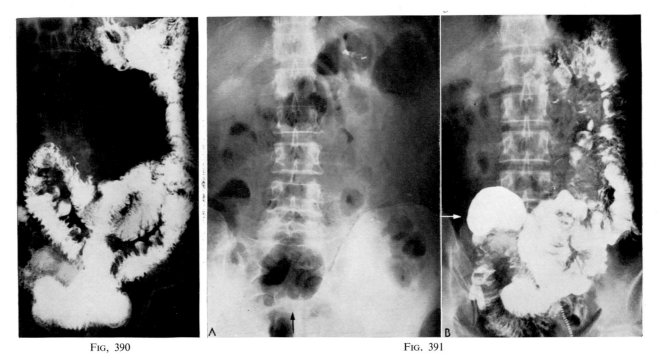

Fig, 390   Fig. 391

Fig. 390. Multiple jejunal diverticula. No clinical evidence of malabsorption. Previous partial gastrectomy.

Fig. 391. Multiple jejunal diverticula—an incidental finding. A: Plain film, erect. The diverticula are outlined with gas and a fluid level is present in some, particularly the largest (arrowed). Thus the appearance at first sight might be mistaken for an obstruction. B: Follow-through of barium meal. Large number of diverticula demonstrated with the largest corresponding to A (arrowed).

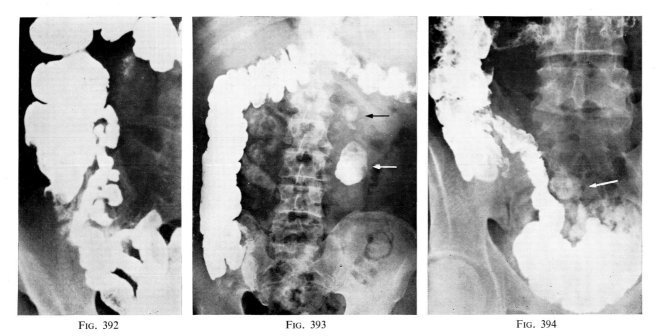

FIG. 392   FIG. 393   FIG. 394

Fig. 392. Multiple congenital diverticula of the terminal ileum—an incidental finding. **Fig. 393.** Congenital diverticula (arrowed) demonstrated on late barium follow-through film. The barium remaining in the diverticula has mixed with normal intestinal content and caused a granular appearance which could be mistaken for calcified lymph nodes. **Fig. 394.** Meckel's diverticulum (arrowed) containing barium and intestinal content, causing a mottled appearance which could readily be mistaken for a calcified lymph node. This diverticulum subsequently caused an intussusception.

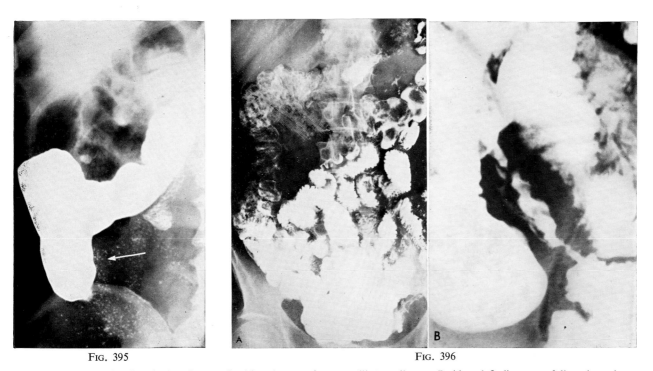

FIG. 395   FIG. 396

Fig. 395. Meckel's diverticulum (arrowed) with a lumen of same calibre as ileum. Incidental finding on a follow-through film. **Fig. 396.** Follow-through of barium meal showing value of fluoroscopy with palpation in examining the terminal ileum. A: Non-specific changes with segmentation and flocculation depicted on over-couch film. B: Following displacement of over-lying loops on fluoroscopy the terminal ileum is clearly seen. It is narrowed with mucosal irregularity strongly suggesting Crohn's disease. This was subsequently confirmed.

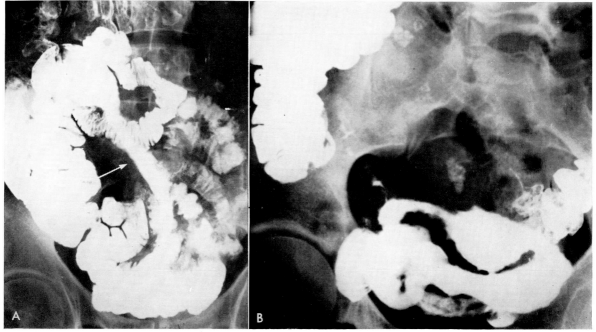

Fig. 397

Fig. 397. Crohn's disease of ileum demonstrated satisfactorily only when aided by fluoroscopy.   A: Three-hour follow-through film.   The terminal ileum is not clearly seen.   There is only one segment (arrowed) which shows mucosal destruction suggesting Crohn's disease.   B: Half an hour later following displacement of overlying loops on fluoroscopy several segments of ileum are clearly seen to be narrowed and ulcerated.   Long 'skip' lesion also of terminal portion of ileum.

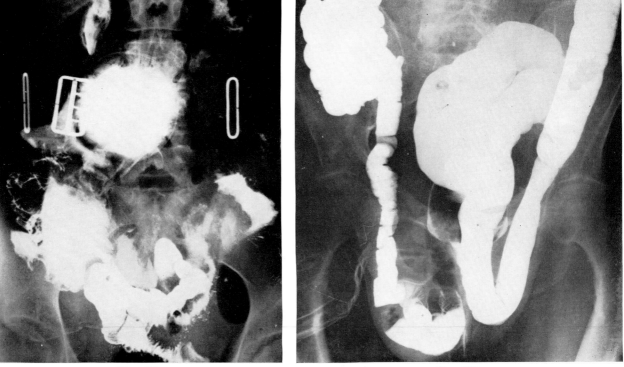

Fig. 398   Fig. 399

Fig. 398. Gross distortion with narrowing of many segments of small bowel resulting from multiple peritoneal adhesions. Previous colectomy for ulcerative colitis followed by widespread peritoneal infection.   **Fig. 399.** Large scrotal hernia containing ileum and part of sigmoid colon demonstrated by barium enema.

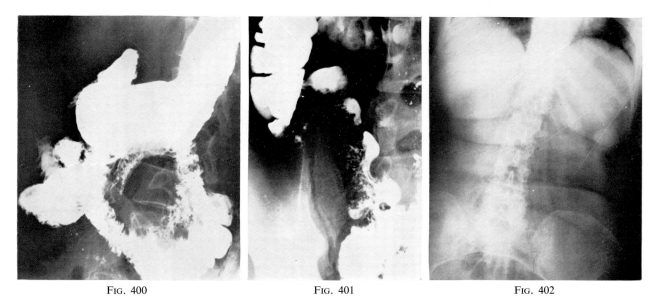

Fig. 400   Fig. 401   Fig. 402

Fig. 400. Displacement of small bowel by a marked lumbar lordosis in a thin patient. Clinically a mass was palpable, considered to be a tumour. On fluoroscopy it was obvious that the palpable mass was in fact the lumbar spine.

Fig. 401. Indentation and displacement medially of terminal ileum by enlarged lymph nodes in a case of glandular fever. Barium meal and follow-through carried out because of abdominal pain.

Fig. 402. Characteristic ground-glass appearance due to profuse watery diarrhoea. Very ill patient who died the following day from a fulminating virus infection. Only a little gas in one or two loops of small bowel in lower abdomen. The horizontal lines are due to skin folds.

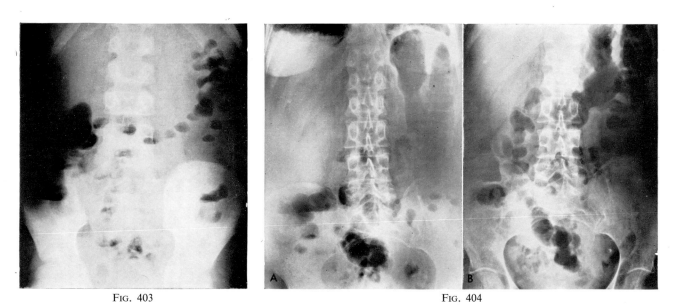

Fig. 403   Fig. 404

Fig. 403. Mild gastro-enteritis. Erect film. Moderate excess of gas in ileum and colon with fluid levels especially in the colonic haustrations. Attack of diarrhoea which settled down satisfactorily.

Fig. 404. Mild gastro-enteritis. Gas-filled loops of small bowel and colon showing a similar degree of distension. Patient presented with a sharp attack of diarrhoea which soon settled down. A: Erect. Some small fluid levels are present, particularly in the terminal ileum. B: Supine.

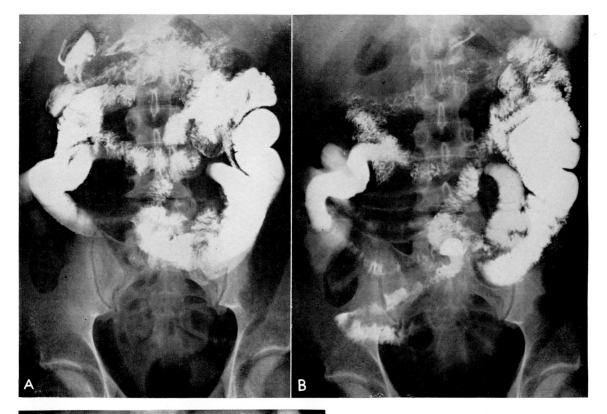

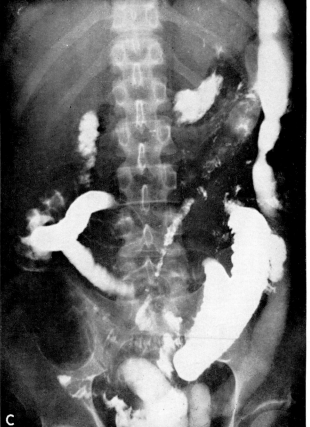

Fig. 405. Severe acute ulcerative entero-colitis. Patient presented with abdominal pain, diarrhoea with blood and mucus. On sigmoidoscopy superficial ulceration in pelvic colon and rectum. A: Half-hour barium follow-through film. The upper jejunum is reasonably normal. The mid-jejunum is dilated with a smooth mucosal pattern—the inflammatory process having ironed out the mucosal folds. B: One-hour film. Abnormal pattern in distal jejunum and in ileum. Some of the loops have a coarse mucosal pattern and are narrowed due to spasm and oedema. Others have a smooth outline as in A. There is some barium in the ascending colon. C: Two-hour film. The abnormal appearances in the ileum are even more obvious. The barium has passed through the colon with great rapidity. Generalised narrowing of the colon with absence of haustrations and abnormally smooth mucosal pattern due to oedema. Recovery from acute illness, but subsequently developed steatorrhoea (36 g. faecal fat excretion in three days). Jejunal biopsy normal.

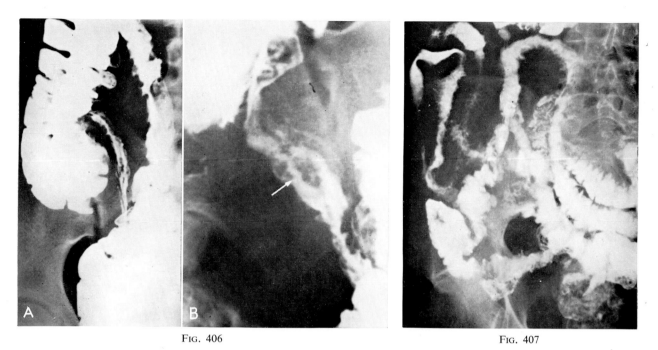

FIG. 406   FIG. 407

Fig. 406. Moderately severe acute entero-colitis in a young adolescent. A: Distortion of mucosal folds with a coarse pattern in the terminal ileum. B: Spot film of terminal ileum showing an enlarged Peyer's patch (arrowed). Complete recovery soon followed. **Fig. 407.** Antibiotic induced entero-colitis. Diffuse narrowing, mucosal swelling and irregularity involving most of the ileum. Rapid transit of the barium. One-hour barium follow-through film.

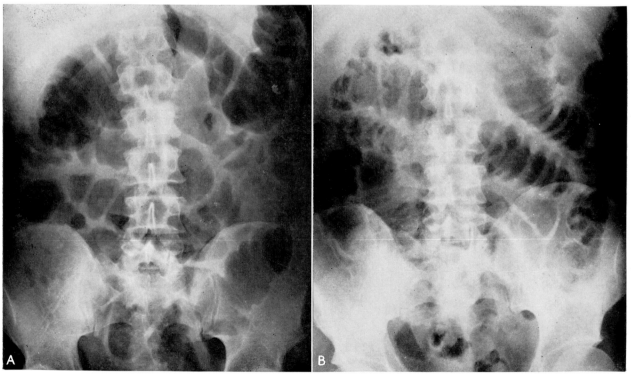

FIG. 408

Fig. 408. Acute entero-colitis following partial gastrectomy. Ill patient with severe diarrhoea with subsequent complete recovery. Supine ward films. A: Markedly distended loops of small and large bowel. The loops in the centre of the abdomen are of the small bowel and these show transverse ridging due to gross mucosal swelling. B: Two days later. Some clinical improvement. Still obviously distended loops, in particular of the jejunum, with gross swelling of the mucosal folds.

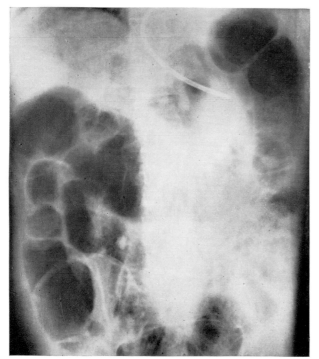

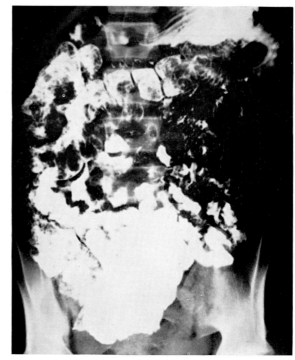

Fig. 409   Fig. 410

Fig. 409. Severe necrotising entero-colitis following operation for inguinal hernia. Considerable distension of both small and large bowel with gas. Branching translucencies in the liver extending out almost to the periphery due to gas in the portal circulation—a grave sign. See also Fig. 889. **Fig. 410.** Subacute gastro-enteritis in a child. Attack of diarrhoea which was slow in settling down. Follow-through of barium meal shows considerable irregularity of the lumen with flocculation and segmentation. Abnormal motility on fluoroscopy with synchronous and frequent ineffective contractions.

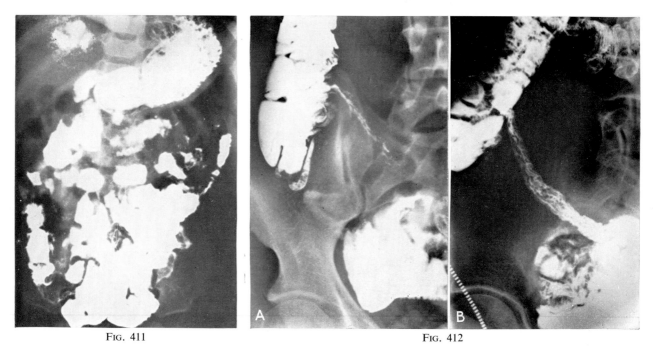

Fig. 411   Fig. 412

Fig. 411. Subacute non-specific gastro-enteritis in a baby. Segmentation of the barium and some dilatation of the loops indistinguishable from coeliac disease. The barium overlying the liver is on the baby's gown—the weave of the fabric being obvious. One-hour barium follow-through. **Fig. 412.** Transient ileitis. A: Dilatation of loops of ileum in the pelvis with a 'skip' lesion and a string sign in terminal ileum. These appearances on first examination could be due to Crohn's disease. Complaint of vague abdominal pain and tenderness in right iliac fossa. B: Three weeks later. Normal appearance. Complete clinical recovery. Crohn's disease thus excluded.

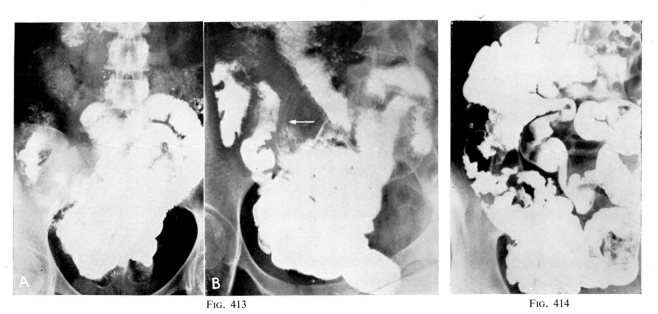

FIG. 413   FIG. 414

Fig. 413. Mesenteric adenitis with palpable lymph nodes in right iliac fossa. Subsequent uneventful recovery. A: Three-hour follow-through film. Some irritability of ileum with incomplete filling and irregularity. Moderate dilatation proximally. B: Half an hour later. The ileum is well filled and there is indentation by lymph nodes (arrowed) near the ileo-caecal valve.

Fig. 414. Subacute gastro-enteritis. Irregularity with spasticity and narrowing of the lumen of segments of terminal ileum. Some dilatation between the narrowed segments. On this one examination Crohn's disease could not be excluded. Three-hour barium follow-through. Subsequent complete recovery with return to normal pattern.

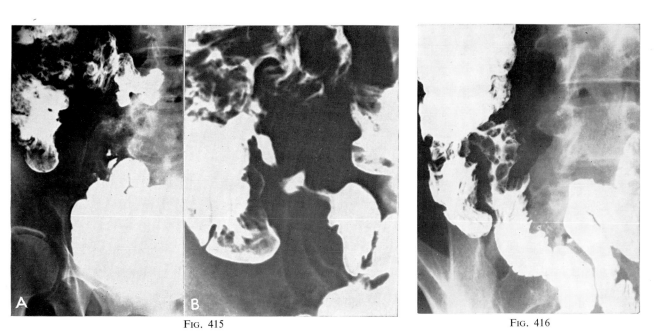

FIG. 415   FIG. 416

Fig. 415. Irritable small bowel (transient ileitis). History of diarrhoea following vagotomy and gastro-enterostomy but which subsequently settled down satisfactorily. A: 'Skip' lesion of terminal ileum with dilatation of loops proximally. Without further investigation a diagnosis of Crohn's disease might be entertained. B: Half an hour later, aided by fluoroscopy. The terminal ileum is filled. It is irritable and spastic but the mucosal pattern is normal.

Fig. 416. Transient ileitis. Patient presented with tenderness and a vague mass in right iliac fossa and generalised abdominal discomfort. Barium follow-through shows irregularity with nodular filling defects in the terminal ileum, probably due to lymphoid hyperplasia. The condition settled down satisfactorily and the patient has remained well.

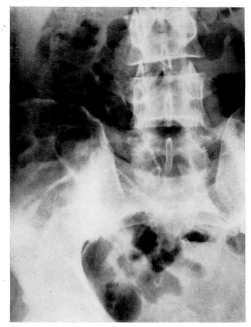
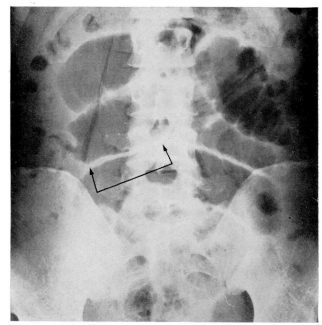

Fig. 417   Fig. 418

Fig. 417. Mesenteric adenitis. Plain film shows gas-filled distended loops of ileum suggesting an inflammatory lesion in the right iliac fossa. Soft tissue shadow opposite right sacro-iliac joint. Acute appendicitis was suspected but at operation a mesenteric adenitis only was present. **Fig. 418.** Acutely inflamed Meckel's diverticulum (arrowed) presenting clinically as an acute appendicitis. (Operative confirmation.) The diverticulum is filled with gas and it has an irregular, narrow connection with the bowel. Markedly dilated gas-filled loops of small bowel due to the local inflammatory process. The lateral border of the right psoas is outlined by gas—presumably due to a local retroperitoneal perforation.

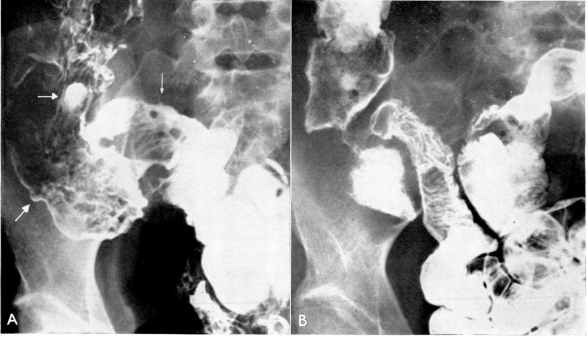

Fig. 419

Fig. 419. Ileo-caecal tuberculosis. A: Irregularity with mucosal destruction and presence of three ulcers (arrowed) in terminal ileum and caecum. Some rigidity of caecum. B: Following six months' chemotherapy, the ileum is now normal. Some residual contraction of caecum and commencement of ascending colon.

(By courtesy of Messrs Butterworths)

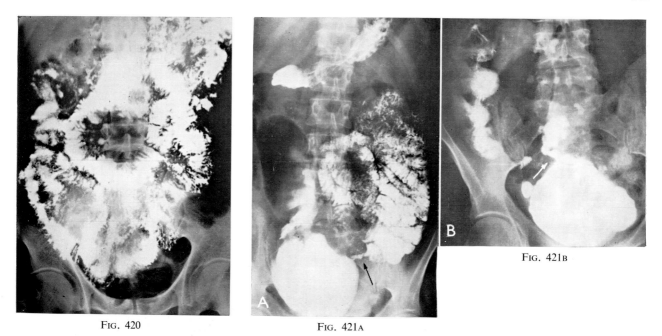

Fig. 420   Fig. 421A   Fig. 421B

Fig. 420. Acute tuberculous enteritis. Irregularity with coarsening of the mucosal pattern and flocculation in jejunum and ileum. Case of advanced pulmonary tuberculosis with diarrhoea and the presence of many tubercle bacilli in the stool.

Fig. 421. Chronic tuberculosis of the ileum with two strictures and a dilated intervening stagnation loop. A: Three-hour barium follow-through film. The proximal stricture (arrowed) causes only minor obstruction. B: Six-hour film. The distal stricture (arrowed) causes considerable obstruction. There is a large stagnation loop between the two strictures. Malabsorption, in particular of vitamin B_{12}.

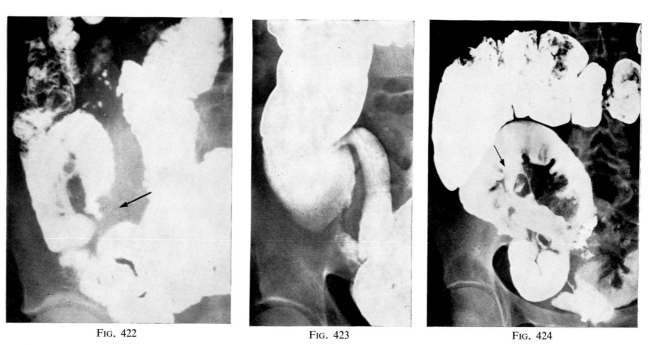

Fig. 422   Fig. 423   Fig. 424

Fig. 422. Old-standing ileo-caecal tuberculosis. Some distortion of the terminal ileum with a narrowed area (arrowed) which was persistent on other films. Some contraction of the caecum. Numerous calcified mesenteric lymph nodes.

Fig. 423. Crohn's disease of terminal ileum causing a smooth, featureless appearance due to superficial mucosal destruction—demonstrated by barium enema but similar appearances on subsequent follow-through. Only minimal symptoms. Laparotomy four years previously when diagnosis of Crohn's disease established.

Fig. 424. Crohn's disease of terminal ileum with some distortion due to matting together of loops of bowel. Ulcer crater (arrowed) also present.

K

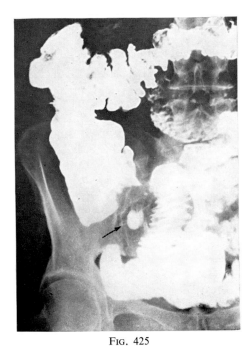

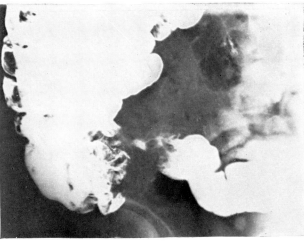

FIG. 426

Fig. 426. Crohn's disease of terminal ileum with a solitary ulcer and a degree of irregular obstruction. As the radiological and clinical diagnosis was uncertain local resection was performed with an ileo-transverse colostomy. The Crohn's disease recurred at the anastomosis six months later. Barium follow-through.

(By courtesy of Messrs Butterworths.)

FIG. 425

Fig. 425. Crohn's disease of terminal ileum. Large ulcer crater (arrowed) in the middle of a large inflammatory mass which displaces the ileum and caecum. The mucosal folds of the ileum adjacent to this mass are swollen due to oedema. Five-hour barium follow-through film. At a subsequent barium enema the terminal ileum could not be filled.

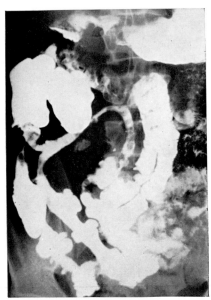

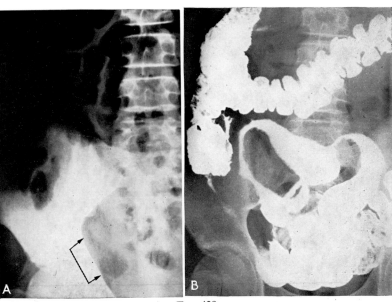

FIG. 427

FIG. 428

Fig. 427. Diffuse Crohn's disease of small bowel with narrowing, mucosal destruction and ulceration. Numerous sacculations also present—an occasional finding. Crohn's disease was also present in the duodenum.

Fig. 428. Crohn's disease. A: Plain film shows terminal ileum (arrowed) outlined by gas. B: Follow-through of barium meal shows gross mucosal destruction with ulceration, narrowing and one or two distended loops of bowel between these narrowed segments. A large area of the ileum is affected and the diseased loop depicted in A is also clearly identified.

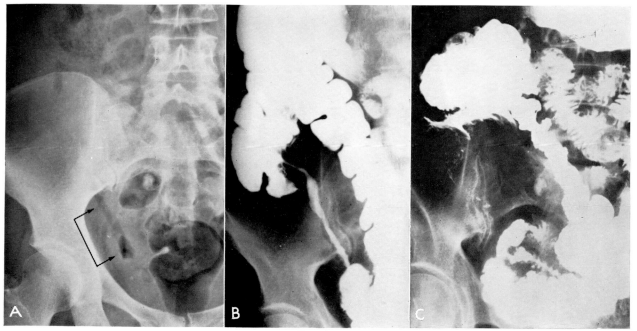

FIG. 429

Fig. 429. Crohn's disease of terminal ileum and caecum. A: Plain film shows a rigid, gas-filled loop of terminal ileum (arrowed). B: Follow-through of barium meal. Rigidity, narrowing and mucosal destruction in terminal ileum—the string sign—corresponding to the arrowed loop in A. Some deformity of caecum also present. C: Second follow-through several months later, when there was clinical deterioration. Increased deformity of caecum and ascending colon. Long 'skip' lesion of terminal ileum. Loops proximal to this are also involved with irregularity and narrowing.

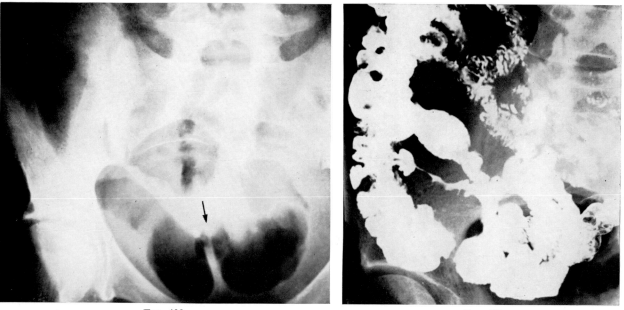

FIG. 430   FIG. 431

Fig. 430. Crohn's disease of ileum. Plain film shows a rigid distended loop of terminal ileum outlined with gas, persistent on other films. Stricture (arrowed) is also clearly seen. Subsequent confirmation by barium follow-through.

Fig. 431. Crohn's disease localised to terminal ileum. Marked narrowing with irregularity and ulceration, and moderate proximal dilatation. Five-year history. The patient was most careful about his food and usually sieved everything. If this was omitted he developed episodes of obstruction.

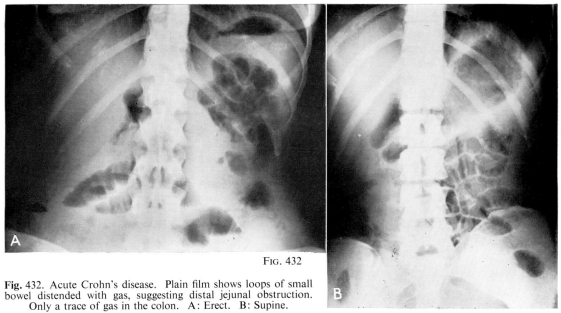

FIG. 432

Fig. 432. Acute Crohn's disease. Plain film shows loops of small bowel distended with gas, suggesting distal jejunal obstruction. Only a trace of gas in the colon. A: Erect. B: Supine.

The distribution of coils of small bowel is more readily appreciated in the supine view. Patient admitted as an emergency with severe abdominal pain, generalised tenderness and abdominal distension. As acute appendicitis with peritonitis was considered the most likely diagnosis, laparotomy was performed and the diagnosis of Crohn's disease established.

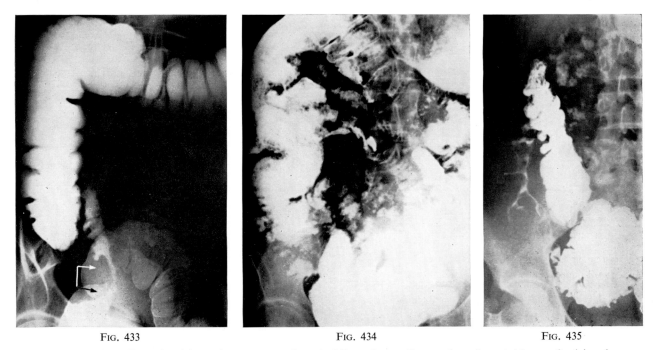

FIG. 433   FIG. 434   FIG. 435

Fig. 433. Crohn's disease involving a short segment of terminal ileum (arrowed), seen through coated loops of pelvic colon. Water contrast barium enema.

Fig. 434. Obstruction of ileum due to Crohn's disease. Considerable dilatation of ileum with flocculation and segmentation proximally. On fluoroscopy obvious writhing movements of bowel proximal to the obstruction. On this film it is impossible to determine the precise nature of the obstructive lesion, but it was proved to be due to Crohn's disease of the terminal ileum.

Fig. 435. Crohn's disease of the ileum, caecum and ascending colon with distortion, irregularity and narrowing. At operation there was only minimal involvement of the colon and the radiological appearances must have been due mainly to spasm.

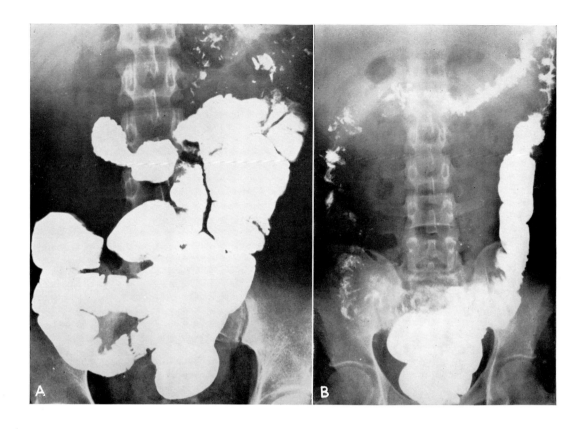

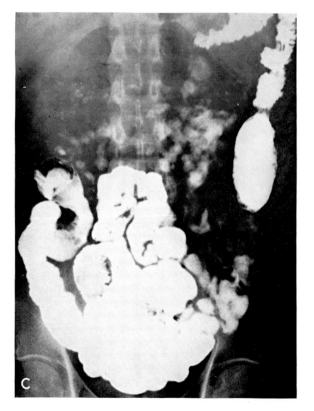

Fig. 436. Acute Crohn's disease of ileum and colon. A: Adynamic ileus of jejunum resulting in dilatation, a smooth outline and almost absent indentation by mucosal folds. Three-hour follow-through film. B: Five-hour film. The meal has passed through the ileum and colon with great rapidity resulting in poor detail in ileum and proximal colon and a long 'skip' lesion. These appearances suggest a severe acute inflammation of the bowel, not necessarily Crohn's disease. Another localised lesion with irregularity in lower part of descending colon. C: After nine months' medical treatment. Five-hour barium follow-through film. Mucosal destruction in terminal ileum. The head of the meal has passed with great rapidity through the colon with a long 'skip' lesion in the ascending and transverse parts of colon indicating persistence of severe inflammatory process here. Operative confirmation of extensive Crohn's disease of ileum and colon.

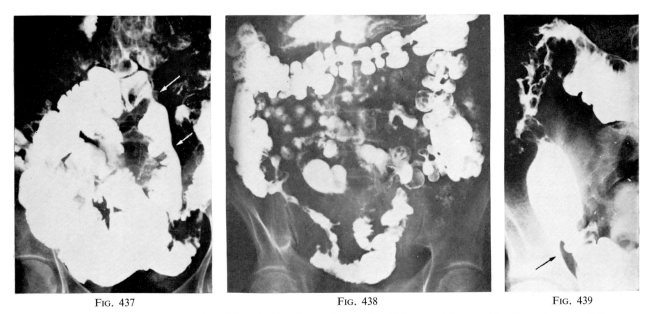

FIG. 437   FIG. 438   FIG. 439

Fig. 437. Chronic Crohn's disease of small bowel with strictures (arrowed), which are mainly eccentric. One or two sacculations also present between these strictures.

Fig. 438. Crohn's disease of ileum. Follow-through of barium meal shows narrowing and mucosal destruction of a long segment of ileum. Some contraction also of caecum and ascending colon. Patient presented with a large abscess in the lower abdomen which was subsequently drained. An initial presumptive clinical diagnosis of diverticulitis with an abscess was made. Subsequent pathological confirmation of the Crohn's disease.

Fig. 439. Crohn's disease of terminal ileum and proximal colon. Deformity with ulcer crater (arrowed) in terminal ileum. Gross shortening with irregularity, narrowing and cobble-stone appearance in the proximal colon.

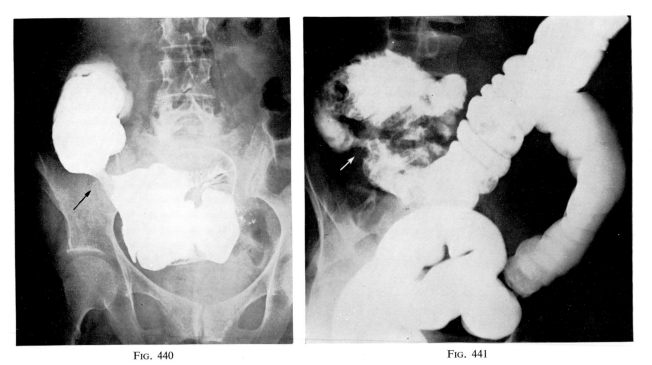

FIG. 440   FIG. 441

Fig. 440. Chronic Crohn's disease of ileo-caecal region. Stricture (arrowed) in terminal loop of ileum. A second stricture adjacent to the ileo-caecal valve but obscured on this film was also present. A little barium has entered the colon but it is almost completely obscured by the dilated terminal ileum. Operative confirmation.

Fig. 441. Recurrence of Crohn's disease (arrowed) in ileum and colon adjacent to an ileo-colic anastomosis causing considerable distortion, narrowing and mucosal destruction. Previous right hemi-colectomy for Crohn's disease. Barium enema.

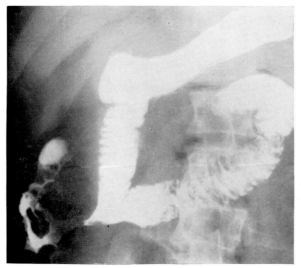

FIG. 442

Fig. 442. Duodeno-colic fistula in a case of Crohn's disease of small bowel and colon. Peaking of duodenum without actual involvement at the site of the fistula. Typical cobblestone appearance of the colon adjacent to the fistula. In spite of the malabsorption, diffuse Crohn's disease and fistula the patient was over weight.

(By courtesy of the Royal College of Physicians of Edinburgh.)

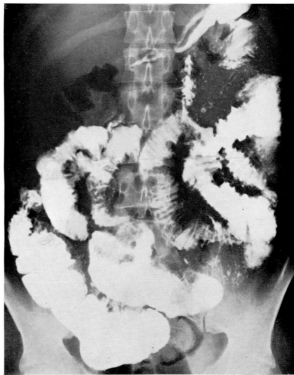

FIG. 443

Fig. 443. Chronic granulomatous enteritis similar to Crohn's disease, but precise nature not finally determined. History of diarrhoea with weight loss for one year. At laparotomy there were non-specific changes of oedema, cellular infiltration and haemorrhages in the mesentery. Follow-through of barium meal shows diffuse changes in small bowel with coarsening of mucosal pattern and areas of spasm and irregularity. Well-marked hypermotility on fluoroscopy.

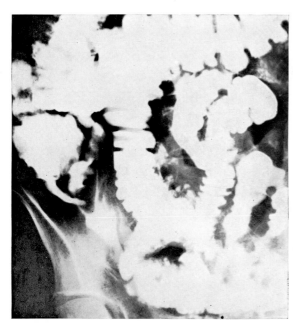

FIG. 444

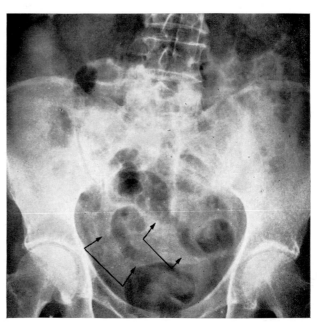

FIG. 445

Fig. 444. Enteritis following radiotherapy for ovarian carcinoma. Narrowing, spasticity and mucosal swelling of ileum, particularly its terminal segment, with irregular dilatation between the narrowed areas. Some spasm of the caecum also present. Well-marked hypermotility on fluoroscopy. Three-hour barium follow-through. **Fig. 445.** Enteritis following radiotherapy for carcinoma of cervix uteri. Plain film shows narrowed segments of ileum (arrowed) with absent mucosal pattern and uniformity of calibre. These appearances can be caused by any form of subacute or chronic inflammation. Complaint of persistent diarrhoea following radiotherapy.

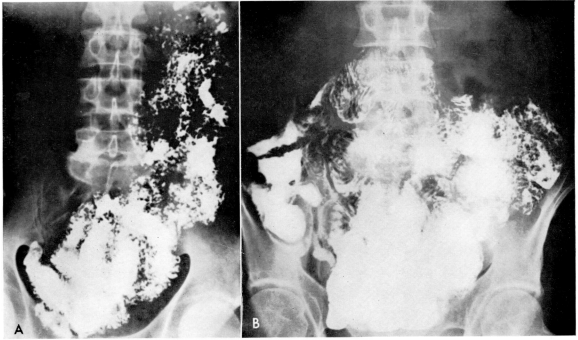

Fig. 446

Fig. 446. Granulomatous lesions in small bowel suggesting sarcoidosis. History of diarrhoea, steatorrhoea, ill health and loss of weight for three weeks. At laparotomy multiple granulomatous lesions throughout the small bowel considered pathologically to represent sarcoidosis. Sarcoid nodules also present in the liver and spleen. A: Coarse mucosal pattern with extensive flocculation of barium in small bowel obscuring detail. One-hour barium follow-through film. B: Flocculation still present. Narrowing of several segments, in particular the terminal ileum with dilatation proximally. These appearances simulate Crohn's disease but it is not possible to make a definite radiological diagnosis. Three-hour follow-through film.

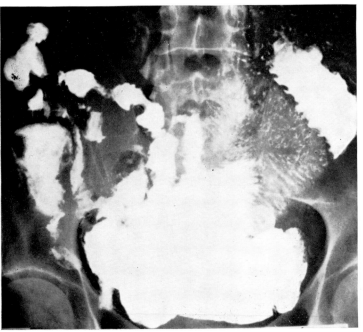

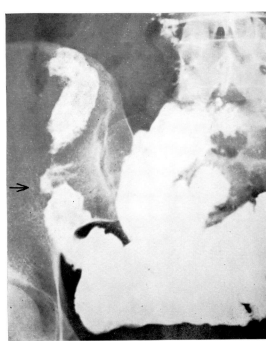

Fig. 447   Fig. 448

Fig. 447. Syndrome with terminal ileitis after Polya partial gastrectomy. Following this operation multiple vitamin deficiencies developed with diarrhoea, steatorrhoea up to 60 g. of faecal fat in three days, peripheral neuritis, marked impairment of B_{12} absorption. Three-hour barium follow-through film shows narrowing with mucosal irregularity of several loops of terminal ileum. A radiological diagnosis of Crohn's disease was made, but at laparotomy only minimal abnormality was present in the ileum and no evidence of Crohn's disease. **Fig. 448.** Paratyphoid fever. Irregularity with ulceration (arrowed) localised to the terminal ileum—considered to be Crohn's disease. The patient was subsequently found to have paratyphoid fever. The abnormality was thus probably at the site of a Peyer's patch. Subsequent follow-through on recovery three weeks later was normal. (By courtesy of Messrs Butterworths.)

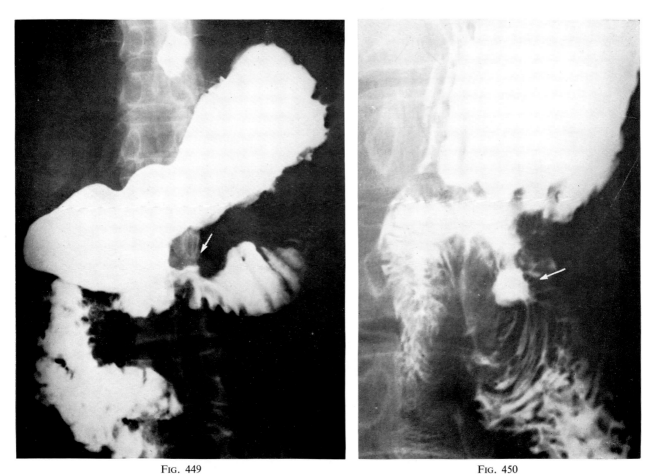

FIG. 449   FIG. 450

Fig. 449. Jejunal ulcer (arrowed) on afferent loop adjacent to the stoma following iso-peristaltic gastro-enterostomy. Some narrowing of the lumen with distortion of the mucosal folds adjacent to the ulcer. **Fig. 450.** Jejunal ulcer (arrowed) demonstrated *en face*, situated on efferent loop about an inch from the stoma. Supine film.

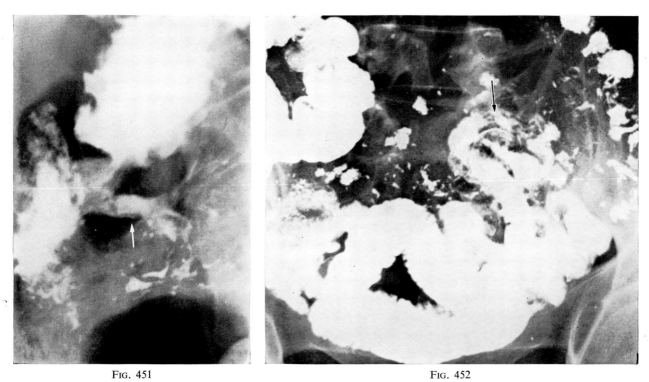

FIG. 451   FIG. 452

Fig. 451. Jejunal ulcer (arrowed) following a Polya gastrectomy. Some narrowing with distortion of the stoma and adjacent part of jejunum. At operation a stitch inserted at the previous operation was present in the floor of the ulcer crater. It is not possible to detect a residual stitch by a barium meal. **Fig. 452.** Ascaris lumbricoides (arrowed) in ileum—showing as a filling defect.

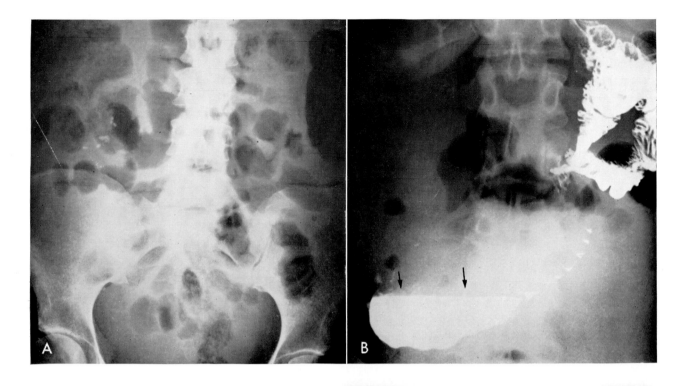

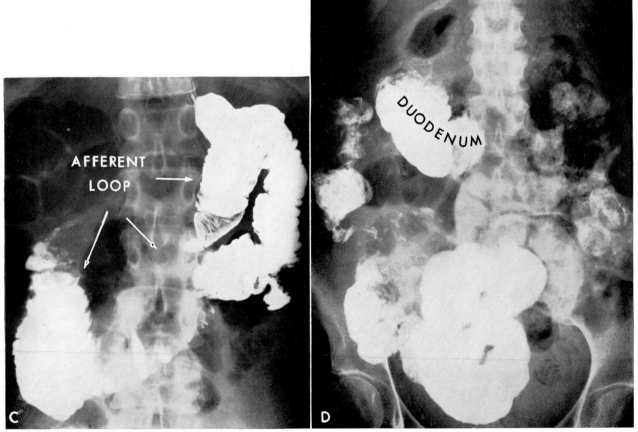

See legends for Figs. 453A-D opposite.

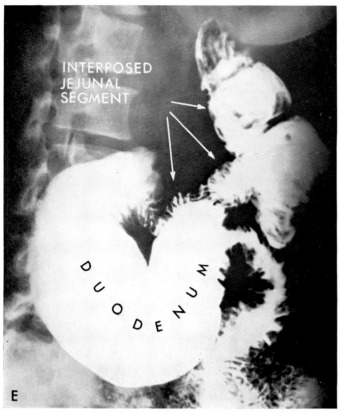

FIG. 453E

Fig. 453. Syndrome resembling kwashiorkor after Polya partial gastrectomy. The patient was emaciated and had a severe malabsorption. Marked jejunal bacterial colonisation also present. A: Plain film (supine). Irregularly dilated gas-filled loops of small bowel with indistinct mucosal pattern—commonly seen in malabsorption. B: Erect. Dilatation of afferent loop which contains a large fluid residue and which acts as a blind loop. The barium and fluid residue cause a fluid level (arrowed). C: Supine. The irregularly dilated afferent loop is clearly seen. D: Eleven-hour film. The barium is in the ascending colon, but there is marked stasis in the small bowel. Considerable residue in duodenal part of afferent loop. Irregularity with narrowing of terminal ileum simulating Crohn's disease and with some dilatation proximally. E: The gastro-enterostomy has been undone and a segment of jejunum interposed between the gastric remnant and the duodenum—resulting in marked clinical improvement. Still residual dilatation of the duodenum but the barium passed satisfactorily into the jejunum.

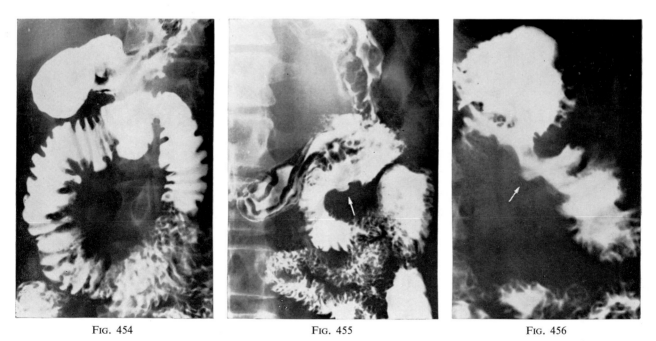

FIG. 454   FIG. 455   FIG. 456

Fig. 454. Coarse mucosal folds in jejunum following gastro-enterostomy—a common appearance. No evidence of ulceration.

Fig. 455. Jejunal ulcer (arrowed) seen in profile opposite gastro-enterostomy stoma.

Fig. 456. Jejunal ulcer (arrowed) situated an inch or so from the stoma on the efferent loop—a common site following a Polya gastrectomy. Some narrowing of the lumen and distortion of the mucosal folds adjacent to the ulcer.

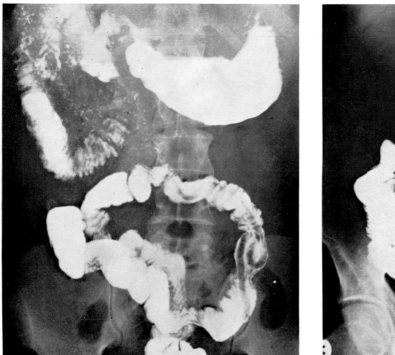

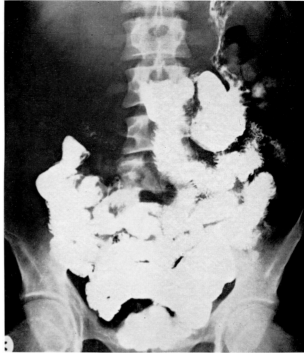

FIG. 457   FIG. 458

Fig. 457. Ascaris lumbricoides in jejunum causing a characteristic smooth filling defect about ten inches long—incidental finding in a patient with a chronic duodenal ulcer. Situs inversus partialis commune mesenterium also present. **Fig. 458.** Hypermotility of small bowel due to a carcinoid tumour and causing a fuzzy outline, particularly in jejunum. The primary tumour was not demonstrated radiologically. Displacement of duodenum and small bowel by an enlarged liver due to metastatic deposits.

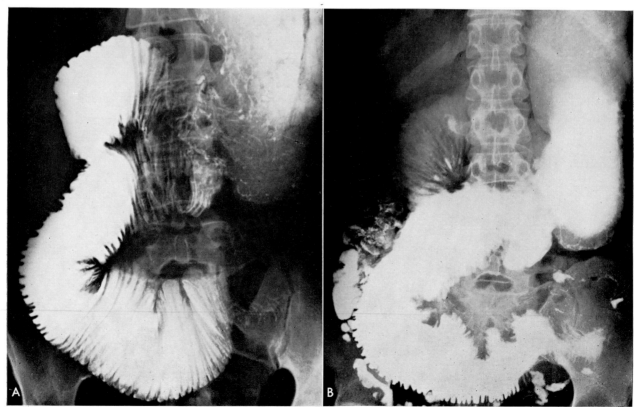

FIG. 459

Fig. 459. Diffuse systemic sclerosis (scleroderma). A: Gross distension of duodenum and jejunum with atony. The mucosal pattern has a sharp outline. Dilatation also of stomach. B: Three hours later. Still large residue of barium in stomach, duodenum and proximal jejunum with dilatation. Some barium has passed onwards and the segmentation distally is due to intermittent transit from the diseased area. Typical changes of diffuse systemic sclerosis were also present in oesophagus and colon.

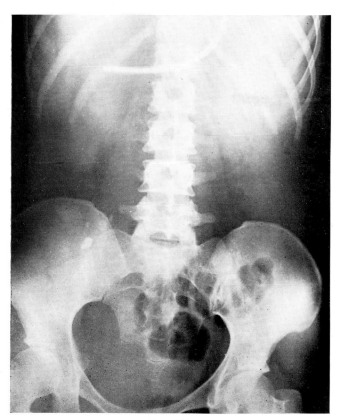

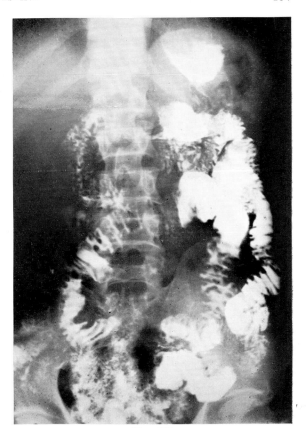

FIG. 460   FIG. 461

Fig. 460. Terminal stage of disseminated lupus erythematosus. Only a few loops of bowel contain gas and these are made obvious by the large ascites. The generalised ground-glass appearance elsewhere is due to the ascites and the large amount of fluid in the bowel lumen. Autopsy confirmation. **Fig. 461.** Dermatomyositis. Very ill patient in the advanced stage of the disease complaining of abdominal pain with diarrhoea. Some segmentation present with coarsening of the mucosal pattern in the small bowel. These appearances are not specific to dermatomyositis. One-hour barium follow-through film.

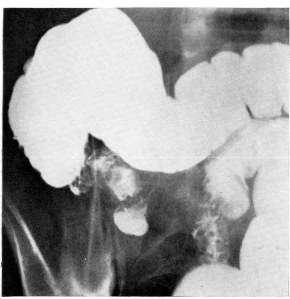
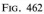

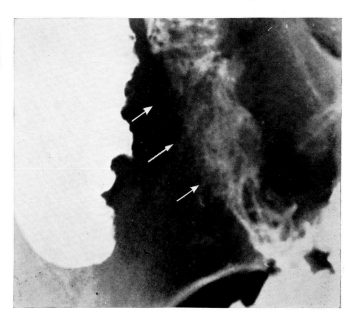

FIG. 462   FIG. 463

Fig. 462. Carcinoid tumour of terminal ileum which had intussuscepted into the colon causing a filling defect. The associated hypermotility of the small bowel probably also predisposed to the intussusception. **Fig. 463.** Henoch-Schönlein purpura. Haematoma (arrowed) in wall of terminal ileum causing blurring of mucosal folds.

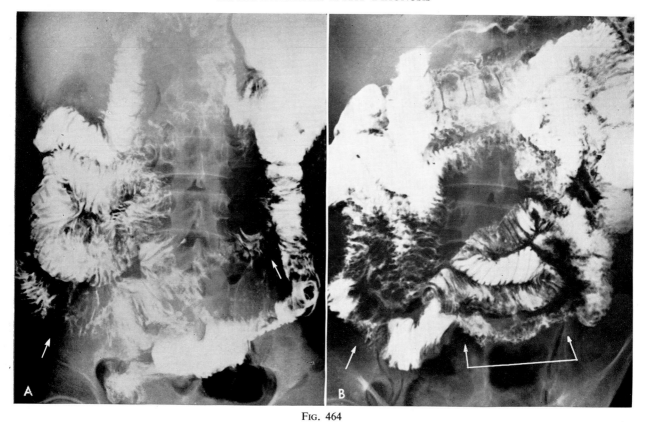

FIG. 464

Fig. 464. Henoch-Schönlein purpura.   A: Filling defects in lumen of small bowel due to blood clot.   Characteristic sharp projections—picket-fence appearance—of one segment (between arrows).   One-hour barium follow-through.   B: Narrowing, irregularity and mucosal distortion of several loops of small bowel—the most extensive being arrowed.   This abnormality is due to diffuse haemorrhage into the bowel wall.   Five-hour barium follow-through.

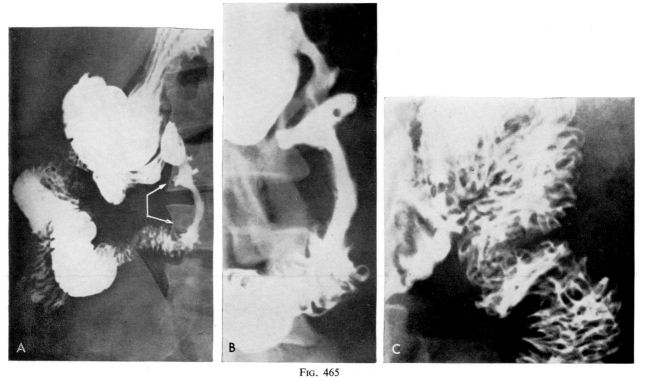

FIG. 465

Fig. 465. Idiopathic thrombocytopenia with haematoma in wall of upper jejunum.   Complaint of severe abdominal pain.   A: Follow-through of barium meal shows narrowing with distortion and abnormal mucosal pattern of a loop of upper jejunum (arrowed).   B: Spot film showing the lesion more clearly.   C: Fourteen days later the pattern is completely normal.   Patient at that time clinically well.

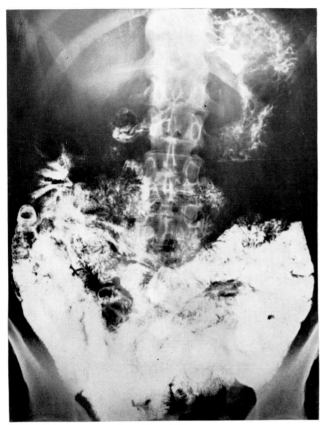

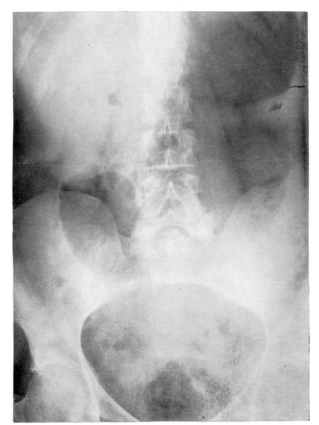

Fig. 466

Fig. 467

Fig. 466. Blood clot in small bowel causing fluffy or streaky filling defects, particularly in jejunum, and thus causing an indistinct mucosal pattern. Absence of deformity of the bowel wall which is of normal calibre. This tends to exclude a Henoch-Schönlein purpura. Case of massive haemorrhage from a gastric ulcer with extensive blood clot in the stomach. **Fig. 467.** Superior mesenteric occlusion with extensive gangrene of small bowel. Subsequent autopsy confirmation. Plain film (supine) shows very little gas in the small bowel since it was gangrenous and filled with fluid. Gross distension of the stomach because of the obstruction.

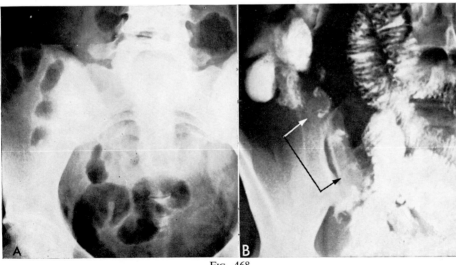

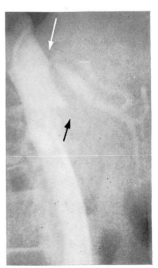

Fig. 468

Fig. 469

Fig. 468. Ischaemia of small bowel. A: Plain film (supine) shows gaseous distension of loops of ileum due to obstruction from an ischaemic segment at a more distal point. B: Follow-through of barium meal. The terminal ileum (arrowed), i.e. the affected part is irritable, spastic and irregular. The loops proximally are distended but are otherwise normal. Severe cardiac angina also present. **Fig. 469.** Vascular occlusion of small bowel. Aortogram shows narrowing of commencement of coeliac axis (top arrow) and obstruction of superior mesenteric artery (lower arrow). Patient complained of typical attacks of abdominal pain after a heavy meal and had steatorrhoea.

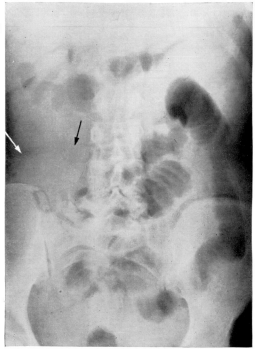

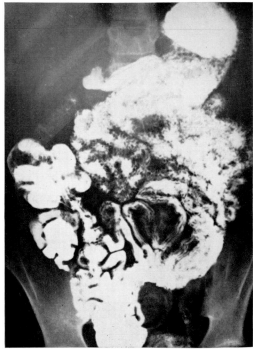

FIG. 470   FIG. 471

Fig. 470. Gangrene of segment of lower ileum from a superior mesenteric embolus in a case of mitral stenosis. Plain film (supine). Loops of lower jejunum and upper ileum distended with gas. Soft tissue shadow (arrowed) containing little gas on the right side. At operation a gangrenous loop of ileum corresponding to the soft tissue shadow was found. The loops distended with gas were proximal to the affected segment. **Fig. 471.** Intestinal hurry. One-hour follow-through film. Some narrowing of the small bowel, in particular the ileum, with increased motility. Normal mucosal pattern.

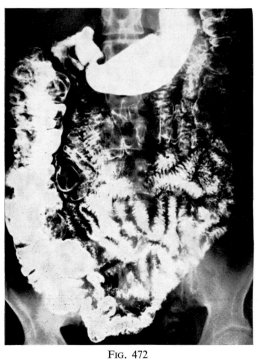

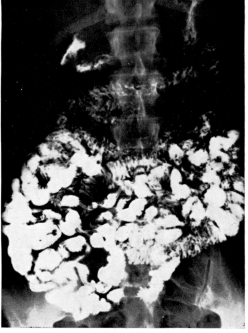

FIG. 472   FIG. 473

Fig. 472. Irritable small bowel. Well marked intestinal hurry—the head of the meal being at the splenic flexure in one hour. Irritability, spasticity and diminution of calibre of most of the loops but absence of segmentation and flocculation. Recent history of abdominal pain and diarrhoea which settled down on simple medical measures. **Fig. 473.** Irritable small bowel. Hyperperistalsis with narrowing of the lumen. Excessive contractions of the circular muscle—very obvious on fluoroscopy. No obvious structural abnormality present. History of diarrhoea with colicky abdominal pain.

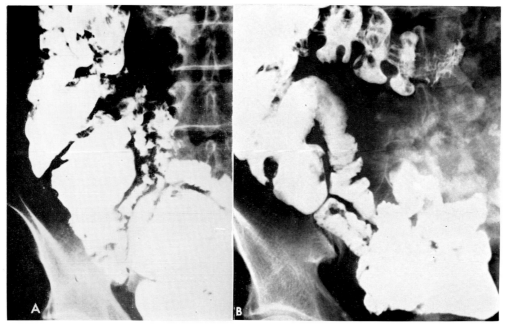

FIG. 474

Fig. 474. Irritable small bowel. Complaint of abdominal discomfort. A: Hypermotility with segmentation and narrowing of the terminal ileum. On this film Crohn's disease is a possibility. B: Half-hour later. The calibre of the ileum is normal. On fluoroscopy still some hypermotility but no ulceration or other evidence of Crohn's disease. The patient recovered satisfactorily and has remained well.

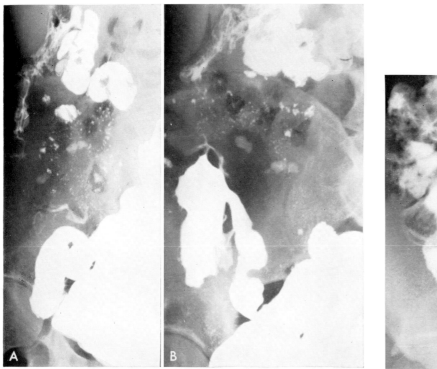

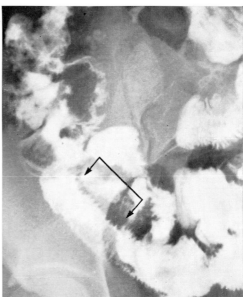

FIG. 475   FIG. 476

Fig. 475. Irritable small bowel and colon showing variability of appearances. A: One-hour follow-through film. Irritability and spasticity with narrowing of the lumen, segmentation, and 'skip' lesions. B: Three-hour follow-through film. The 'skip' lesions previously noted in the ileum are not now evident. These loops are now outlined by barium, but irritability obviously persists with increased peristalsis but no persistent narrowing or ulceration in the ileum itself. Marked spasticity of the ascending colon resulting in absence of filling and a 'skip' lesion at the moment the film was taken. Short history of abdominal pain and diarrhoea which settled down satisfactorily. Subsequent examination of the colon by barium enema showed no structural abnormality. **Fig. 476.** Irritable small bowel. Some blurring of loops of terminal ileum due to hypermotility. Saw-tooth margin of one loop (arrowed)—due to excessive contractions of the muscularis mucosae. Complaint of some abdominal pain and diarrhoea. Rapid recovery on simple medical measures. One-hour barium meal follow-through.

L

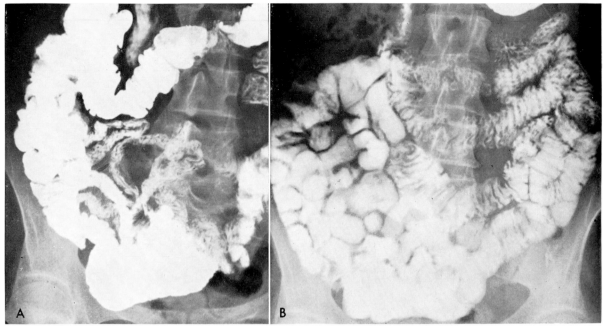

FIG. 477

Fig. 477. Disaccharidase deficiency.   Young woman complaining of attacks of vomiting, diarrhoea, and abdominal distension.
A: Normal barium follow-through.   Three-hour film.   B: One-hour follow-through after addition of lactose to the barium.
Marked intestinal hurry with dilution of the barium and some distension of the loops.

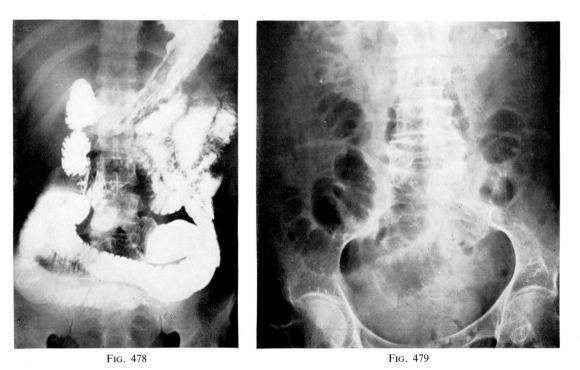

FIG. 478   FIG. 479

Fig. 478. Subacute obstruction of ileum following adhesions from an appendix abscess and with an unusual degree of
atony.   Barium was used as the patient was not acutely ill and had little pain.   The barium has become uniformly dispersed in the loops of ileum because of the fluid content and the intestinal atony.

Fig. 479. Obstruction of terminal ileum (right-sided femoral hernia).   No gas in the colon.   Supine film.

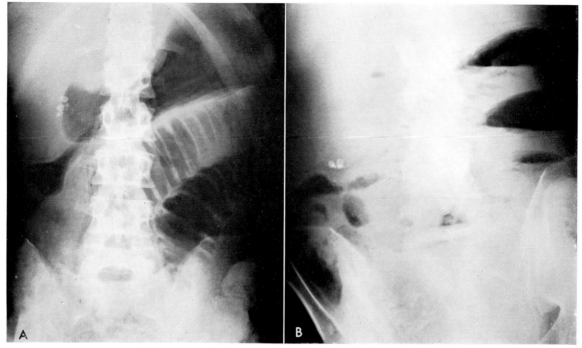

FIG. 480

Fig. 480. Obstruction of jejunum. Case of gross Crohn's disease with multiple strictures. A: Supine film. Grossly distended jejunal loops with characteristic cross-hatching. B: Erect film. Distended loops of jejunum with fluid levels. Multiple tiny fluid levels due to small pockets of gas caught up in the mucosal folds of loops which are grossly distended with fluid. Large fluid levels also present. Gall-stones also seen, having changed their relative positions between the two films.

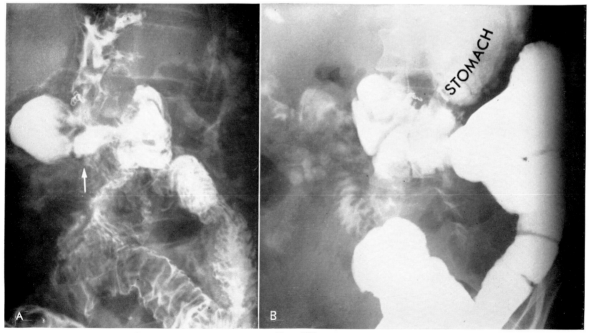

FIG. 481

Fig. 481. Jejunal ulcer with perforation into the colon causing a gastro-jejuno-colic fistula. Polya gastrectomy 17 years previously. Recent history of diarrhoea and weight loss. A: Barium meal shows large jejunal ulcer (arrowed) opposite the stoma, but no fistula to the colon demonstrated. B: Barium enema reveals immediate filling of jejunum and stomach when the barium has reached the transverse colon.

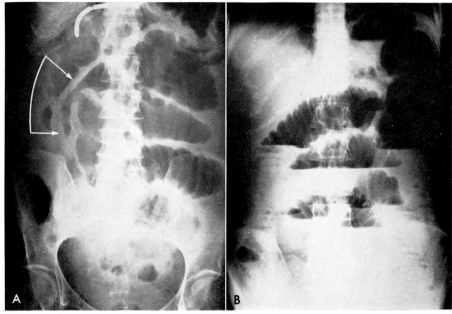

F<small>IG</small>. 482

Fig. 482. Obstruction of small bowel due to Crohn's disease. A: Supine. Gross distension particularly of jejunum with characteristic cross-hatching. An obviously narrowed, rigid segment (arrowed) due to Crohn's disease is present in upper jejunum. It was this segment that gave the clue to the underlying disease. B: Erect. Obvious fluid levels, including a number of tiny ones, due to small pockets of gas caught up in mucosal folds in loops distended with fluid. The patient regurgitated his naso-gastric tube between films A. and B.

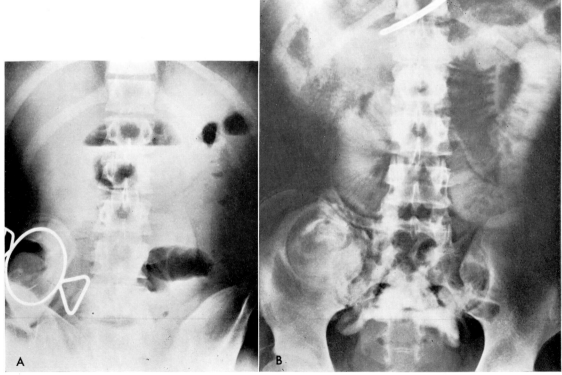

F<small>IG</small>. 483

Fig. 483. Obstruction of small bowel by an adhesion (operative proof). Previous colectomy for ulcerative colitis. A: Erect. Dilatation of small bowel with fluid levels. B: Supine. Eighty-minute film following Gastrografin. Dilatation of the jejunum to a point near the middle of the small bowel with marked dilution of the Gastrografin. Beyond this the bowel is collapsed and the lumen obviously narrowed.

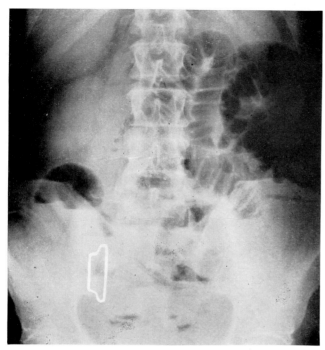

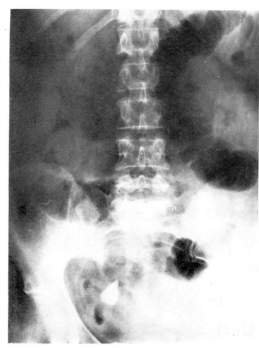

FIG. 484   FIG. 485

Fig. 484. Obstruction due to prolapse of terminal ileum into the anterior abdominal wall in a patient with an ileostomy. Distended loop with fluid levels in right iliac fossa. Tiny fluid levels in pelvis in grossly distended loops of ileum. These appearances are due to a large amount of fluid but little gas. Erect film. **Fig. 485.** Enterolith in ileum causing acute intestinal obstruction. At operation it was impacted in an old fibrous stricture and had formed between two such strictures in a stagnation loop. These strictures were presumably caused by old healed tuberculous lesions.

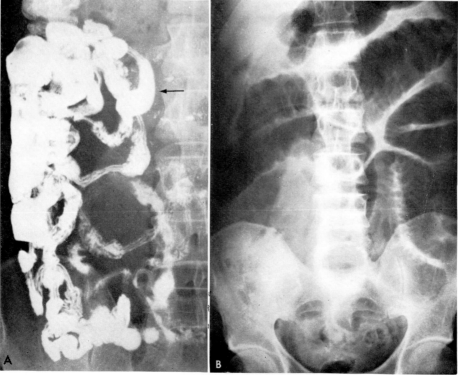

FIG. 486

Fig. 486. Meckel's diverticulum. A: Diverticulum (arrowed). Incidental finding on barium follow-through. B: Five months later. Patient presented with acute intestinal obstruction. Plain film shows gross distension of proximal small bowel with a large soft tissue mass in right iliac fossa. At operation a loop of bowel had become twisted around an adhesion between the diverticulum and the umbilicus.

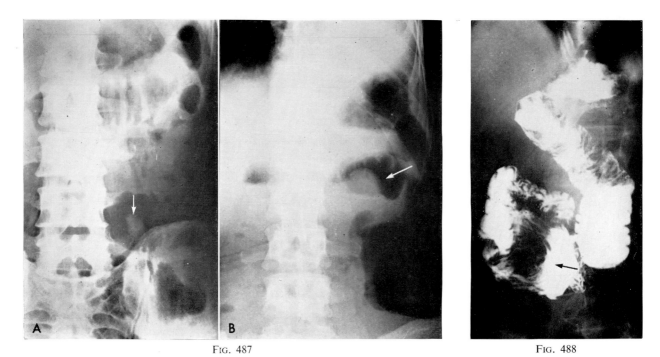

FIG. 487   FIG. 488

Fig. 487. Obstruction due to intussusception by a polyp which is not seen on the films. A: Supine film. Distension of loops of jejunum. A second polyp (arrowed) is shown as a soft tissue opacity surrounded by gas in a distended loop at a higher level. B: Erect. The polyp (arrowed) is again demonstrated.

Fig. 488. Intussusception of Roux-en-Y loop (arrowed) into the jejunum causing a characteristic whorled filling defect.

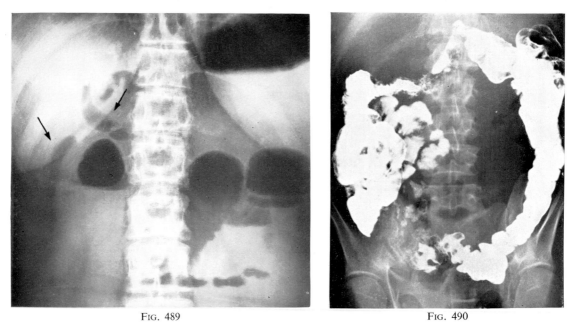

FIG. 489   FIG. 490

Fig. 489. Gall-stone ileus. Erect film. Distension of loops of jejunum with fluid levels due to an obstruction in lower jejunum. Gas in biliary tract—seen also on supine film though not so clearly. At operation a large gall-stone (not obvious on the films) had become impacted in lower jejunum. Gall-bladder and common hepatic duct (arrowed).

Fig. 490. Adhesions affecting terminal ileum and caecum. The loops of bowel are matted together and on fluoroscopy with palpation could not be separated. History of peritonitis with abscesses one year previously. Seven-hour follow-through.

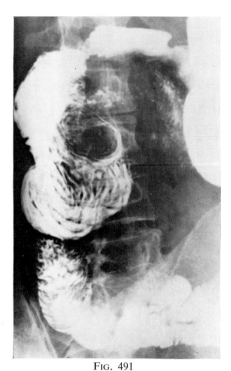

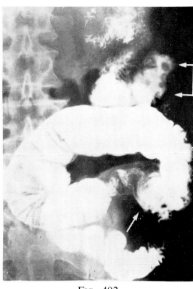

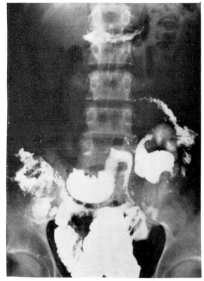

FIG. 492

FIG. 493

FIG. 491

Fig. 491. Intermittent retrograde jejuno-duodenal intussusception. Duodeno-jejuno-stomy 40 years previously (by the late Sir David Wilkie) for duodenal ileus. Dilatation of duodenum with typical whorled filling defect caused by the intussusception. Recent history of abdominal pain and vomiting. Operative confirmation.

Fig. 492. Intussusception in upper jejunum due to a large pedunculated polyp (arrowed). Only minimal obstruction. Several other small polypi (arrowed) in jejunum at a higher level. **Fig. 493.** Adhesions involving ileum (previous appendicectomy) causing irregularly narrowed areas with dilatation between the stenoses. Operative confirmation. Three-hour barium follow-through film. On this one examination Crohn's disease could not be excluded.

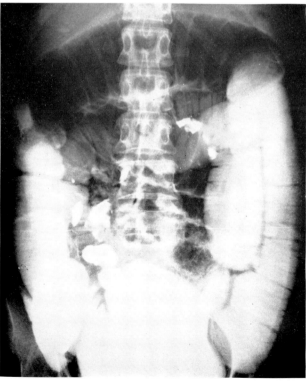

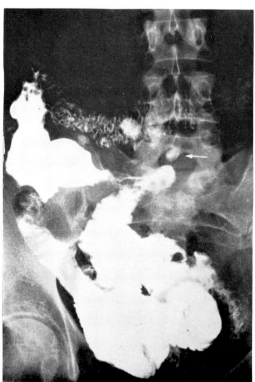

FIG. 494

FIG. 495

Fig. 494. Gross obstruction in ileum from extension of a carcinoma of uterus. An unusual degree of intestinal atony has supervened. Barium meal carried out three weeks previously as the degree of obstruction was not obvious clinically. Because of the dilatation and diminished motility the barium is evenly interspersed in the fluid with very little clumping. **Fig. 495.** Adhesions to a calcified mesenteric lymph node (arrowed) causing obvious kinking of an adjacent loop of ileum with localised narrowing.

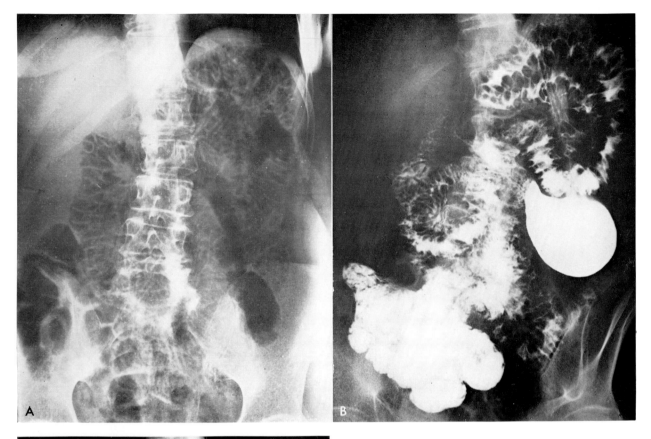

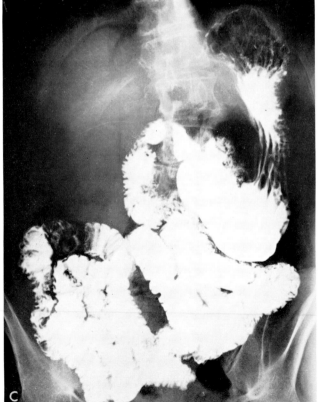

Fig. 496. Pneumatosis cystoides intestinalis affecting the small bowel. A: Plain film. The large number of cysts containing air in the small bowel are clearly seen. At first the appearance simulates an obstruction with a coarse mucosal pattern. B: Follow-through of barium meal. The translucencies due to the cysts cause extensive thumb-printing and distortion, especially in upper part of jejunum. No cysts present in the colon. C: Follow-through of barium meal seven months later—normal.
(By courtesy of Dr. J. G. Duncan.)

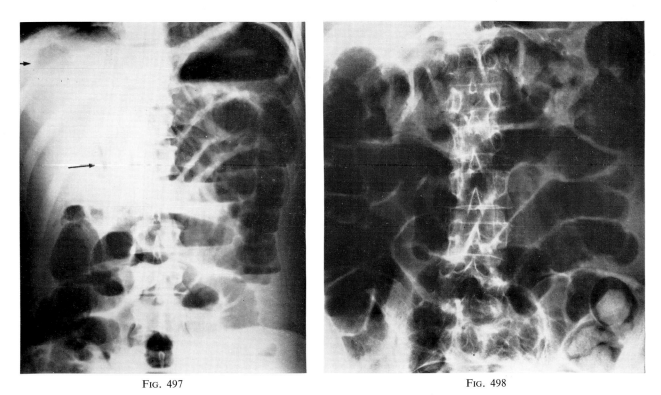

Fig. 497   Fig. 498

Fig. 497. Post-operative adynamic ileus with abdominal distension and absent bowel sounds. Considerably dilated loops of small bowel with fluid levels. Recent perforation of a duodenal ulcer with a residual inflammatory mass below the liver in which there is a small loculation (arrowed). Subphrenic abscess (arrowed) also present under the right dome of diaphragm. **Fig. 498.** Gross adynamic ileus due to hypokalaemia. Patient admitted with marked muscular weakness. Subsequent recovery following substitution therapy.

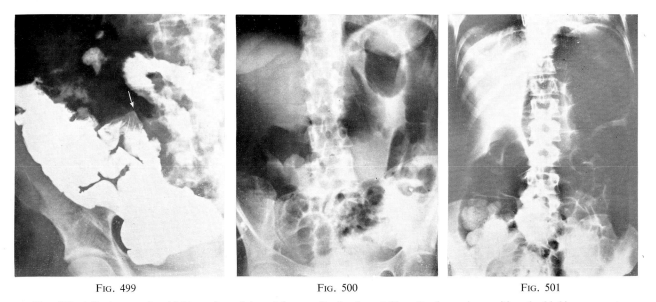

Fig. 499   Fig. 500   Fig. 501

Fig. 499. Adhesion causing kinking of small bowel (arrowed). Semi-erect film. In the supine position the kinking was not obvious. **Fig. 500.** Ileus of small bowel and colon—due to a retro-peritoneal haemorrhage. Bleeding subcutaneously and also from the bowel and renal tract. Complaint of severe back pain. Patient being treated with anticoagulants. **Fig. 501.** Generalised ileus of small and large bowel due to a severe virus infection—clinically simulating acute appendicitis. Appendix removed but normal at operation.

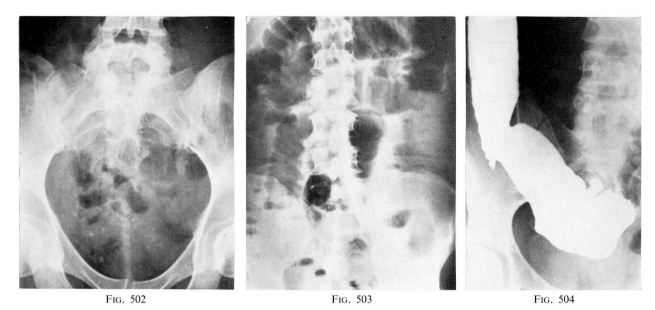

FIG. 502   FIG. 503   FIG. 504

Fig. 502. Ileus from a mild salpingitis and parametritis. Loops of ileum distended with some gas, similar to findings in acute appendicitis. Barium follow-through subsequently showed no intrinsic small bowel lesion.

Fig. 503. Adynamic ileus in a very stout man six days after operation for left inguinal hernia. Grossly distended loops of small and large bowel. The small fluid levels in the flanks are in colonic haustrations—the lumen of the colon in these areas being filled with fluid.

Fig. 504. Gross dilatation with stasis in ileum in a case of chronic ulcerative colitis. Gross contraction of caecum. The ascending colon is smooth and shows lack of haustrations. Widely patent ileo-caecal valve. Seven-hour follow-through film.

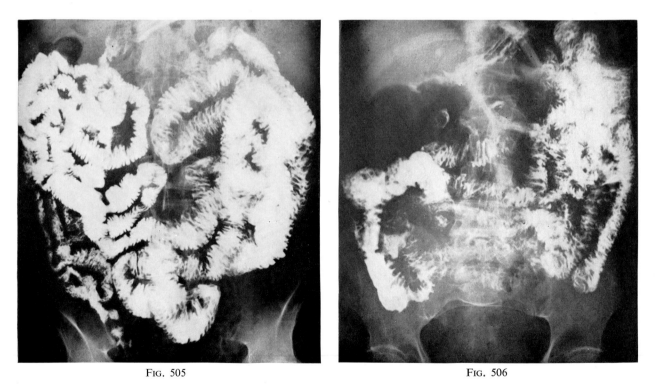

FIG. 505   FIG. 506

Fig. 505. Chronic oedema of wall of small bowel. Case of portal hypertension with hepatic encephalopathy. Large gastric and oesophageal varices were present. Follow-through of barium meal shows coarsening of the mucosa of jejunum and upper ileum. No obvious ascites—unusual at this stage.

Fig. 506. Chronic myxoedema with generalised coarsening and irregularity of mucosal folds throughout the small bowel. Some colonic distension also present—a common finding in myxoedema.

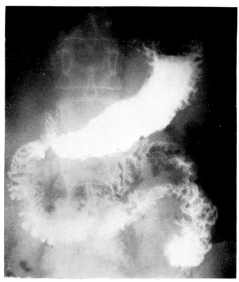

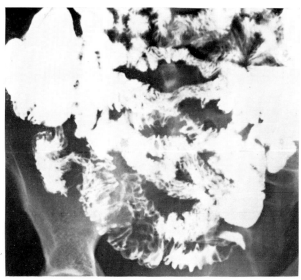

Fig. 507   Fig. 508

Fig. 507. Chronic oedema of wall of jejunum with coarsening and thickening of mucosal folds. Case of gross cirrhosis of the liver with oesophageal and fundal varices and gross ascites.

Fig. 508. Oedema of terminal ileum due to lymphatic obstruction. Marked coarsening and thickening of mucosal folds. Radiotherapy 18 months previously for carcinoma of the cervix.

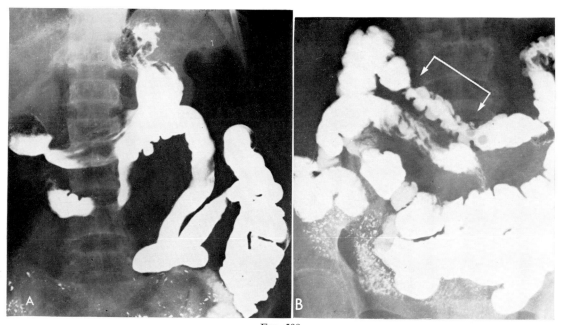

Fig. 509

Fig. 509. Non-specific enteropathy affecting the entire small bowel. Four-year history of attacks of vomiting, abdominal pain, diarrhoea alternating with constipation. Generalised weakness and malaise. Pale offensive stools containing undigested food. At laparotomy during acute exacerbation an acute jejunitis with areas of ulceration found. Patient subsequently developed iron deficiency anaemia and gross steatorrhoea. Jejunal biopsy showed infiltration with inflammatory cells, mainly eosinophils, and with total villous atrophy. Osteomalacia and Looser's zones also present. A: Barium meal and follow-through during relatively quiescent phase. Gross mucosal destruction of jejunum with smooth outline and absence of normal mucosal pattern. Marked loss of motility on fluoroscopy. B: Some dilatation of the ileum with similar atrophic mucosal changes. Sacculations (arrowed) also present.

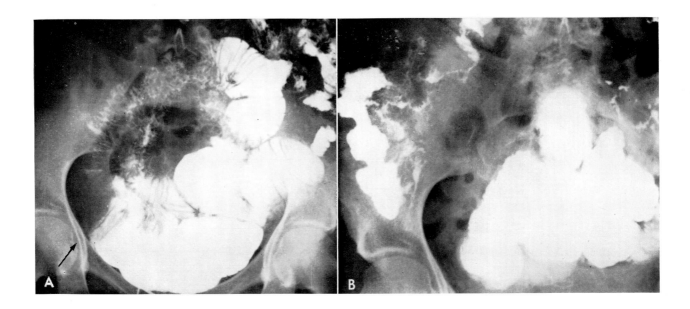

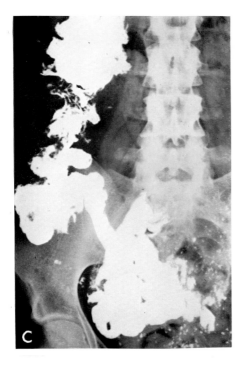

Fig. 510. Non-specific enteropathy. History of pulmonary sarcoidosis one year previously. Complaint of diarrhoea for three months. A: Obstruction (arrowed) in terminal ileum with some dilatation proximally. Two-hour film. B: 'Skip' lesion present in terminal ileum with stasis proximally. Three-hour film. On these two films the radiological diagnosis of Crohn's disease was made. At laparotomy an extensive area of small bowel, in particular the terminal ileum, was heavy and oedematous, but no evidence of Crohn's disease or actual ulceration. Subsequently the patient developed well-marked steatorrhoea. Treatment by prednisolone, but with frequent relapses. C: Two and a half years later. Follow-through of barium meal shows the small bowel, including the terminal ileum, to be normal. Treatment by gluten-free diet and prednisolone with temporary improvement, but subsequent relapse.

The patient is still under observation with the final diagnosis uncertain.

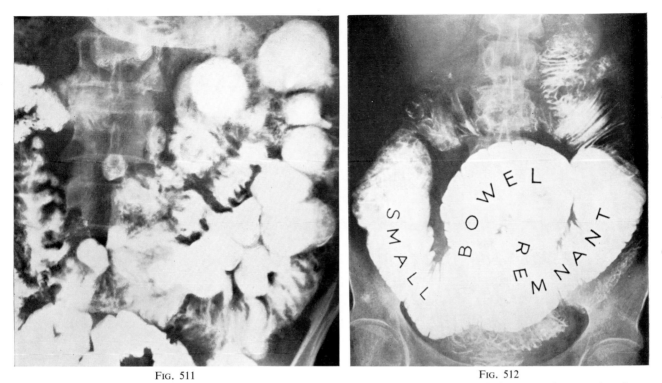

FIG. 511   FIG. 512

Fig. 511. Diverticulosis of small bowel causing malabsorption. Two-hour barium follow-through shows a very large number of diverticula. Patient complained of episodic diarrhoea with bulky foul-smelling stools. **Fig. 512.** Gross malabsorption due to an extremely short small bowel. Previous extensive resection of the small bowel, the remainder becoming dilated in order to act as a reservoir. Well-marked associated osteomalacia. (By courtesy of the Royal College of Physicians, Edinburgh.)

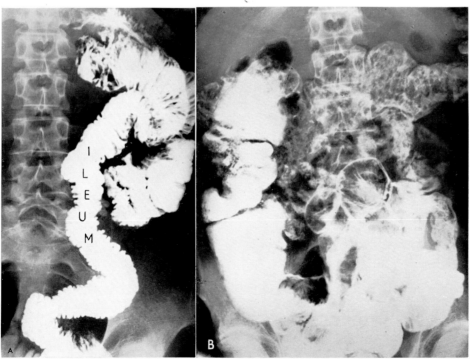

FIG. 513

Fig. 513. Previous partial gastrectomy of Polya type for duodenal ulcer with an inadvertent gastro-ileal anastomosis. This was followed by diarrhoea, steatorrhoea and weight loss. A: Follow-through of barium meal shows that the stomach had been anastomosed to the ileum, causing a long blind loop of jejunum. The absence of flocculation and segmentation is presumably due to the otherwise normal small bowel including motility. B: Three-hour barium follow-through. Mottled appearances in the transverse colon due to barium mixed with excessive fat. At a second operation the anastomosis was undone and gastro-jejunostomy performed with cure.

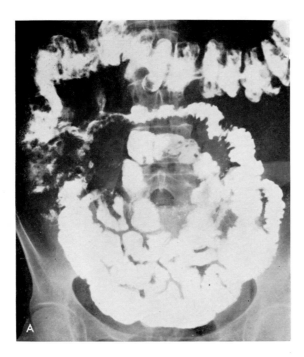

Fig. 514. Non-specific enteropathy particularly affecting the jejunum. Complaint of diarrhoea, loss of weight, abdominal pain with some vomiting, for several months. A: Three-hour follow-through film. Irregularity with some dilatation and coarsening of mucosal pattern of most of small bowel due to oedema.

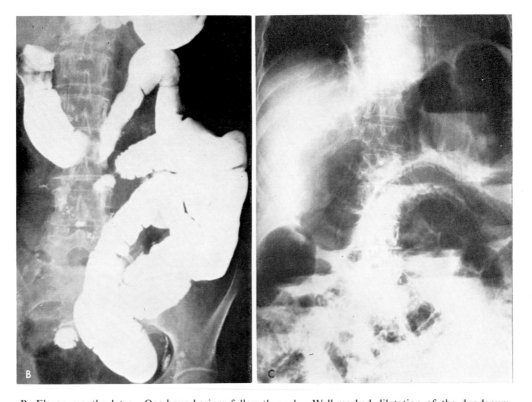

B: Eleven months later. One-hour barium follow-through. Well-marked dilatation of the duodenum, jejunum and upper ileum with smooth outline and absence of normal mucosal pattern. Greatly diminished motility on fluoroscopy with some rigidity. At laparotomy the bowel was heavy, oedematous, thickened and congested. Enlarged lymph nodes present with petechial haemorrhages in the mesentery. Total villous atrophy and infiltration of bowel wall with plasma cells. Patient recovered from this acute attack but developed steatorrhoea with impaired absorption also of folic acid. C: One month later. Plain erect film of abdomen shows marked distension of small and large bowel with fluid levels. At this time the patient complained of abdominal distension with profuse watery diarrhoea.

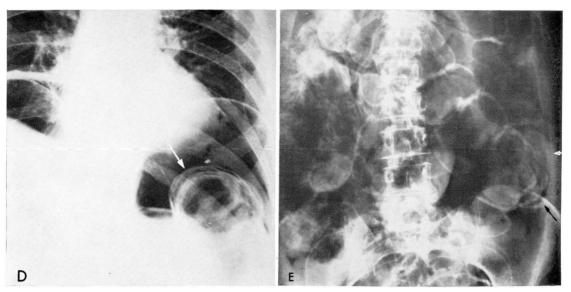

D: Three weeks later. Patient admitted to hospital as an acute abdominal emergency with severe pain and generalised abdominal tenderness. Erect film shows large amount of gas under both domes of diaphragm with gas below the serous coat of the splenic flexure of colon (arrowed). E: Supine film of abdomen at the same time shows gross distension of coils of small and large bowel whose outline is clearly depicted because of the large pneumo-peritoneum. Gas present (arrowed) along lateral border of descending colon. At laparotomy large amount of gas in the peritoneal cavity. Considerable gas in the wall of the jejunum, transverse colon and in the falciform ligament. No significant free fluid. Patient recovered from the operation in spite of no specific surgical procedure apart from a colostomy.

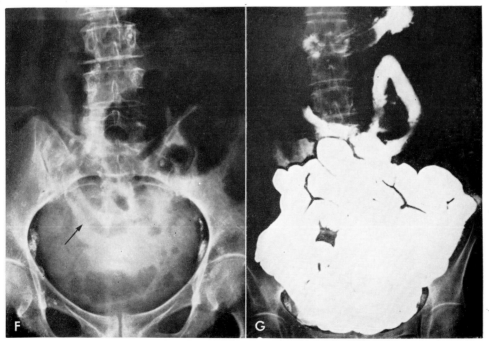

FIG. 514

F: Seven months later. Recurrence of diarrhoea and generalised abdominal pain. Plain film shows narrowed, rigid loops of ileum (arrowed) indicating structural disease. G: One week later. Three-hour follow-through of barium meal shows a well-marked moulage sign with smooth mucosal pattern. Gross steatorrhoea persistently present.

This patient has been followed up for four years and the precise diagnosis has not yet been established.

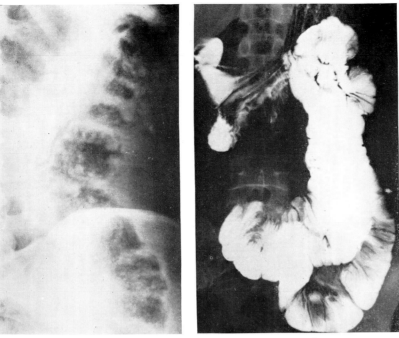

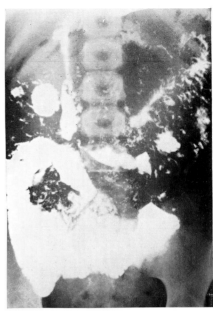

FIG. 515   FIG. 516   FIG. 517

Fig. 515. Excessive fat in faeces causing characteristic mottled appearance in colon on a plain film. Gross malabsorption present.
Fig. 516. Gluten-sensitive enteropathy. Smooth sharp outline with atony causing the moulage or plaster-cast appearance in small bowel. Jejunal biopsy showed villous atrophy. Remarkable improvement within days of starting gluten-free diet.
Fig. 517. Coeliac disease. Typical disordered X-ray pattern with segmentation, flocculation and dilatation. Two-hour barium follow-through.

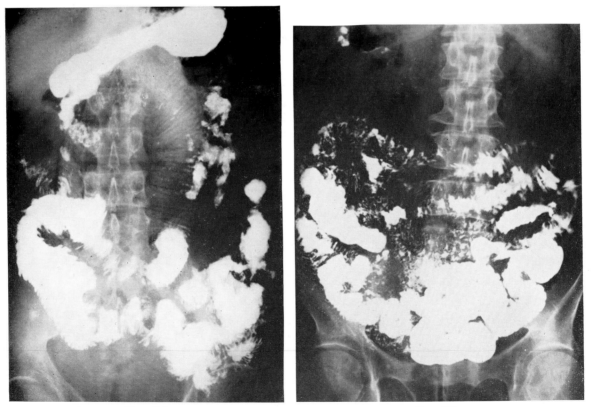

FIG. 518   FIG. 519

Fig. 518. Gluten-sensitive enteropathy. Typical disordered X-ray pattern with segmentation, flocculation, dilatation and coarsening of mucosal pattern. Abnormal motility on fluoroscopy. Clinical cure on gluten-free diet. **Fig. 519.** Malabsorption due to several causes including chronic pancreatitis, sclerosing cholangitis with irregular dilatation of the intrahepatic ducts. Previous Whipple's operation. Gross steatorrhoea (faecal fat excretion of 140 g. in three days). Jejunal biopsy showed total villous atrophy. Some improvement on pancreatic substitution therapy. Follow-through of barium meal shows grossly disordered X-ray pattern with segmentation, flocculation and coarsening of the mucosal pattern. Gas in the biliary tract due to the choledocho-jejunostomy.

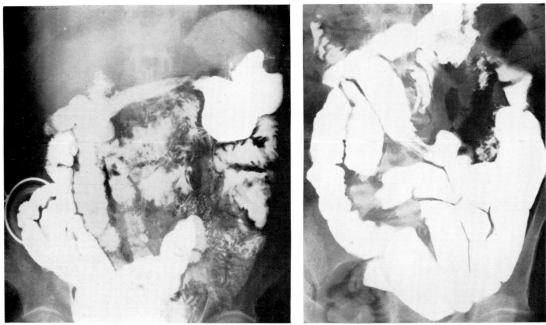

FIG. 520   FIG. 521

Fig. 520. Malabsorption associated with gross jejunal bacterial colonisation. Dilatation of jejunum and ileum with slow transit, coarsening of the mucosal pattern and some segmentation and flocculation. Previous procto-colectomy for ulcerative procto-colitis. Normal mucosa on jejunal biopsy. No response to gluten-free diet but some response to antibiotics.

Fig. 521. Tropical sprue developed in the Far East. Two-hour follow-through film shows gross atrophy of the mucosa with smooth outline—the moulage sign.

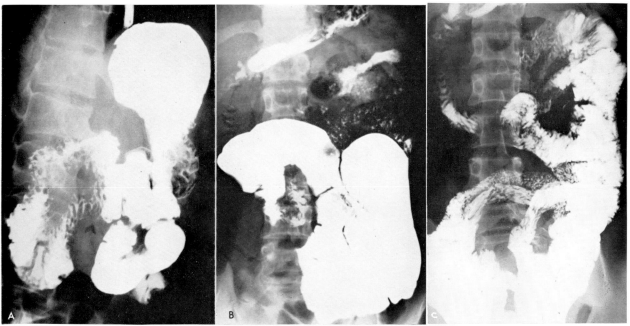

FIG. 522

Fig. 522. Gluten-sensitive enteropathy. A: Coarse mucosal pattern in duodenum and uppermost loop of jejunum. B: Dilatation with smooth outline in lower jejunum and upper ileum—the moulage sign. C: Return to normal pattern with clinical cure after six months' gluten-free diet.

M

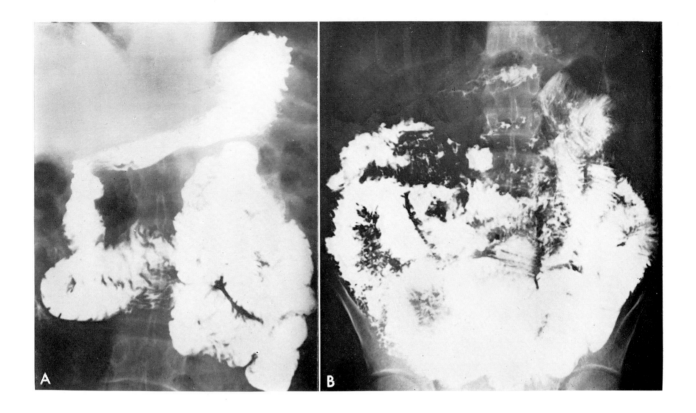

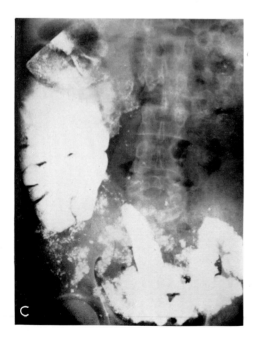

FIG. 523

Fig. 523. Idiopathic steatorrhoea proceeding to reticulosis. A: Some dilatation of jejunum with coarsening of mucosal pattern. B: One-hour follow-through film. Dilatation of small bowel with well-marked flocculation, some segmentation and coarsening of mucosal pattern. C: Three-hour film. Obvious segmentation and flocculation. On this film there is the appearance of a 'skip' lesion of the terminal ileum and Crohn's disease could not be excluded. This segment, however, was filled on other films taken under fluoroscopic control. Case of severe malabsorption for years with osteomalacia and Looser's zones. Total villous atrophy. Did not respond adequately to gluten-free diet or when steroids were subsequently added. White count 15,000 per c. ml. Night sweats. Because of suspicion of malignancy laparotomy was performed but no abnormality detected except brown pigmentation of the bowel wall. One year later patient died of perforation of a lymphosarcoma of small bowel.

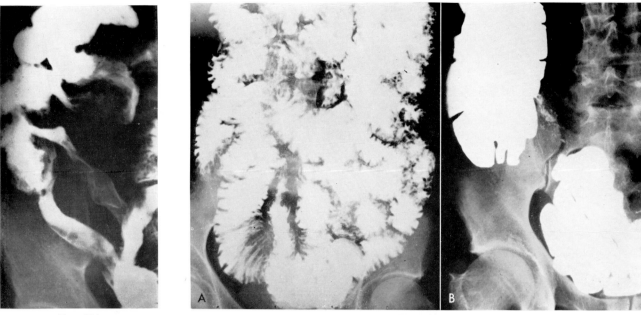

FIG. 524   FIG. 525

Fig. 524. Malabsorption with up to 36 g. faecal fat excretion in three days. Follow-through of barium meal shows smooth mucosal pattern of an extensive area of ileum due to diffuse mucosal destruction or atrophy. Patient presented one month previously with an acute episode of abdominal pain and diarrhoea which improved slowly. Careful follow-up maintained. Case similar to others classified under non-specific enteropathy. **Fig. 525.** Whipple's disease. A: One-hour follow-through film. Dilatation of jejunum and ileum with coarsening of mucosal pattern. B: Three-hour film. 'Skip' lesion of terminal ileum with some dilatation proximally. These appearances on a single examination are not specific to any one intestinal disorder but in this case ultimately proved to be due to Whipple's disease. History of fever, joint pains, marked diarrhoea, weight loss and steatorrhoea. Treated with tetracycline with satisfactory result and the patient has remained well.

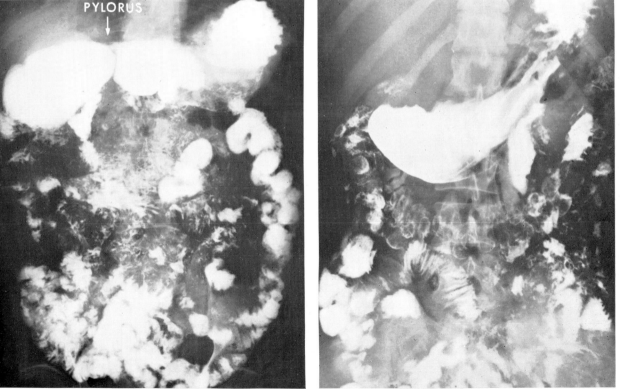

FIG. 526   FIG. 527

Fig. 526. Disordered pattern simulating malabsorption. Marked segmentation and flocculation in small bowel due to intermittent passage of barium through a stenosed area of the duodenum—due to adhesions from a previous cholecystectomy. Gross dilatation of the first part of the duodenum. Five-hour barium follow-through. **Fig. 527.** Disordered X-ray pattern from a very high acid output (basal output 30 mEq/hr.). Gross segmentation with flocculation and coarsening of mucosal pattern in jejunum and ileum. The patient was subsequently discovered to be a case of the Zollinger-Ellison syndrome. Duodenal ulcer also present. One-hour barium follow-through.

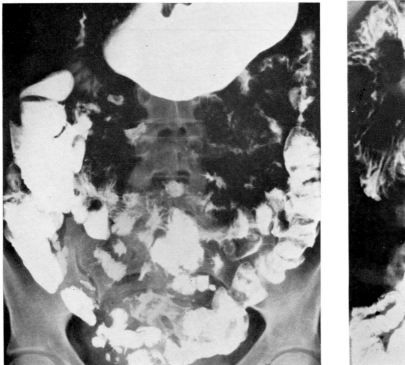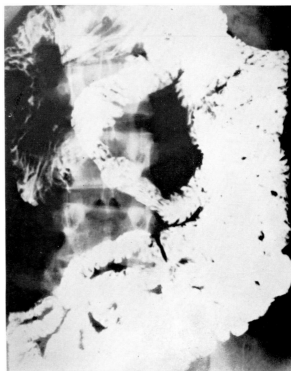

FIG. 528   FIG. 529

Fig. 528. Diabetic enteropathy.   Disordered X-ray pattern with segmentation and marked intestinal hurry—the head of the meal being in the rectum in one hour.   Case of severe diabetes which was difficult to control and was associated with intermittent diarrhoea and steatorrhoea.   One-hour barium follow-through film.

Fig. 529. Intestinal allergy to salmon.   At the time of this barium follow-through the patient had almost completely recovered. Now only some residual coarsening of the mucosal pattern in duodenum and jejunum.

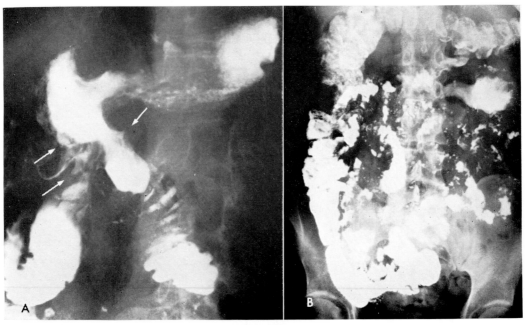

FIG. 530

Fig. 530. Partial gastrectomy for chronic duodenal ulceration in a case which was subsequently discovered to be of the Zollinger-Ellison syndrome.   Very high acid output.   A: Three jejunal ulcers (arrowed).   Gross coarsening of mucosal pattern of jejunum.   At operation seven ulcers were found.   B: Grossly disordered X-ray pattern with segmentation and flocculation in jejunum and ileum.   Three-hour barium follow-through.

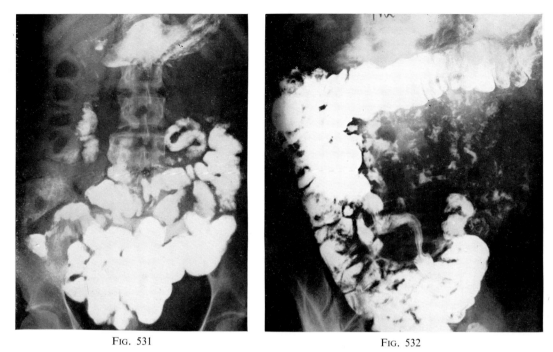

Fig. 531   Fig. 532

Fig. 531. Zollinger-Ellison syndrome with very high acid output (basal output 29 mEq/hr.). Segmentation and dilatation with poorly depicted mucosal pattern in small bowel. Duodenal ulcer also present with grossly deformed duodenal bulb. One-hour barium follow-through.

Fig. 532. Peptide secreting tumour with predominance of carcinoid features. One-hour barium follow-through shows marked intestinal hurry with narrowing and hypermotility of small bowel. The head of the meal is at the splenic flexure in one hour.

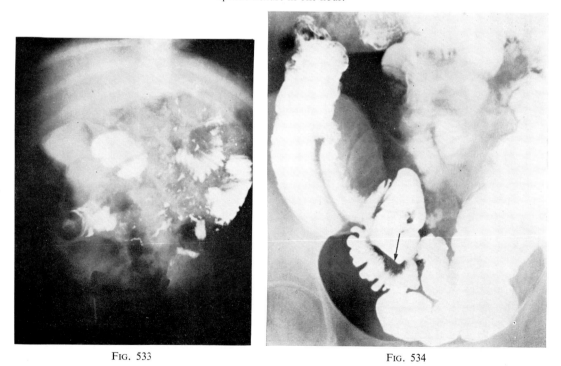

Fig. 533   Fig. 534

Fig. 533. Milk allergy in a seven-month-old baby. Well-marked flocculation and segmentation of the barium with coarsening of the mucosal pattern. One-hour barium follow-through. Recovery on a milk-free diet.

Fig. 534. Endometriosis involving small bowel. Infiltration of a segment of ileum (arrowed) showing a ragged outline with mucosal destruction.

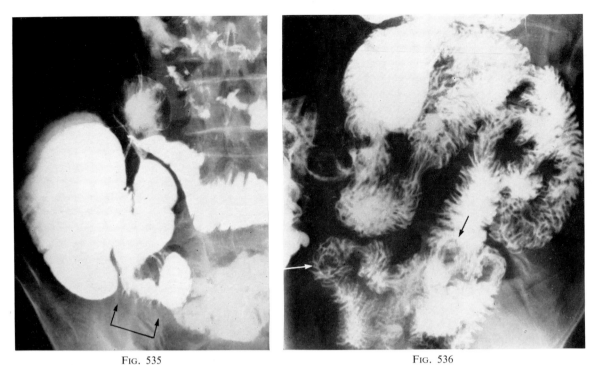

FIG. 535   FIG. 536

Fig. 535. Neurofibromatosis involving terminal ileum. The segment affected (arrowed) is narrowed with deep penetrating ulcers—indistinguishable from Crohn's disease. (By courtesy of Dr. Eric Samuel.) **Fig. 536.** Peutz-Jeghers syndrome. At least two polypi are seen (arrowed). History of severe attacks of abdominal pain resulting on a previous occasion in intussusception of a polyp and which required resection of a segment of jejunum.

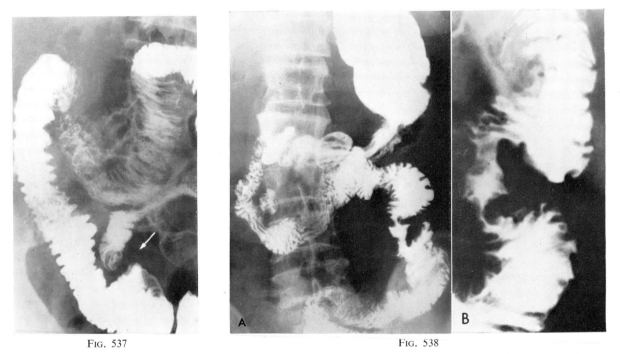

FIG. 537   FIG. 538

Fig. 537. Carcinoma of ileum causing a napkin ring type of stricture (arrowed). The bowel proximal to the tumour is dilated and the mucosal pattern is coarse due to oedema. At operation a tumour was found and the bowel proximally was heavy and oedematous. (By courtesy of Messrs Butterworths.) **Fig. 538.** Carcinoma of jejunum. A: Irregular filling defect distal to duodeno-jejunal flexure. Patient presented with vague indigestion and with provisional clinical diagnosis of carcinoma of stomach. This emphasises the importance of examining the upper jejunum at the end of a barium meal. B: Spot film of the tumour showing the narrowing and mucosal destruction more clearly.

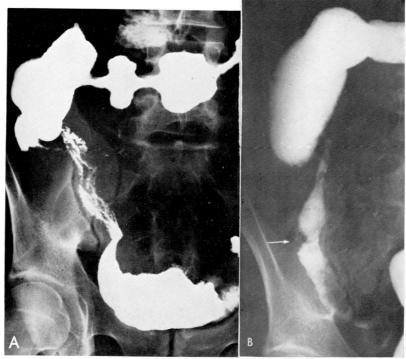

FIG. 539

Fig. 539. Carcinoma of ileum in a case of chronic ulcerative procto-colitis of over 10 years' duration. A: A little distortion with coarsening of mucosal pattern of terminal ileum indicating a mild back-wash ileitis. Diffuse changes of chronic ulcerative procto-colitis in colon. Follow-through of barium meal. B: Eight years later. Changes in colon more marked. Now mucosal destruction of terminal ileum with the presence of a moderately large filling defect (arrowed). Procto-colectomy performed and the filling defect in the ileum was proved to be due to a carcinoma. No carcinoma in the resected colon. (By courtesy of Mr. J. M. Ross, Roodlands Hospital.)

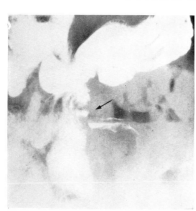

FIG. 540

Fig. 540. Leiomyosarcoma of jejunum with ulcer (arrowed) which had perforated. Escape of barium into an abscess cavity which contains gas.

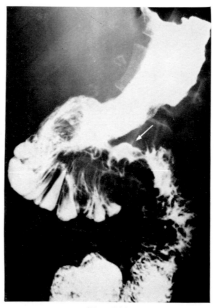

FIG. 541

Fig. 541. Diffuse recurrence of carcinoma of stomach in jejunum adjacent to the stoma —an uncommon occurrence. Large ulcer crater present (arrowed). The stomach is also diffusely infiltrated with the tumour. Previous partial gastrectomy with gastro-jejunostomy for antral carcinoma.

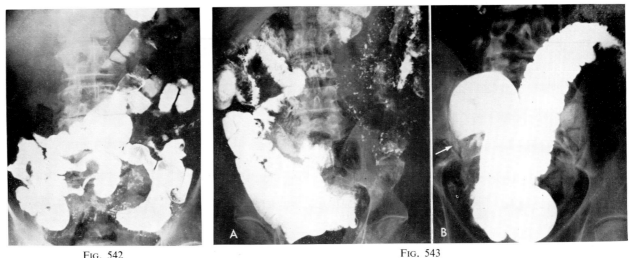

FIG. 542   FIG. 543

Fig. 542. Reticulosis mainly involving mesenteric lymph nodes causing displacement and narrowing of several segments of small bowel.

Fig. 543. Lymphosarcoma of small intestine. Known case of steatorrhoea presumed initially to represent a gluten-sensitive enteropathy. Gluten-free diet did not result in complete recovery. Leucocytosis with persistently high E.S.R. A: Only minor changes of a disordered X-ray pattern with some dilatation and coarsening of mucosal pattern. Three-hour barium follow-through film. Laparotomy performed but on multiple biopsies no tumour was found. B: Six months later. Patient presented with abdominal pain. Three-hour barium follow-through film shows obstruction in ileum (arrowed) with dilatation proximally. At laparotomy the obstruction proved to be due to a lymphosarcoma which had developed at the site of a previous biopsy identified by the presence of a stitch. Diffuse malignant infiltration elsewhere in the small bowel.

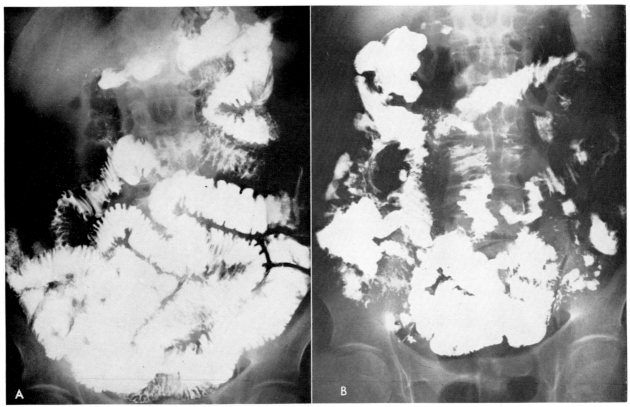

FIG. 544

Fig. 544. Reticulosis (Hodgkin's disease) of small bowel. A: Dilatation of loops with coarsening of mucosal pattern. One-hour follow-through film. B: Three-hour follow-through film. The changes are more marked with segmentation and flocculation. The disordered X-ray pattern is usually more obvious on later films, not only in reticulosis but in malabsorption from other causes. Two hours later an ulcer in the ileum perforated and the diagnosis of a form of Hodgkin's disease was made at laparotomy.

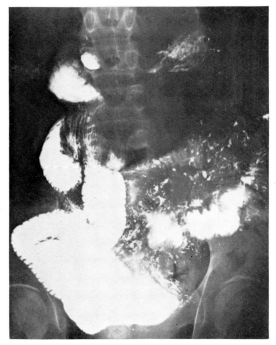

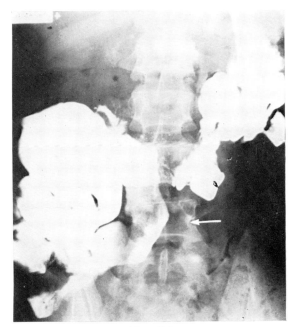

FIG. 545   FIG. 546

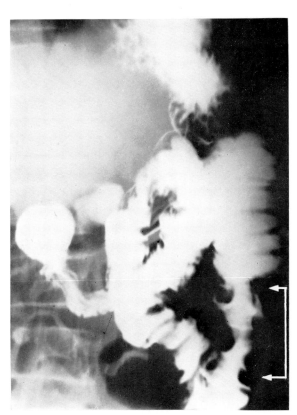

Fig. 545. Plasmacytosis involving the small bowel—proved at laparotomy with biopsy. Dilatation of loops of small bowel with some segmentation and flocculation. These appearances are non-specific and can be due to many causes. Two-hour barium follow-through.

Fig. 546. Reticulosis (Hodgkin's disease) of the small bowel. Biopsy proof. Moderate dilatation with absent mucosal pattern. Rigidity of the loops, particularly the one (arrowed) which has straight borders. Previous partial gastrectomy for a duodenal ulcer. One-hour barium follow-through.

(By courtesy of Messrs Butterworths.)

Fig. 547. Malignant lymphoma. Diffuse infiltration of a segment of upper jejunum (arrowed) with narrowing and mucosal destruction. Perforation occurred at another tumour lower down the small bowel a few weeks later.

FIG. 547

CHAPTER VI

THE APPENDIX

RADIOLOGY has much to offer in the investigation of suspected disease of the appendix. Even although no abnormality of the appendix itself is revealed other intra-abdominal conditions may be diagnosed or excluded.

RADIOLOGICAL METHODS OF INVESTIGATION

Plain Films. Erect and supine films are necessary in both acute and chronic cases. It is also advisable to take a film of the chest.

A follow-through of a barium meal is, of course, contra-indicated in suspected acute appendicitis. It is of value in subacute and chronic cases when the diagnosis is uncertain and for the purpose of precisely localising calculi or a palpable mass in the right iliac fossa. In other instances a clinical suspicion of Crohn's disease has prompted the barium meal.

A barium enema is usually performed because of the presence of a palpable mass in the right iliac fossa or in the pelvis and in cases with localised tenderness in the right iliac fossa.

CLINICAL RADIOLOGY

NORMAL APPEARANCES

Plain films sometimes show the presence of lead shot in the appendix from ingested game.

Absence of filling of the appendix by a barium follow-through or enema is of no significance. When the appendix does fill, especially by barium enema, translucencies due to faeces may be demonstrated, but these are usually of no significance. Barium may remain in an appendix for four or more weeks.

The site and length of the appendix are variable and need no further description. Generally speaking, it is not fixed and it can be displaced by palpation.

CALCULI (CALCIFIED CONCRETIONS)

These may be single or multiple and are commonly densely calcified and laminated. They differ from the granular appearance of calcified nodes but may be mistaken on a plain film for stones in the renal or biliary tract or in a Meckel's diverticulum. A barium meal or enema reveals the calculi closely related in the tip of the caecum.

INFLAMMATORY CONDITIONS

Acute Appendicitis

Plain films are of considerable value and show gaseous dilatation of the terminal ileum with fluid levels in the erect position. Sometimes the gas-filled caecum is conical in shape due to spasm. These appearances are in no way specific to acute appendicitis and can be caused by any local inflammatory process, e.g. Crohn's disease, salpingitis, etc.

A soft-tissue shadow may also be seen in the right iliac fossa. A linear streak of gas in this soft-tissue shadow due to gas in the appendix indicates gangrene. A careful search should also be made for calculi. In rare instances gas is present under the diaphragm so that a perforation is suspected.

If the infection settles down and the appendix is not removed adhesions may form to adjacent structures, in particular to the ileum or caecum. These may precipitate another acute attack. In such cases on fluoroscopic examination on a barium follow-through the appendix is obviously adherent to the ileum or caecum. In other cases the appendix is kinked and may not fill completely. Occasionally a faecolith may be present causing obstruction.

Appendix Abscess

This is indicated by a soft-tissue shadow in the right iliac fossa or pelvis and it may contain gas with a fluid level. In the absence of gas the deformity caused by an abscess frequently cannot be distinguished from a carcinoma at one examination. Following a short course of antibiotics, however, the soft-tissue shadow and bowel deformity become substantially less obvious.

Calculi may be present. There is also a variable degree of gaseous distension of the jejunum and ileum depending on the acuteness of the infection and degree of obstruction.

A barium meal or enema localises the soft-tissue shadow and there is usually also deformity of the caecum, especially the tip. In the great majority of cases the appendix does not fill with barium. Very occasionally a little barium enters the proximal part of its lumen. If an abscess is present in the pelvis, the pelvic colon and rectum are displaced backwards.

Subacute Appendicitis

This is a most unsatisfactory radiological diagnosis. When the caecum is localised by barium, tenderness over its apex suggests that the appendix is inflamed. Sometimes on a barium follow-through some distortion and irritability of the terminal ileum may be noted.

Crohn's Disease

This is usually the result of spread from the caecum causing some narrowing and deformity of the base of the appendix.

Mucocoele

This is a rare finding and cannot be diagnosed with certainty. Sometimes a soft-tissue shadow is present indenting the caecum or the terminal ileum. Occasionally the wall of a mucocoele becomes calcified and calculi may also be present.

Post-operative Appearances

After appendicectomy or drainage of an appendix abscess some deformity of the apex of the caecum may persist. In other cases the invaginated appendix stump causes a small filling defect.

TUMOURS OF THE APPENDIX

These can rarely be demonstrated radiologically. A carcinoid tumour may be associated with intestinal hurry.

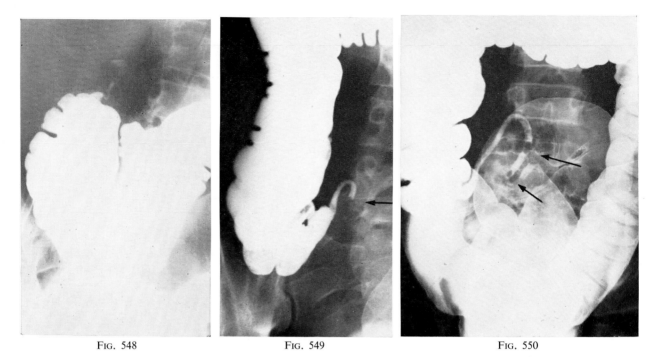

FIG. 548   FIG. 549   FIG. 550

Fig. 548. Subhepatic appendix demonstrated by barium enema. On fluoroscopy the appendix could be mistaken for a carcinoma of hepatic flexure of colon. In doubtful cases the post-evacuation film is very helpful.

Fig. 549. Faecolith (arrowed) in appendix causing obstruction—demonstrated by barium enema. History of pain and some localised tenderness in right iliac fossa. Clinical diagnosis of subacute appendicitis.

Fig. 550. Appendix with faecoliths (arrowed) demonstrated by water contrast barium enema. Incidental finding. The coated loops of pelvic colon do not obscure the appendix.

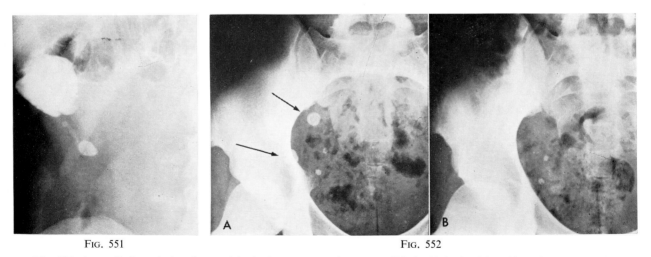

FIG. 551   FIG. 552

Fig. 551. Appendicular calculus diagnosed by barium enema. The caecum (filled with barium) is subhepatic. On the plain film there was some doubt as to the nature of the calcified opacity because of its abnormally high position.

Fig. 552. Acute appendicitis. A: Two large laminated calculi (arrowed). A little ileus of terminal ileum—not so marked as is sometimes seen. B: After appendicectomy. Plain film shows that the calculi have been removed.

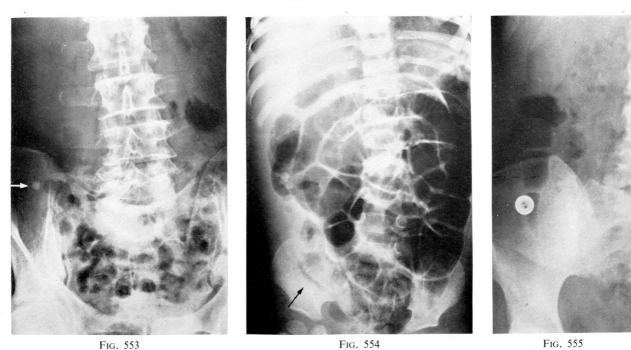

FIG. 553   FIG. 554   FIG. 555

Fig. 553. Acute appendicitis. Some distension of terminal ileum with gas—a common finding. Calculus (arrowed) present in appendix. **Fig. 554.** Acute gangrenous appendicitis. Generalised ileus of small bowel with an inflammatory mass in right iliac fossa. The lumen of the appendix (arrowed) is outlined by gas suggesting that the appendix has become gangrenous. Operative confirmation. **Fig. 555.** Acute appendicitis with an inflammatory mass. Soft-tissue shadow in right iliac fossa displacing and indenting the caecum which is unfortunately partially obscured by a button.

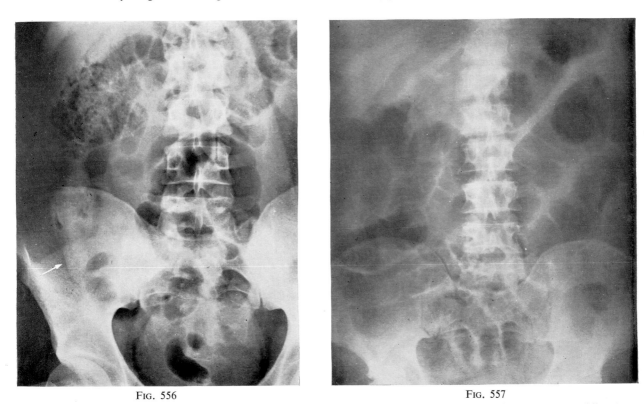

FIG. 556   FIG. 557

Fig. 556. Acute appendicitis. Soft-tissue shadow in right iliac fossa (arrowed). Well marked ileus of a long segment of ileum. **Fig. 557.** Acute appendicitis in a case of situs inversus. Operative confirmation. Plain film shows gaseous distension of ileum which is situated on the right side of the abdomen. Some distension also of the colon which is on the left-side of the abdomen. Typical history and clinical findings of acute appendicitis with the exception of left-sided signs and symptoms.

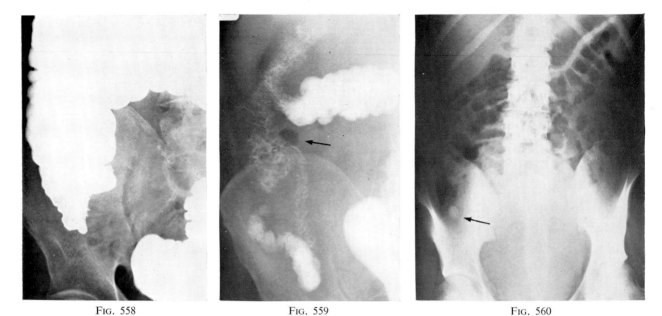

Fig. 558   Fig. 559   Fig. 560

Fig. 558. Chronic appendix abscess causing a large filling defect in caecum suggesting a carcinoma—demonstrated by barium enema. **Fig. 559.** Chronic appendix abscess. Localised collection of gas (arrowed) adjacent to caecum. After evacuation film of barium enema with filling also of the terminal ileum. The gas is obviously outside the bowel lumen. **Fig. 560.** Very large appendix abscess, clinically suggesting an ovarian cyst. Soft-tissue shadow arising out of pelvis and extending upwards towards umbilicus. Calculus (arrowed) in appendix.

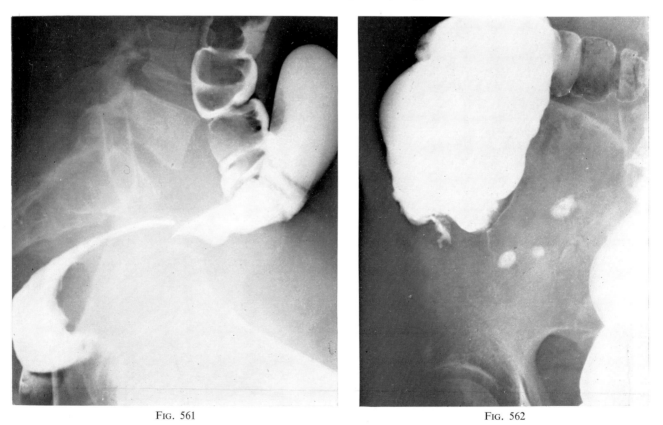

Fig. 561   Fig. 562

Fig. 561. Large appendix abscess in pelvis causing a large soft-tissue shadow. Barium enema shows backwards displacement with compression of pelvic colon. **Fig. 562.** Appendix abscess. Barium enema shows deformity of caecum and the presence of three appendicular calculi. Complaint of several episodes of colicky abdominal pain during the previous year. Clinically a mass was palpable in the right iliac fossa considered to represent a carcinoma.

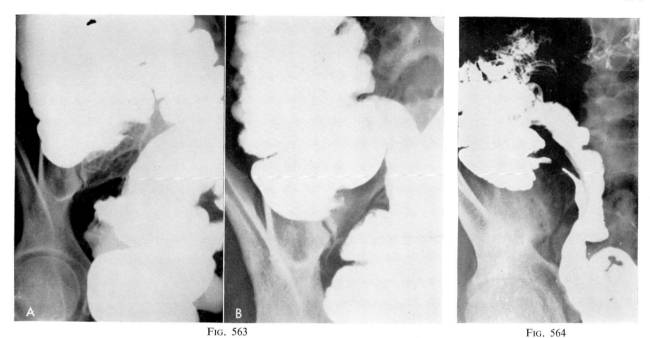

FIG. 563   FIG. 564

Fig. 563. Appendix abscess demonstrated by barium enema. A: Filling defect indenting the caecum. Some irregularity, distortion and displacement of adjacent loop of pelvic colon. Clinically a mass was present in the right iliac fossa. Treatment by antibiotics instituted. B: Three months later the abscess has substantially resolved and only a little irregularity present at the apex of the caecum, and in adjacent loop of pelvic colon. Diminution in distance between caecum and pelvic colon when compared with Fig. A.

Fig. 564. Appendicular adhesions. The appendix is adherent to terminal ileum and could not be separated from it by palpation during fluoroscopy. It is also incompletely filled. No symptoms referable to the appendix. Follow-through of barium meal.

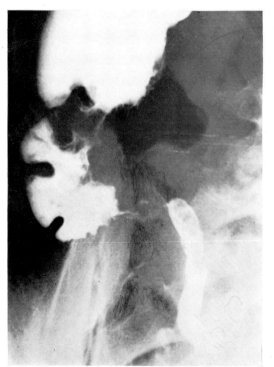

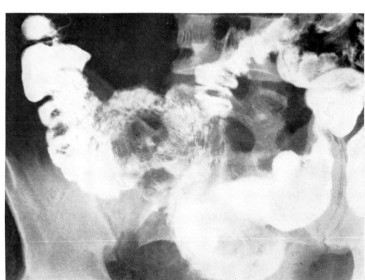

FIG. 566

Fig. 566. Subacute appendicitis with inflammatory mass. Clinical suspicion of Crohn's disease. Complaint of vague ill-health with abdominal pain and fever for a few weeks. Palpable mass in right iliac fossa. Follow-through of barium meal shows some distortion and displacement of terminal ileum, but normal mucosal pattern.

FIG. 565

Fig. 565. Crohn's disease of appendix due to extension from the caecum and ascending colon which show deformity—demonstrated by barium enema. Irregular stricture in the appendix adjacent to the caecum with gross dilatation of the lumen. No filling of terminal ileum.

CHAPTER VII

THE COLON

RADIOLOGICAL METHODS OF INVESTIGATION

Plain Films

These are required particularly in cases of intestinal obstruction, ulcerative colitis and Crohn's disease especially when toxic dilatation of the colon is suspected, perforations, and for the purpose of excluding other disease. Erect and supine films are necessary—the erect film must include the diaphragm. Except in suspected perforations and gall-stone ileus the supine view is of greater value. If the patient cannot sit a lateral decubitus view may be taken. In all cases the films should be obtained before a cleansing enema is given as air may be insufflated into the colon distal to an obstruction, masking its site.

Barium Enema

This is the standard method of examining the colon. Most experienced radiologists have developed a satisfactory method of their own. However, the author's technique is described in detail for the benefit of more junior colleagues and as an aid to the interpretation of many of the subsequent illustrations.

Preparation. A laxative should be taken two days and one day beforehand. On the day of examination a cleansing enema containing a colonic actuator (Veripaque*—one vial containing 3 g. dissolved in 2 litres of water is most satisfactory) should be given three hours before the examination but it may be omitted in outpatients. The laxative and cleansing enema should also be omitted in active ulcerative colitis and in babies and young children.

Technique. The quality of the barium is of supreme importance.

Two parts of warm water to one part of Micropaque suspension and well stirred.

Finger put in barium suspension to see that it is lukewarm.

Two containers lashed together, hung preferably from the ceiling—one for barium, the other for lukewarm water (again tested with the finger).

Plastic Micropaque containers with the bottom cut off and turned upside down are most satisfactory. Equipment shown (Fig. 567).

Controls set with exposure for lateral view of pelvic colon and rectum (100 to 110 kV, 40 to 60 milli-ampere-seconds in an average case).

Patient lies in right lateral position with knees bent up.

Barium run through to see that the system is clear.

Foley catheter (100 ml.) lubricated and introducer inserted into its distal aperture and pulled slightly taut. Satisfactory introducer is part of frame of a stainless-steel developing hanger approximately 9 in. long with the ends rounded.

Catheter introduced into rectum with great care by the radiologist himself. If catheter is felt to slip off introducer, they are both withdrawn and reintroduced. Balloon now carefully inflated.

Barium run into the bowel. Level of barium in container approximately two feet above table top. If flow too slow, examination speeded up by raising the containers a little.

True lateral 12 in. by 10 in. film of pelvic colon centred on pelvi-rectal junction when barium is seen to enter descending colon. Second almost true lateral 12 in. by 10 in. film taken as soon as assistant can change the cassette. Flow of barium stopped and water run in when head of barium is in middle of transverse colon. This is done by changing the clip on the tubing leading from the water container to the tubing from the barium container. Most important that flow of barium or water is never stopped,

---

* Manufactured by The Bayer Products Co., Surbiton upon Thames, England.

otherwise the tube may block. In other cases the colon may prematurely contract and the enema be evacuated.

14 in. by 14 in. film taken of splenic flexure with

This is important as changes in ulcerative colitis are not so obvious during the water contrast phase.

Patient now lies on his back.

14 in. by 14 in. film taken of pelvic colon when it

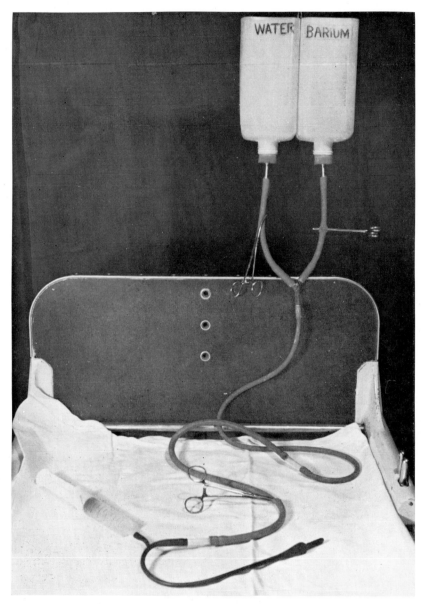

FIG. 567

patient supine and left side raised so that this flexure clearly seen. 80 to 90 kV preferable. This film includes the splenic flexure, descending colon, upper sigmoid colon and part of the transverse colon.

Thus, so far, films of the whole of the distal colon containing barium suspension alone have been taken.

is seen to be less dense. Less penetration, 70 to 80 kV is usual.

Commonly slight hold-up at junction of caecum and ascending colon. In all cases the caecum must be positively identified either by seeing the appendix or observing reflux into the ileum.

N

Flow of water now stopped.

14 in. by 14 in. film taken to include the caecum, ascending colon, hepatic flexure and as much of the rest of the colon as conveniently possible. Film taken with right side raised to open out the hepatic flexure.

Tube disconnected at the glass connection in the middle. Water plus barium run from the patient into a bucket beside the table.

Evacuation aided by placing two hands firmly on the patient's abdomen. These are taken away from time to time to permit fluoroscopy.

Evacuation may occur more readily if the balloon of the Foley catheter is deflated.

Films taken of any area which arouses suspicion at any time during the examination.

14 in. by 14 in. P.A. film taken particularly to show the pelvic colon. Application of compression pad sometimes advisable to displace the ileum from the pelvic colon.

Abdomen carefully palpated with gloved hand under fluoroscopic control.

Catheter deflated and removed and patient goes to the toilet.

Subsequently 17 in. by 14 in. post-evacuation film in prone position. Occasionally fluoroscopy with palpation of colon repeated and further films taken if necessary.

The technique is modified depending upon the nature of the lesion found.

If a complete or almost complete obstruction is encountered, the radiologist should not persist too long in an attempt to overcome it. No harm results except that the patient may prematurely evacuate the enema.

If the patient is frail and the anal sphincter lax, the enema may be given with advantage prone with slight traction applied to the catheter, and with a large pad of cotton-wool between the thighs. When the colon is completely filled, as much of the enema as possible should be run into the bucket in the normal way without deflating the catheter until the patient has turned to lie on his back.

If premature ejection of the catheter occurs, films are taken if possible, the examination discontinued and repeated later if necessary.

In babies and young children, adequate sedation is necessary.

To demonstrate the distal colon in presence of a colostomy, the barium enema should be given per rectum. This is not merely more convenient but safer if an obstruction is present.

For examination of the proximal colon in presence of a colostomy the Foley catheter is inserted into the proximal opening and the balloon inflated carefully. The balloon is kept in place by a pad of cotton-wool pressed over the colostomy by one of the patient's hands.

Gastrografin Enema

In the newborn, Gastrografin diluted with equal parts of warm water is used.

30-ml. Foley catheter introduced into rectum and partially inflated.

Gastrografin is injected using a 50-ml. syringe.

In adults, diluted Gastrografin sometimes used in cases of rectal and lower pelvic colon fistulae, sinuses, and stenoses when examination of distal bowel only is required.

Sometimes diluted Gastrografin run down through distal opening of a colostomy to show sinuses, etc.

Double Contrast Barium Enema (Barium Air Contrast Enema)

Indications

1. When a polyp has been seen on sigmoidoscopy in order to detect the possible presence of others proximally.

2. Doubtful lesions seen on a conventional water contrast enema.

3. When there is clinical suspicion of the presence of a tumour or polyp and the water contrast barium enema is negative.

4. Cases of unexplained haemorrhage.

5. When polypi have been found at operation for resection of a carcinoma.

This is an impressive list but in practice the number of patients requiring a double contrast barium enema is relatively small. In acute ulcerative colitis this examination is contra-indicated because of the danger of perforation.

Preparation

1. Two days' preparation with a laxative.

2. A cleansing enema containing Veripaque is given preferably by a specially trained nurse attached to the X-ray Department.

Following evacuation of cleansing enema intravenous injection of 30 mg. Buscopan to produce
relaxation of colon. Alternatively delay double
contrast examination for one hour.

Equal parts of Micropaque suspension and water
(lukewarm mixture) put into container of Pneumo-
colon device.* Patient supine. Barium run into colon
as far as splenic flexure.

Left side now slightly raised.

Air insufflated under careful fluoroscopic control.
Film taken of pelvic colon when distended with air.

Patient turned on his face and more air insufflated
under fluoroscopic control.

Three 14 in. by 14 in. films taken. One centred on
pelvic colon, one centred on splenic flexure, one
centred on hepatic flexure.

Patient turned on his back. Additional films of
pelvic colon and proximal colon taken.

Thus films of all areas in both supine and prone
positions have been obtained. The areas obscured
by a pool of barium when supine are seen in
double contrast when prone, and vice versa. One
or two vertical films are taken following tilting the
table.

Finally, over couch 17 in. by 14 in. films taken
supine and prone.

Occasionally difficulty is encountered in filling
the caecum, and this is one reason why a conventional barium enema is desirable prior to air
contrast.

Perforations are rare but this examination should
not be carried out in acute ulcerative colitis.

Follow-through of Barium Meal

This is not recommended as a means of radiological investigation of the colon. Some lesions,
e.g. tumours, diverticulitis, etc., can be detected
but it is wise to confirm an abnormality by barium
enema.

Aortography

This is sometimes employed when a vascular lesion
of the colon is suspected. It is of limited value as
stenosis of the superior and inferior mesenteric
arteries and their branches is occasionally seen when
an aortogram is performed for other reasons and in
the absence of bowel signs or symptoms.

CLINICAL RADIOLOGY

NORMAL APPEARANCES

It is not proposed to discuss the normal appearances at length, but the following features are worth
stressing.

Water Contrast Barium Enema

The initial two lateral views or one true lateral
and one slightly oblique are of the greatest value.
Frequently, an area of spasm or a faecal mass may
simulate a carcinoma in one film while its absence
in the other effectively excludes a tumour. Normally,
the pelvic colon and rectum are parallel to the curvature of the sacrum, and the posterior wall is separated
from the sacrum by no more than 2 cm. Any increase
in this distance must be looked upon as significant.
The translucency of the air-filled balloon is clearly
seen in the lateral view.

The margins of the colon are smooth apart from
sharp indentations caused by the haustrations.
Occasionally, in partially contracted segments fine
marginal spiculation is present. This is caused by
contractions of the muscularis mucosae and must
not be mistaken for multiple tiny ulcers. An error
should be avoided as they disappear on distension.

Sometimes the lips of the ileo-caecal valve are
extremely prominent but they are usually more or
less symmetrical. Only rarely is this enlargement of
significance.

Occasionally the colon is indented by the costal
margin or the spine especially in thin individuals.
The cause of the deformity, however, is obvious
especially on palpation during fluoroscopy.

The post-evacuation film is of particular value in
demonstrating tumours of the ascending colon.
Otherwise its main purpose is to confirm a lesion
already suspected.

Double Contrast (Air Contrast)

The main difficulty as in a conventional enema, is
to differentiate residual faecal material from tumours
or polypi and thus the colon should be as clean as
possible. Faeces, however, can usually be displaced
and thus should not be mistaken for polypi even
when pedunculated.

* Manufactured by Barnes-Hind Barium Products, Sunnyvale, California, U.S.A.

Sometimes the descending colon has a dark double contour. This can also be seen on a conventional enema though less clearly and is due to pericolic fat. In the case of a double contrast enema, the radiologist must not be alarmed by the initial impression of a perforation.

TECHNICAL FAULTS AND DIFFICULTIES

If left to an inexperienced assistant the catheter may be inserted in error into the vagina. When this happens it is immediately obvious as a complete obstruction to the flow of barium is soon encountered. The enema should be stopped immediately, the catheter removed and inserted properly into the rectum. Usually no treatment is required and it is remarkable how soon the vagina becomes clear of barium.

Sometimes the end of the catheter doubles back so that the barium runs in initially distal to the balloon. If the patient can retain the enema the balloon ascends into the pelvic colon and a tumour may be erroneously suspected on fluoroscopy. The balloon should be deflated and the catheter re-introduced properly.

If a barium enema is carried out immediately after a sigmoidoscopy with biopsy, bleeding may be provoked causing streaky filling defects in the column of barium. In other cases localised spasm is caused simulating a distal ulcerative procto-colitis. It is permissible to perform a barium enema immediately following a sigmoidoscopy provided no biopsy has been taken and no air insufflated.

CONGENITAL ANOMALIES

The hepatic flexure of the colon sometimes becomes interposed between the liver and the diaphragm and this may be intermittent, especially in children. It must not be mistaken for free gas under the diaphragm indicating a perforation. The interposed loop is usually anterior to the liver but very occasionally it is posterior.

In situs inversus partialis commune mesenterium the colon is usually completely on the left side. The appendix is also on the left side but occasionally the hepatic flexure is in its normal position in the right hypochondrium.

Sometimes the caecum is low down in the pelvis or high up under the costal margin.

In some cases the ileum enters the colon from the lateral aspect.

Sometimes an accessory loop of pelvic colon lies between the lower pelvic colon and the sacrum.

Congenital diverticula which are often large occur usually in the proximal colon and may contain scybala.

A congenital fistula occasionally occurs to the bladder or vagina. In these cases ano-rectal atresia may be present.

Retroposition of the transverse colon is a rare anomaly. In this abnormality, the transverse colon lies below and behind the small bowel which mainly occupies the upper and left half of the abdomen.

DISPLACEMENTS

The colon may be displaced by enlargement or tumours of various abdominal and pelvic organs and the cause is usually obvious. Sometimes a retroverted uterus gives rise to a smooth localised indentation on the anterior wall of the pelvic colon. This returns to normal when the displacement is rectified. A large tumour of the head of the pancreas may displace the right half of the transverse colon downwards—the hepatic flexure remaining in its normal position.

IRRITABLE OR SPASTIC COLON

Plain films are rarely helpful. Occasionally slight excess of gas is present in an obviously narrowed colon.

When examined by barium enema the colon fills rapidly, its outline is smooth and the lumen narrowed especially in the distal colon. The haustrations are less prominent than usual, but there is no shortening and the retro-rectal space is normal. Sometimes regular transverse ridges due to excessive contractions of the circular muscle are seen. Strings of mucus may be present causing long linear translucent filling defects in the filled colon. They may be coated with barium on the post-evacuation film causing long worm-like structures. Commonly there is very little residual barium on the post-evacuation film.

If fluoroscopic examination is carried out when the barium on a follow-through examination is in the colon, a rapid peristaltic rush may be observed. Contractions of the longitudinal muscle behind the bolus of barium then cause a curious spiky or 'picket-fence' outline which must not be mistaken for ulceration.

INFECTIVE AND INFLAMMATORY CONDITIONS

Non-specific Infective Colitis

This term is applied to cases of diarrhoea occurring sporadically and usually with complete recovery in a few days. Commonly the small bowel is also affected so that the term entero-colitis might be more appropriate. Radiological investigation is unnecessary unless symptoms persist or the clinical features are unusual.

Plain films show excessive gas in the colon and sometimes also in the ileum. The calibre of the colon is diminished. Broad transverse ridging, due to contraction of the circular muscle and probably also some mucosal oedema, may be obvious especially in the transverse colon. The colon is not shortened as in ulcerative colitis or Crohn's disease and no pseudo-polypi are seen. In the erect position fluid levels are present particularly in the haustrations of the ascending colon. In the descending colon these fluid levels may be saucer-shaped owing to the less prominent haustrations.

In a few instances when the diagnosis is uncertain, a barium enema is necessary. Usually the colon is irritable and the barium enema is carried out with some difficulty and with discomfort to the patient. The barium may be diluted by excessive fluid contained in the colon. Occasionally there is dilatation of the colon with multiple small filling defects due to semi-liquid faeces.

In cases with a gastro- or entero-colic fistula a form of colitis generally occurs. A barium enema reveals an irritable spastic colon with excess of mucus and with swollen mucosa.

Ulcerative Colitis

Radiology plays a most important part in the investigation of this disease but the pathological changes in the bowel are often more extensive and severe than would appear from a barium enema. Ulcerative colitis usually starts in the distal colon and extends proximally in a continuous manner without intervening normal areas.

Plain Films. In the early stage these are not helpful but when the disease is more advanced there may be excessive gas present and the lumen of the bowel is narrowed with transverse ridging. Commonly, in chronic cases, the proximal colon is considerably dilated and contains large smooth faecal masses with excess of gas.

In severe cases toxic dilatation may occur, especially of the transverse colon—a most serious complication. Usually a large number of pseudo-polypi are present showing as filling defects. A search should be made for gas under the liver or diaphragm to detect a possible perforation. The bowel wall is usually thin but the distance between the stomach and colon may be increased by thickened omentum wrapped round the transverse colon.

Barium Enema. This is the standard method of radiological investigation but, of course, should not be carried out in severely ill patients. Special care should be taken in the insertion of the catheter. The balloon must be inflated slowly and carefully and it may not take the full 100 ml. The lateral views of the pelvic colon are of particular importance.

No abnormality may be detected in an early case even when changes are present on sigmoidoscopy. The earliest radiological signs are narrowing of the distal colon and rectum with obvious spasm on fluoroscopy and with increase in the space between the bowel and sacrum, i.e. more than 2 cm. The colon is also smooth with lack of haustrations. Ulcers may be noted showing as projections beyond the normal contour. They must not be mistaken for the fine, uniform spiculation which is sometimes normally seen in the partially contracted colon and which disappears on distension (p. 195).

As the disease progresses it extends proximally with narrowing, shortening, and obvious ulceration. Sometimes the ulcers are deep and of the collar-stud type so that the colon has a shaggy or double contour. Pseudo-polypi may subsequently develop and these are seen as multiple filling defects. Sometimes multiple small pseudo-polypi cause a cobble-stone appearance simulating Crohn's disease.

In the late chronic stage the colon is shortened and smooth owing to mucosal destruction and with absent haustrations—the hose pipe or inverted 'U' colon. Barium usually floods into the terminal ileum which may show a featureless appearance simulating mucosal destruction. This is because the pre-existing colonic content mixes with the barium which inadequately coats the mucosa of the ileum. These appearances simulate a 'back-wash ileitis'— a mild superficial inflammation which occasionally affects the terminal ileum. A barium follow-through is necessary for precise diagnosis. In cases where the distal colon is considerably narrowed the proximal colon is dilated and smooth and filled with large solid scybala.

Strictures may develop at any point. They may be either fusiform or of string stricture type in which case a carcinoma may be suspected. Stasis is marked so that barium may persist in the colon for weeks or even months. This also happens if barium has been given for a follow-through. Some of the 'strictures' noted at barium enema are not evident at laparotomy and the radiological appearances thus must have been due to spasm.

In chronic ulcerative colitis of many years' duration malignancy not uncommonly develops. It is worth stressing that a tumour may originate in the unaffected part of the colon in non-total colitis. A carcinoma is the commonest type, but a lymphosarcoma may also occur and multiple tumours may be present. Their detection is relatively easy when the colon is smooth and shortened, but sometimes is made difficult by large faecal residues.

In some cases ulcerative colitis is associated with disseminated lupus erythematosus, rheumatoid arthritis, Raynaud's phenomenon or in rare instances sclerosing cholangitis. Only rarely do ulcerative colitis and Crohn's disease co-exist. Ankylosing spondylitis may also occur in ulcerative colitis.

See also section on Small Intestine for differentiating features from Crohn's disease (p. 127).

Crohn's Disease

See section on Small Intestine (p. 127).

Amoebic Colitis

Amoebic colitis is occasionally seen in Britain amongst subjects who have never been abroad. Thus this disease must be borne in mind when an ulcerative form of colitis presents unusual features.

A barium enema is the radiological method of examination of choice.

In the early stage the disease is usually restricted to the caecum and commencement of ascending colon and manifests itself by narrowing, hyper-motility, spasticity and perhaps obvious ulceration. After treatment some contraction usually remains.

In some cases the amoebic infection is localised, i.e. an amoeboma, which may simulate a carcinoma. Multiple amoebomata may be present.

When the colon is extensively involved it is shortened, rigid, shows lack of haustrations and sometimes active ulceration. There may be diffuse mucosal destruction. Strictures may develop sometimes with sacculations. The small bowel is not involved.

The liver should be examined for enlargement due to an amoebic hepatitis. In the acute stage the right dome of diaphragm is elevated and shows impaired movements. There are also some inflammatory changes at the base of the right lung. Subsequently the wall of an abscess may calcify.

Actinomycosis

This disease is rare and generally follows an existing chronic inflammation, e.g. Crohn's disease. The affected area of the colon is grossly deformed with areas of stenosis. Fistulae are common and there may be soft-tissue shadows due to inflammatory masses. Only rarely can a pre-operative diagnosis be made.

Tuberculosis

Ileo-caecal tuberculosis is not now common but cases occur from time to time. The radiological appearances closely simulate Crohn's disease which is the usual initial diagnosis. Tuberculosis, however, tends to be localised to the ileo-caecal region with involvement particularly of the caecum and ascending colon and to a lesser degree the terminal ileum. (See also section on Small Intestine (p. 125).

Swelling or Prominence of the Lips of the Ileo-caecal Valve

Occasionally the lips are very obvious but this is generally of no significance. Rarely a chronic inflammatory fibro-fatty mass arises from one of the lips and may simulate a carcinoma.

X-irradiation Procto-colitis

This most commonly follows radiotherapy for an ovarian or uterine carcinoma. In the acute stage the colon and rectum are narrowed and distorted with swelling of the mucosal folds due to oedema. As the loops may be filled with gas the deformity is sometimes obvious on a plain film. This can be confirmed by barium enema and superficial ulceration may also be seen. The ileum is usually also involved and fistulae may occur especially to the vagina.

Ultimately the mucosa becomes atrophic and in rare cases malignancy develops after an interval of many years.

TUMOURS OF THE COLON

SIMPLE TUMOURS

Adenomatous Polypi

These may be sessile or pedunculated and are commonly multiple, especially in familial cases. An air contrast barium enema is usually necessary for diagnosis. Sometimes the conventional post-evacuation film is helpful, especially if a polyp has partially intussuscepted.

On double contrast barium enema, polypi show as persistent smooth filling defects with a surface coating of barium. Sometimes the stalk is similarly coated. In all cases a search must be made for a carcinoma.

Diverticula seen *en face* are differentiated only with difficulty. Oblique views are of great help as the diverticula are then seen in profile extending beyond the lumen of the bowel. In addition, some distortion of the bowel is usually present. If enough barium is in the colon erect films are diagnostic as diverticula contain fluid levels.

Villous Papillomata

These are less common and are usually found in the pelvic colon or rectum. They tend to be large, bulky, fungating tumours and are readily detected by a barium enema.

MALIGNANT TUMOURS

An adenocarcinoma is by far the commonest malignant tumour, but lymphosarcomata and other forms of reticulosis and secondary tumours also occur.

Plain films are of limited value and are usually taken when a patient presents with obstruction. In such cases the bowel proximally is dilated and the tumour may be identified if it indents the gas-filled lumen.

Perforation may occur and it may cause either a generalised peritonitis or a localised abscess.

Only rarely is a malignant tumour calcified.

A follow-through of a barium meal is, of course, contra-indicated because of the danger of precipitating a complete obstruction. In rare cases when atony has supervened, barium if given by mouth becomes evenly dispersed throughout the small and proximal part of the large bowel and may persist for weeks.

A barium enema is the standard method of radiological investigation.

The tumour may cause a stricture either of the string or napkin-ring type, or an irregular filling defect if of the fungating type. Sometimes mucosal destruction with a flat featureless appearance may be seen if superficial ulceration is the predominant macroscopic feature. Occasionally, a diffuse superficial carcinoma may extend over a considerable length of bowel and closely resemble ulcerative colitis. The post-evacuation film is of limited value except in tumours of the ascending colon or when a tumour has intussuscepted.

A double contrast enema is usually necessary to detect small tumours and/or polypi.

DIFFERENTIAL DIAGNOSIS

1. Diverticular disease. The colon is more extensively involved even in the initial stages. Diverticula are present by the time there is any doubt and in the late stage there is distortion with a zig-zag appearance, i.e. when a true diverticulitis is present. The point of greatest narrowing is usually in the middle of the affected segment. In some cases the obstruction caused by a carcinoma of the pelvic colon predisposes to the development of diverticular disease proximally. In these cases the area of greatest narrowing is at the distal end of the abnormal segment and when this is seen, the suspicion of malignancy should always be aroused.

2. Lymphosarcoma and other forms of reticulosis tend to be bulkier than carcinomata and have a greater tendency to perforate.

3. Endometriosis is uncommon. It may cause displacement and infiltration of the pelvic colon. The diagnosis is usually easy because of a previous history of endometriosis.

4. Strictures in the late stages of ulcerative colitis and Crohn's disease. In some cases differentiation from malignant strictures is impossible.

5. Tuberculosis only rarely causes difficulty in the caecum and ascending colon.

6. Deformity of the tip of the caecum following invagination of the appendix stump gradually diminishes but may not entirely disappear.

7. An appendix abscess causes a soft-tissue shadow which may indent the caecum. The shadow may contain a loculation of gas with a fluid level in the erect position. There is usually also distortion of the terminal ileum and pelvic colon. A careful search should be made for an appendix calculus.

8. Obstruction of ascending colon by a congenital band causing a narrow string-like stricture.

9. Intussusception. In most cases in an adult there is an underlying polyp or carcinoma.

10. Faeces in the colon causing filling defects. They are usually multiple, and obviously move when different films are compared. In doubtful cases a repeat barium enema following further preparation should be performed.

11. Adhesions from operations.

12. Ischaemic colitis. The splenic flexure of the colon is most commonly affected and a considerable segment of bowel is usually involved. Sometimes in the subacute stage, differentiation from a carcinoma by barium enema is impossible as a complete obstruction may be encountered.

13. Post-X-irradiation colitis. The stricture is over a considerable segment and usually involves the pelvic colon and rectum.

14. Torsion of an appendix epiploica causes a string stricture with a typical 'signet ring' appearance.

15. Physiological 'sphincters'. During the filling stage of a barium enema temporary hold up may occur at certain points (physiological 'sphincters')—the most common being at the junction of the caecum and ascending colon. No confusion should occur as the spasm disappears with further filling. These appearances are only rarely seen in the distal colon if the technique of continuous flow of water or barium is adopted.

After resection of a tumour a stricture may develop at the anastomosis. When simple, that is, due to fibrosis, it is usually smooth with clear-cut margins but occasionally a chronic inflammatory mass causes a filling defect at the suture line. A malignant recurrence usually causes an irregular stricture or a local filling defect.

VASCULAR OCCLUSION

Ischaemia of the colon, especially of the distal half, is becoming increasingly recognised as a cause of an acute obstruction or rectal bleeding. The most common site is the splenic flexure and if an inflammatory lesion or ulcerative form of colitis is localised to this region, ischaemia is the most likely cause.

In acute severe cases the patient is seriously ill with pain, shock and bloody diarrhoea. Plain films show a soft-tissue shadow due to the affected part of the colon being filled with fluid and containing only traces of gas. The bowel proximally however is distended with gas.

Gangrene may supervene and streaks of gas may be noted in the bowel wall. Gas may subsequently be present in the portal vein and its tributaries in the liver, extending out almost to the periphery.

In other cases especially in the distal colon the appearances clinically resemble a mechanical obstruction and a barium enema is requested. A filling defect causing obstruction is encountered and the erroneous diagnosis of a carcinoma may be made.

In acute cases of less severity a soft-tissue swelling is present around the affected area. The lumen is narrowed and outlined by gas. Transverse ridging, possibly due to oedema but more probably to spasm of the circular muscle, is present. There may be obvious thumb-printing due to local oedematous swellings. At this stage a barium enema is contra-indicated. After ten days or so, provided there has been sufficient improvement, the diagnosis should be confirmed by barium enema. The changes noted on the plain film are more obvious—transverse ridging, thumb-printing, narrowing of the lumen and soft-tissue swelling. Ulcers are sometimes also noted.

Subsequently, depending upon the severity of the ischaemia, the bowel may return to normal or strictures especially of the fusiform type may develop sometimes with sacculations. In some instances the disease resembles a localised Crohn's disease or ulcerative colitis.

ADYNAMIC ILEUS

This has been described in the section on the Small Intestine (p. 131).

An adynamic ileus particularly affecting the colon is sometimes seen following the use of tranquillisers.

DIVERTICULAR DISEASE

It is now realised that the underlying pathology is generally but not always thickening of the circular muscle with the subsequent development of diverticula. Infection commonly supervenes and the term diverticulitis is then appropriate. The infection may extend beyond the bowel wall causing peri-diverticulitis. The pelvic colon is usually initially involved and the disease tends to spread proximally even as far as the ascending colon.

Radiological Appearances

On plain films of the abdomen, diverticula filled with gas or opaque material, e.g. bismuth or barium, are occasionally seen. If obstruction supervenes, the colon proximally is dilated with fluid levels in the erect position.

A barium enema is the standard method of examination, but commonly the disease can be well recognised on a follow-through of a barium meal. However, detail in the latter is not sufficient to exclude a carcinoma.

In the early stage the affected segment is hypermotile, narrowed and spastic, and filling of the colon may be achieved only with difficulty. Transverse ridging is present with a regular 'saw-tooth' or ripple border. At the summit of a 'saw-tooth' a diverticulum subsequently develops and thus initially the diverticula are extremely regular in disposition. A barium enema usually causes only a proportion of the diverticula to fill with barium, whereas more are filled on a follow-through. Sometimes a diverticulum presents a flask-like appearance when it contains a faecal mass coated on its surface with barium.

Ultimately if fibrosis occurs, indicating diverticulitis, the affected part of the bowel becomes distorted and narrowed with a zig-zag appearance. A peri-colic abscess may occur and may rupture into the ileum or bladder causing a fistula. Gas in the bladder on a plain film or barium following a barium enema indicates a fistula. These are inconstant findings and to demonstrate a fistula it may be necessary to insufflate air into the rectum at sigmoidoscopy and thereby cause some to enter the bladder.

Elongation of the necks of the diverticula has been stated to indicate diverticulitis. In some cases infection has the opposite effect and the diverticula become engulfed in a fibrous reaction.

Intense spasm sometimes occurs during the barium enema resulting in complete obstruction and a precise diagnosis cannot thus be made. The enema should be repeated with prior injection of 30 mg. Buscopan intravenously to relieve the spasm. Usually the colon can then be filled and the diagnosis established.

On a double contrast examination diverticula *en face* can look like polypi. In some cases the regular linear distribution of diverticula makes the diagnosis obvious. Oblique or erect views are valuable as previously mentioned (p. 199).

In the presence of diverticular disease, if the point of greatest narrowing is at the extreme distal end, an underlying carcinoma or a distal ulcerative colitis is likely.

HIRSCHSPRUNG'S DISEASE

The characteristic radiological appearance in babies as depicted by barium enema is a localised narrowing in the pelvic colon or rectum. Proximal to this the colon is dilated, often markedly so with a large faecal residue. Occasionally most of the colon is narrowed causing one form of micro-colon.

IDIOPATHIC MEGACOLON

In this condition the colon and rectum are dilated and atonic—the dilatation usually extending down to the anus. On plain films and barium enema the colon contains large faecal residues.

In some cases only the pelvic colon and rectum are affected, occasionally to a gross degree. There may be a sharp demarcation between the normal and abnormal bowel or the one may gradually merge into the other. The bladder is generally atonic and dilated.

DIFFUSE SYSTEMIC SCLEROSIS

When the colon is affected the diagnosis has frequently been established by characteristic features elsewhere. Strictures and sacculations are the predominant features.

PNEUMATOSIS CYSTOIDES INTESTINALIS

This disease is more common than was at one time thought and there is no doubt that in the past some cases were mistaken for ulcerative colitis. It is frequently associated with obstructive airways disease. The splenic flexure is usually affected but the disease may extend proximally and distally.

Plain films can be diagnostic. The gas-filled cysts with absence of fluid may be seen following the line of the colon. Sometimes streaks of gas are noted in the wall of the colon following rupture of a cyst. A barium enema shows that the colon is narrowed and distorted with thumb-printing due to the gas-filled cysts, which vary in size from a pea to a tennis ball. Strings of mucus are generally present. The enema is usually performed with great difficulty due to marked irritability and spasticity of the colon.

TRAUMA

The pelvic colon or rectum may be damaged by foreign bodies or by procedures such as enemata or the removal of polypi. If the tear is below the peritoneal reflection, gas is generally present in the retroperitoneal tissues—if above, a pneumoperitoneum results.

ABNORMALITIES OF THE APPENDICES EPIPLOICAE

Calcification may occur presumably due to degeneration or torsion. As the hepatic flexure is a common site they look remarkably like gall-stones or stones in the renal tract and are usually considered as such until excluded by further investigation of the appropriate system. The calcified appendix may become detached and gravitate into the pelvis where it simulates a bladder or ureteric stone on a plain film.

Sometimes an appendix epiploica undergoes torsion causing an acute or subacute obstruction. On barium enema this causes a string or annular type of stricture with a filling defect at one side—the 'signet-ring' appearance.

OBSTRUCTION

Plain erect and supine films show a variable degree of distension with fluid levels in the erect position.

When air and fluid are trapped in haustrations the fluid levels are small especially in the ascending colon. It must be remembered that a cleansing enema should not be given before the radiological investigation as air and fluid are inevitably retained causing confusion as to the site of the obstruction.

In the supine position in cases where there is a large amount of fluid and relatively little gas, an initial impression of minimal distension may be formed. This is because the gas floats on the fluid and does not extend across the entire width of the bowel.

Caecal distension can be a serious complication. When perforation occurs there is usually a very large amount of gas in the peritoneal cavity together with filling defects due to faeces.

Except in acute emergencies, e.g. suspected perforations, toxic dilatation of the colon, a barium enema is safe and is the standard radiological procedure.

There are many causes of obstruction, in particular carcinoma, diverticular disease, distal ulcerative procto-colitis, but only the following need further elaboration.

A congenital band occasionally compresses the ascending colon immediately proximal to the hepatic flexure. It is usually mistaken for a carcinoma.

Malignant infiltration of the mesentery sometimes causes narrowing over a length of colon—presumably due to interference with its blood supply.

Adhesions sometimes cause obstruction in the colon but less frequently than in the small bowel. Obvious matting together or peaking may be seen.

Scybala are usually secondary to obstruction of the distal colon but sometimes to chronic constipation alone. They are particularly common in chronic ulcerative colitis and Crohn's disease.

Occasionally a solid faecal mass forms in the caecum or in a large congenital diverticulum of the proximal colon. It may progress distally and if of considerable size may obstruct the descending or pelvic colon. If it has been present for some time it may show fine concentric rings of calcification.

A volvulus of the sigmoid colon, less commonly of the caecum, sometimes occurs. In the case of the sigmoid colon its presence is suspected on the plain film by gaseous distension of the affected part with approximation and tapering of the extremities. If the volvulus is subacute or chronic the distension may be gross and the sigmoid colon may almost fill the abdomen.

On barium enema examination the approximation, narrowing and tapering of the ends of the volvulus are even more obvious and sometimes a definite twist of the bowel is seen. Occasionally a subacute or chronic volvulus can be undone by a barium enema.

A meconium plug in the newborn is a common cause of colonic obstruction. A Gastrografin enema provides the diagnosis showing a long smooth worm-like filling defect in the colon. The plug is usually passed during evacuation of the Gastrografin with relief of the obstruction.

Intussusception occurs both in babies and in adults but the underlying pathology is different.

In babies the predisposing cause is mobility of the ileo-caecal region, in some cases without any intrinsic abnormality, in others associated with a local inflammatory condition of the bowel. A barium enema is helpful in diagnosis and treatment. Sometimes pre-existing faecal material in the distal colon driven ahead of the barium reduces the intussusception and the bowel thus appears normal. A gentle attempt should be made to reduce the intussusception but undue pressure or persistence must never be used.

The radiological appearances are characteristic. The entering loop (intussusceptum) causes an elongated filling defect with curvilinear streaking due to a coating by barium. The receiving loop (intussuscipiens) is usually wider than the normal colon.

In the adult the predisposing cause is usually a tumour or polyp but occasionally a Meckel's diverticulum. The appearances are similar to those found in babies but it is not usually possible to reduce the intussusception.

The underlying cause of an intussusception cannot usually be determined by radiological means.

OEDEMA

Oedema of the bowel may be due to lymphatic obstruction from malignant glands but sometimes results from portal hypertension. A barium enema shows the colon, especially the distal colon, to be narrowed with an extremely coarse mucosal pattern and transverse ridging. A large ascites is usually present.

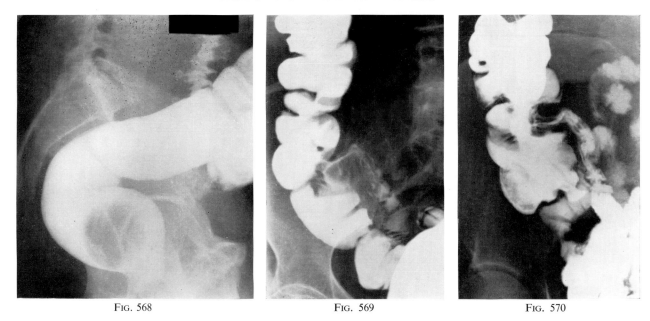

FIG. 568   FIG. 569   FIG. 570

Fig. 568. Normal pelvic colon and rectum following the curve of the sacrum and separated from the latter by only a short distance. The translucency above the anus is the balloon of the Foley catheter. Diverticular disease of the descending colon.

Fig. 569. Ileo-caecal valve seen in profile. It is larger than usual but is within normal limits. Normal filling of terminal ileum.

Fig. 570. Normal ileo-caecal valve seen in profile. Characteristic smooth outline. Normal filling of terminal ileum.

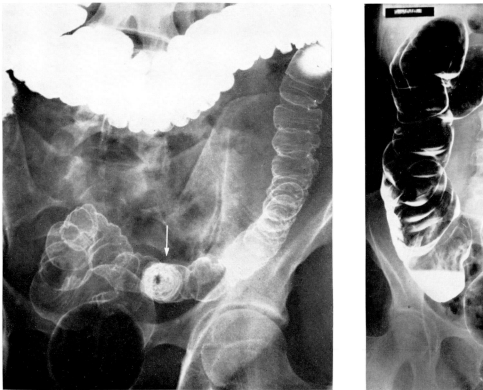
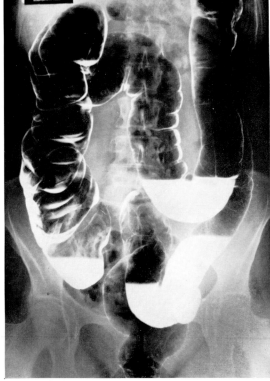

FIG. 571   FIG. 572

Fig. 571. Normal water contrast barium enema. A loop of upper pelvic colon (arrowed) is seen *en face*, giving an 'onion layer' appearance with concentric circles.

Fig. 572. Normal double contrast barium enema. Erect film.

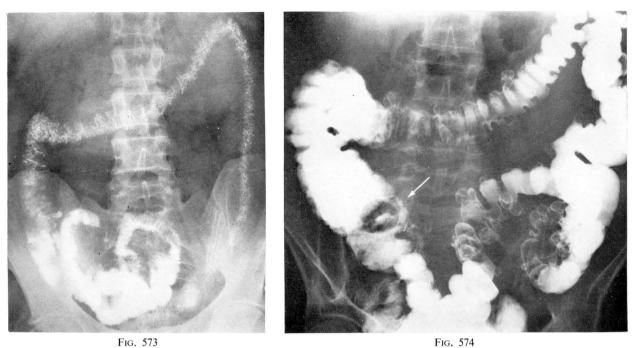

Fig. 573   Fig. 574

Fig. 573. Normal post-evacuation barium enema film showing characteristic feathery mucosal pattern. It is not common to obtain such a good pattern using the water contrast technique. Considerable filling of terminal ileum—the usual finding.

Fig. 574. Normal ileo-caecal valve (arrowed) seen *en face* demonstrated by barium enema. The lips of the valve cause an obvious filling defect, but cause no obstruction as there is filling of the ileum. Extensive diverticular disease in the colon, especially the sigmoid colon.

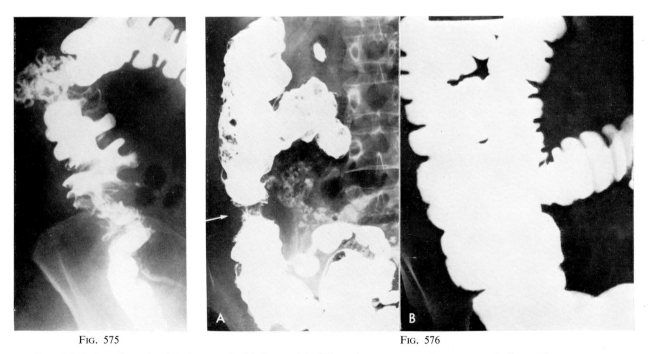

Fig. 575   Fig. 576

Fig. 575. Follow-through of barium meal with incomplete filling of caecum—a not uncommon finding. The caecum was normal when examined by barium enema. A suspected abnormality on a follow-through must be confirmed by barium enema.

Fig. 576. Physiological 'sphincter' in ascending colon. A: Five-hour barium follow-through film. The sphincter (arrowed) cannot be distinguished with certainty from a carcinoma. B: Barium enema shows this area to be normal.

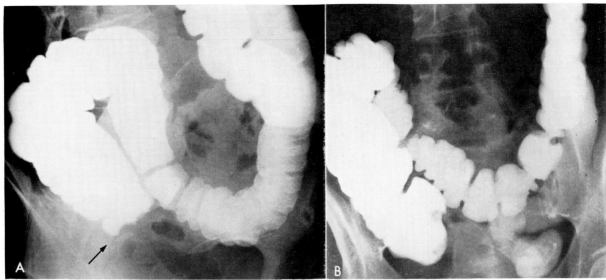

FIG. 577

Fig. 577. Physiological sphincter in ascending colon opposite ileo-caecal valve causing temporary obstruction during a barium enema. A: Obstruction (arrowed) initially simulating a carcinoma. B: With continuing flow of barium, the caecum is filled and no abnormality detected. To be certain that the caecum has filled either the terminal ileum or the appendix should, if possible, be outlined. In all cases the right iliac fossa must be carefully palpated.

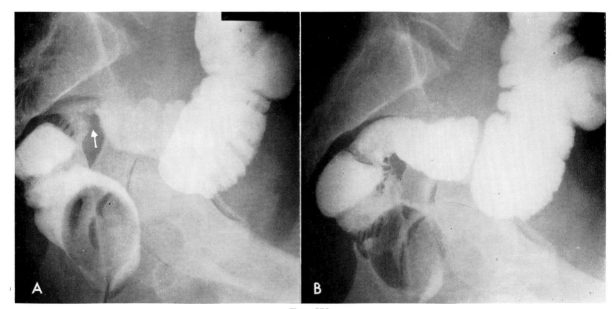

FIG. 578

Fig. 578. Barium enema showing value of two lateral views of pelvic colon. A: First film. Abnormality (arrowed) near pelvi-rectal junction due to spasm and faeces, but a carcinoma cannot be excluded. B: Half a minute later. Most of the faecal material has been driven onwards by the continuous flow of barium. The filling defect is not now seen.

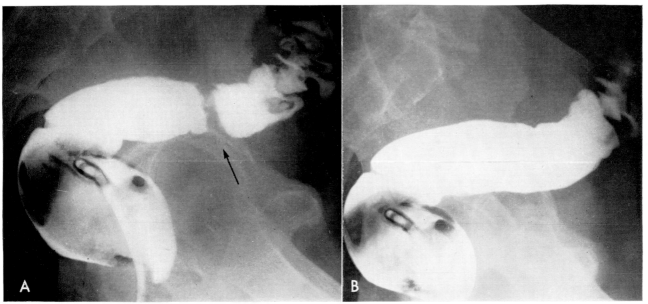

FIG. 579

Fig. 579. Barium enema showing value of two lateral views of pelvic colon. A: Localised narrowing (arrowed) presumably a physiological sphincter in pelvic colon. A 'string' stricture type of carcinoma cannot be excluded. B: Second film half a minute later and with continuous flow of barium. The narrowing is no longer seen and was thus due to localised spasm. Diverticular disease at a higher level.

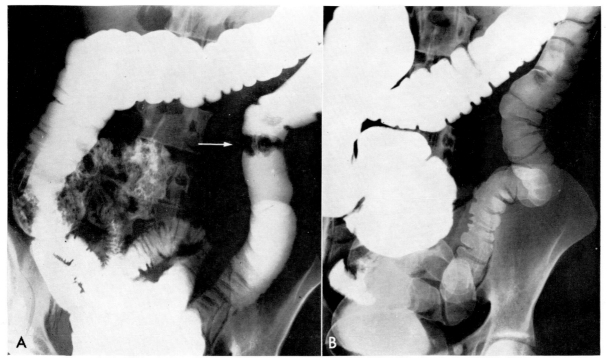

FIG. 580

Fig. 580. Physiological sphincter in descending colon. A: The narrowed area (arrowed) simulates a napkin-ring type of carcinoma. B: Normal appearance of descending colon with continuous flow of barium during filling.

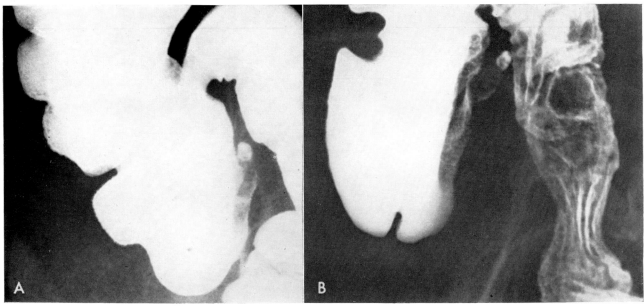

FIG. 581

Fig. 581. Normal colon.   A: Fine uniform spiculation due to contractions of the muscularis mucosae especially affecting lateral wall of caecum and ascending colon.   B: Film with compression.   The spiculation is now absent.   Note normal mucosal pattern of terminal ileum disposed in longitudinal folds at the site of a peristaltic wave.   Smooth filling defect due to intestinal content.

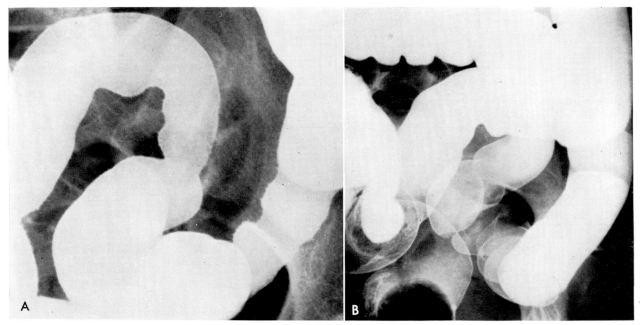

FIG. 582

Fig. 582. Normal sigmoid colon.   A: Fine spiculation due to contractions of the muscularis mucosae.   Because of the regularity and uniformity, ulceration should not erroneously be diagnosed (magnified print).   B: With further distension the contractions have disappeared and the colon now has a smooth outline.

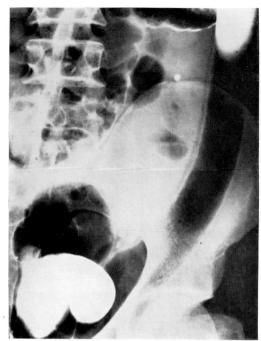

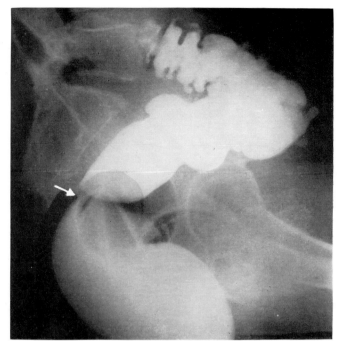

FIG. 583

FIG. 584

Fig. 583. Double contour of descending colon due to peri-colic fat. Air contrast barium enema. At first sight a perforation might be suspected. A double contour can also be seen on a conventional enema, though not so clearly. **Fig. 584.** Technical fault on barium enema using a Foley catheter. The catheter has doubled back on itself so that the balloon (arrowed) causes an obstruction and the rectum distal to the balloon fills initially. This fault should be noted during fluoroscopy as the balloon being filled with air is clearly seen at an abnormally high level. As soon as this is noted the balloon should be deflated and the catheter re-introduced. Diverticular disease higher up in the pelvic colon.

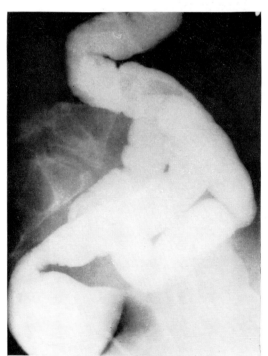

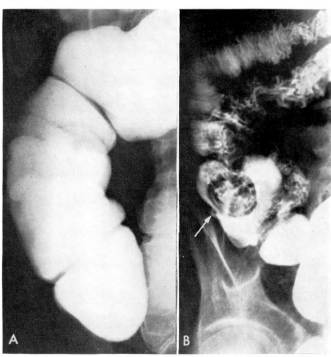

FIG. 585

FIG. 586

Fig. 585. Spasm at pelvi-rectal junction due to recent sigmoidoscopy and biopsy (of a polyp) simulating a localised proctitis. If a sigmoidoscopy is carried out immediately before a barium enema, no biopsy should be performed and no air insufflated. **Fig. 586.** Films of technical interest to show how an obvious structure—normal or abnormal—can be masked in the filled ascending colon. A: Filled caecum and ascending colon. B: After most of the barium has been evacuated the lips of the ileo-caecal valve (arrowed) are revealed. The lips are more prominent than usual but are still within normal limits. Normal filling of the terminal ileum.

O

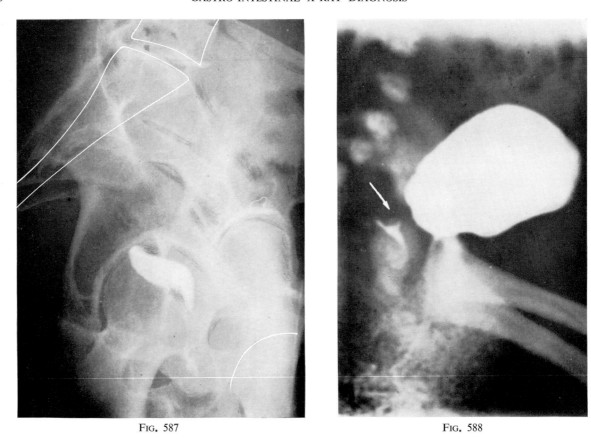

Fig. 587   Fig. 588

Fig. 587. Technical fault during barium enema.   The tube inadvertently had been inserted into the vagina.   The barium is obviously too far forwards and an obstruction (the cervix uteri) has been encountered.   If the fault is not appreciated an erroneous diagnosis of carcinoma of the rectum may be made.   **Fig. 588.** Congenital recto-vesical fistula demonstrated by a cystogram.   Trace of medium in rectum with narrow fistulous tract (arrowed).

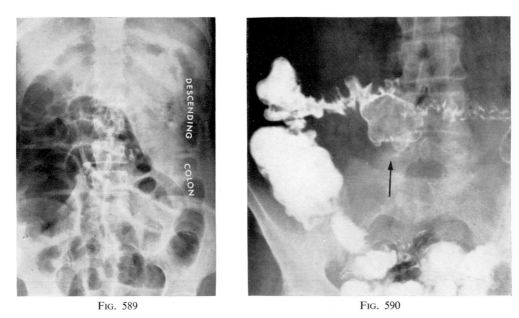

Fig. 589   Fig. 590

Fig. 589. Plain film (supine) of abdomen in a case of obstruction at splenic flexure by a carcinoma.   A cleansing enema had inadvertently been given prior to the X-ray examination causing insufflation of gas into the distal colon and masking the site of the obstruction.   **Fig. 590.** Large congenital diverticulum of transverse colon (arrowed) containing a faecolith.

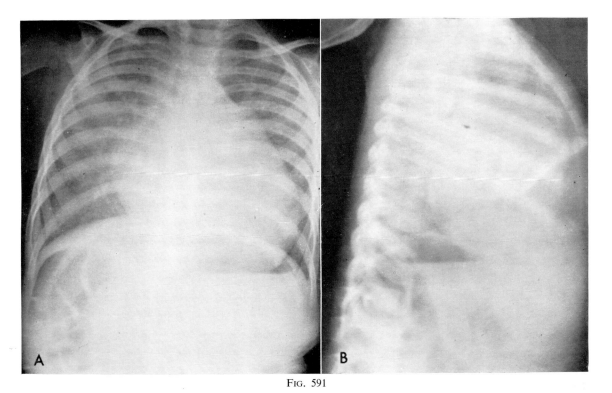

Fig. 591

Fig. 591. Interposed colon—the hepatic flexure being posterior to the liver—less common than anterior. Incidental finding in a case of congenital heart disease. A: P.A. view. B: Lateral view. The air fluid level, superimposed on the colon, is the gastric air bubble.

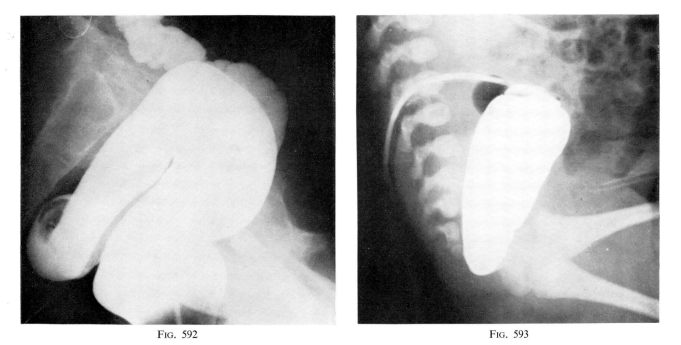

Fig. 592   Fig. 593

Fig. 592. Accessory loop of pelvic colon lying posteriorly. Incidental finding and of no significance.

Fig. 593. Anal atresia. Dilute Gastrografin instilled down distal loop of a colostomy demonstrating complete obstruction at anus.

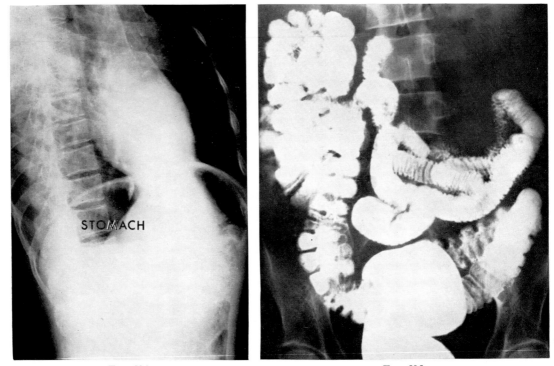

FIG. 594   FIG. 595

Fig. 594. Interposed colon—the hepatic flexure being in front of the liver—the common position.

Fig. 595. Retro-position of the transverse colon which lies below and behind the small bowel—a very rare congenital anomaly.   Incidental finding on a barium enema.

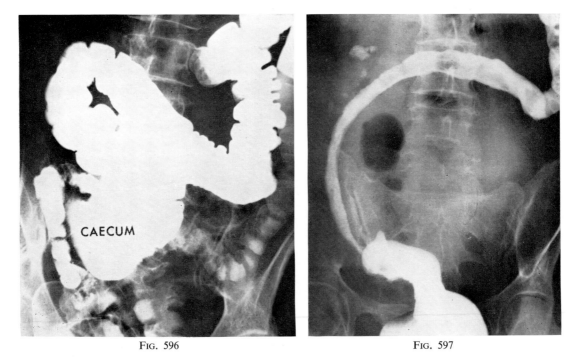

FIG. 596   FIG. 597

Fig. 596. The terminal ileum entering the colon on its lateral aspect—an unusual congenital anomaly.

Fig. 597. Displacement and stretching of pelvic colon by a large ovarian cyst.   The cyst is more or less in the midline and obviously arises from the pelvis.   The bowel wall is smooth and not infiltrated.

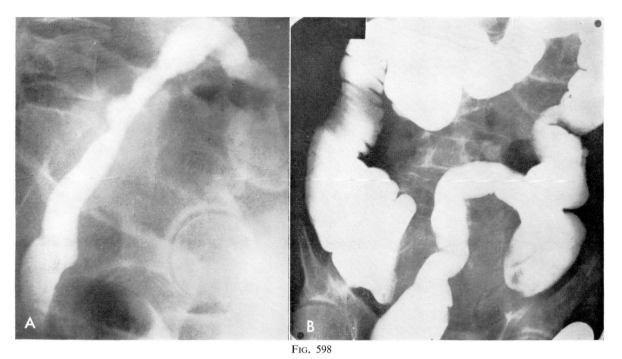

FIG. 598

Fig. 598. Displacement of colon and rectum by an enormously distended bladder. A: Lateral view. The pelvic colon and rectum are compressed and displaced backwards. B: Postero-anterior view. Smooth indentation on caecum. Impression of flattening of pelvic colon by the soft-tissue shadow of the bladder.

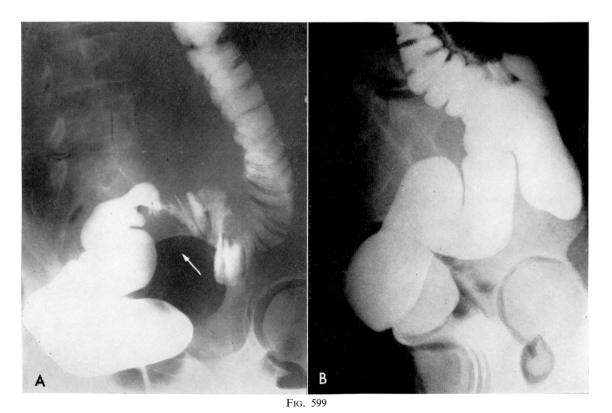

FIG. 599

Fig. 599. Displacement of pelvic colon by a retroverted uterus. A: Typical smooth indentation of anterior wall (arrowed) B: Normal appearances after the retroversion has been corrected.

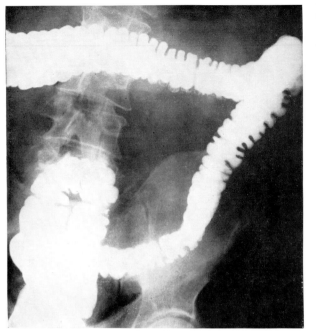

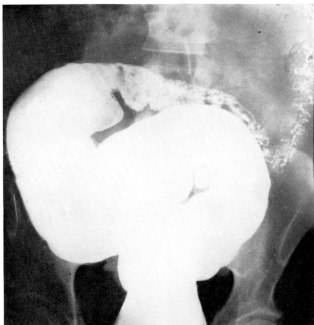

FIG. 600   FIG. 601

Fig. 600. Unusually severe irritable spastic colon. The barium flowed with great rapidity to the caecum. The colon shows multiple deep haustration-like contractions and has a more or less uniform calibre. Nervous introspective individual. Very little barium remained in the colon on the post-evacuation film.

Fig. 601. Post-dysenteric colonic irritability and spasticity. During the course of the barium enema the descending and upper pelvic colon went into a most marked spasm resulting in evacuation of the enema and inability to complete the examination.

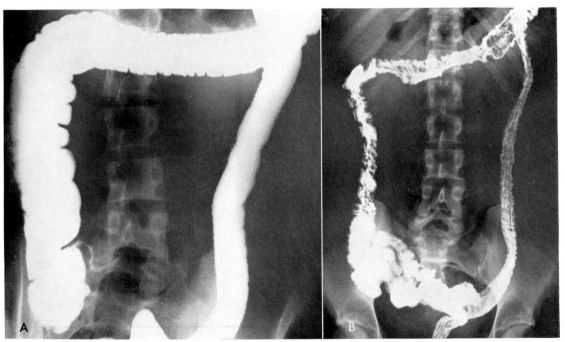

FIG. 602

Fig. 602. Spastic colon. Extremely nervous, introspective woman complaining of attacks of diarrhoea. A: Uniform narrowing with relative absence of normal haustrations and smooth outline. The colon filled extremely quickly. B: Post-evacuation film. The distal colon shows a coarse mucosal pattern due to oedema. No clinical or sigmoidoscopic evidence of ulcerative colitis.

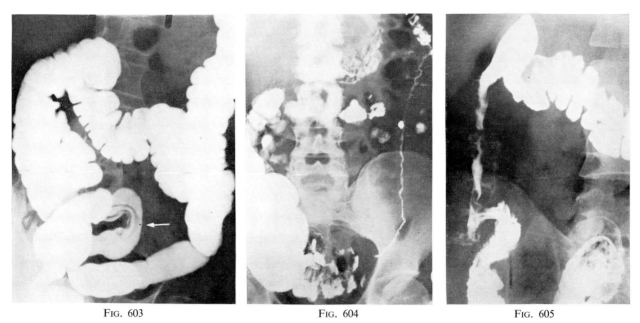

FIG. 603   FIG. 604   FIG. 605

Fig. 603. String of mucus (arrowed) in pelvic colon causing a linear filling defect. Irritable spastic colon. **Fig. 604.** Long string of mucus coated with barium in the descending colon causing a worm-like appearance. Follow-through of barium meal. **Fig. 605.** Right-sided granulomatous colitis (probably of the Crohn type). The caecum, ascending colon and hepatic flexure are affected with irregularity, shortening and mucosal destruction. Follow-through of barium meal. Pathological examination of resected specimen showed superficial malignant change.

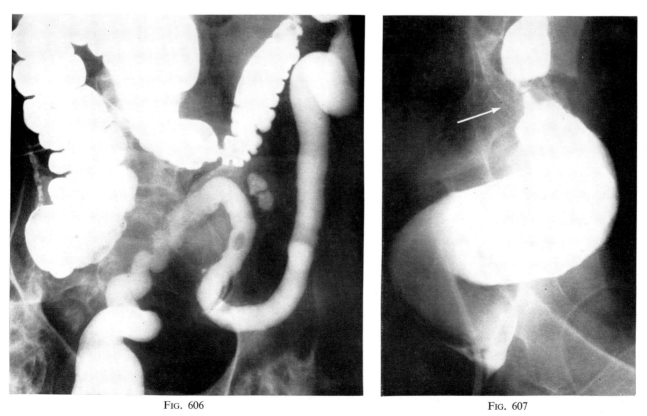

FIG. 606   FIG. 607

Fig. 606. Irritable and spastic colon. Clinical diagnosis of diverticular disease. The distal colon is smooth and narrowed, but no evidence of shortening ulceration or diverticular disease. The appendix contains faecoliths and is situated behind and lateral to the caecum and ascending colon—an incidental finding. **Fig. 607.** Stricture of sigmoid colon (arrowed) due to Crohn's disease—indistinguishable from a scirrhous carcinoma.

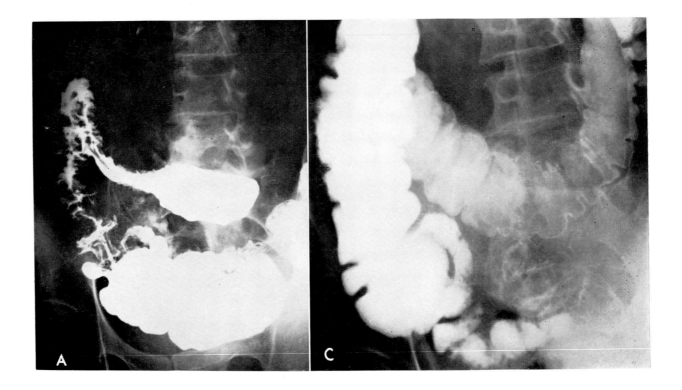

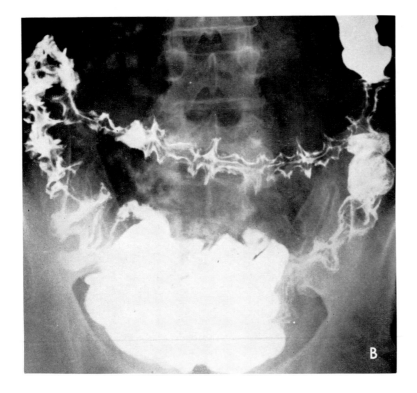

Fig. 608. Irritable spastic colon. A: Follow-through of barium meal after three hours. Marked spasticity of proximal colon. On fluoroscopy a rapid peristaltic rush was noted in the transverse colon at the moment the film was taken. B: A few seconds later, the head of this bolus of barium had reached the splenic flexure. Curious spikiness of the transverse colon due to excessive contraction of the longitudinal muscle causing a concertina-like or picket-fence appearance. This must not be mistaken for ulceration. C: Barium enema reveals a structurally normal colon.

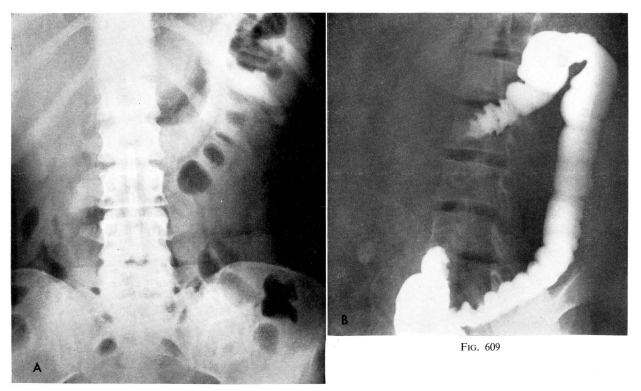

Fig. 609

Fig. 609. Acute infective colitis. Patient severely ill for five weeks with diarrhoea and some blood in the stool. A: Plain film of abdomen showing gas with some narrowing of the lumen and obvious contractions of the circular muscle particularly of left half of transverse colon producing pseudo-haustrations. B: Barium enema. Extreme irritability of the colon. The proximal colon went into marked spasm during the course of the enema and filling could not be completed.

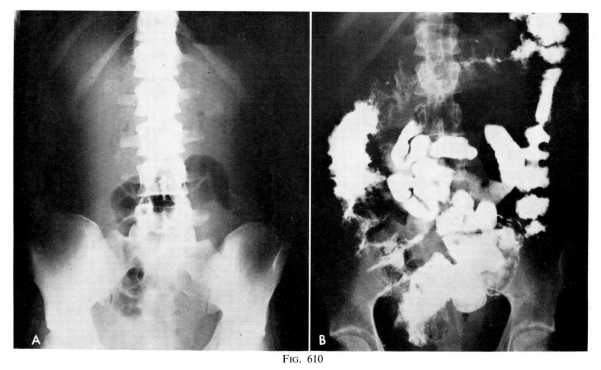

Fig. 610

Fig. 610. Acute non-specific entero-colitis. Complaint of abdominal pain with profuse watery diarrhoea for a few days. Some tenderness in lower abdomen. A: Plain film shows distended loops of ileum. Very little gas in the colon because of marked irritability and spasticity. B: Follow-through of barium meal four days later. Marked irritability and spasticity of terminal ileum, the proximal half of the ascending colon and the transverse colon. The radiological diagnosis was some form of acute entero-colitis—Crohn's disease being a possibility. The condition however settled down satisfactorily within two weeks and the patient has remained well.

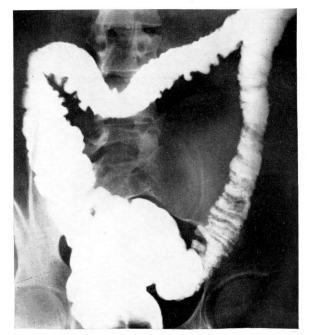

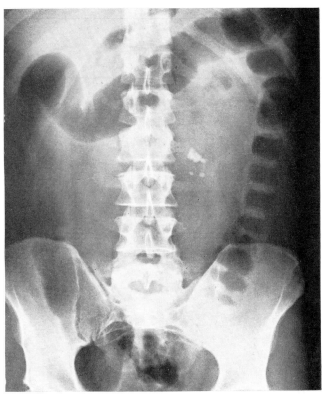

FIG. 611

FIG. 612

Fig. 611. Ulcerative form of colitis still unclassified. The colon is shortened with lack of haustrations. Sacculations present in ascending and transverse colon. Treated first of all as possibly tuberculous owing to Mantoux test $+++$ but without effect. Still undecided whether this is Crohn's disease or ulcerative colitis clinically and following rectal biopsy. **Fig. 612.** Mild chronic ulcerative colitis for five years. The proximal colon is outlined by gas and is smooth with lack of haustrations. Transverse ridging in distal colon due to spasm of circular muscle. The thickness of the ridges distinguishes them from normal haustrations. Calcified lymph nodes to left of spine.

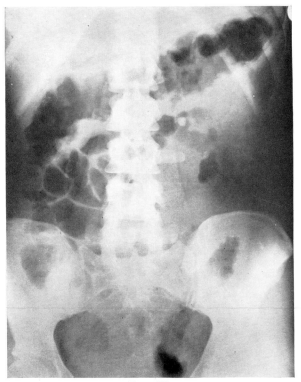

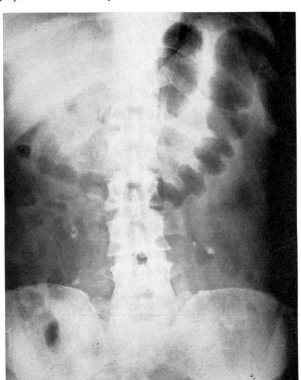

FIG. 613

FIG. 614

Fig. 613. Chronic ulcerative colitis with gaseous distension not amounting to toxic dilatation and with marked irregularity of contour of the transverse colon. Acute exacerbation superimposed upon chronic disease. Obvious pseudo-polypi at the hepatic flexure causing filling defects. Some spasm of ascending and descending parts of colon. **Fig. 614.** Chronic ulcerative colitis with acute exacerbation. Plain film shows characteristic changes in transverse colon with spasticity, narrowing and transverse ridging due to an abnormal form of contractions superficially resembling haustrations.

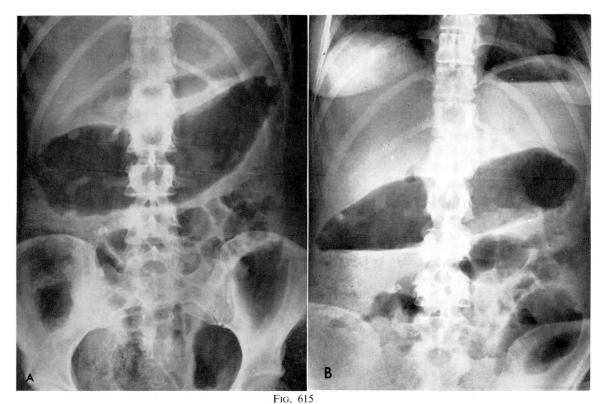

Fig. 615

Fig. 615. Ulcerative colitis with toxic dilatation.   The transverse colon—the commonest site—is particularly involved. Numerous pseudo-polypi are seen causing filling defects when seen *en face* and marginal thumb-printing when seen in profile. A: Supine.   B: Erect.

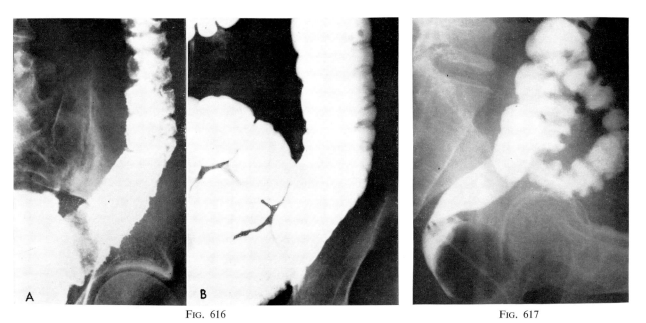

Fig. 616   Fig. 617

Fig. 616. Mildly active ulcerative procto-colitis.   Barium enema (no tannic acid or other actuator used) showing fine spiculation which disappears when colon distended.   A: Multiple tiny projections (due to contractions of the muscularis mucosae) arising from the lower descending and upper sigmoid colon.   Partially filled colon.   B: Colon distended.   Projections are not now present.   This fine spiculation is slightly more common in ulcerative colitis than in a normal colon.   Granular appearance of mucosa sigmoidoscopically but no actual ulceration.   **Fig. 617.** Early distal ulcerative procto-colitis.   Smooth contraction at the pelvi-rectal junction.   Slight increase in the retro-rectal space.   History of passage of blood and mucus for one month.

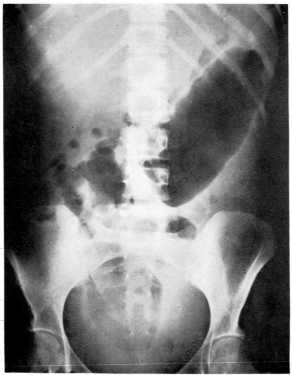

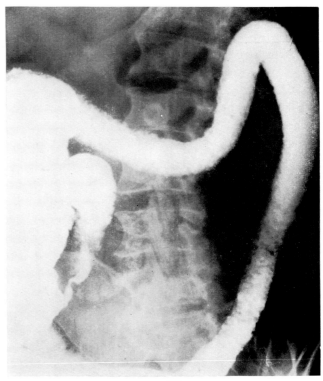

FIG. 618   FIG. 619

Fig. 618. Toxic dilatation of colon in severe acute ulcerative colitis.   First admission to hospital.   The transverse colon and to a lesser degree the pelvic colon are affected—the common sites.   The short distance between the distended transverse colon and the gas in the stomach indicates the thinness of the wall of the colon. **Fig. 619.** Extensive chronic ulcerative colitis with large numbers of pseudo-polypi of the same size giving a cobble-stone appearance.   The colon is shortened with lack of haustrations.

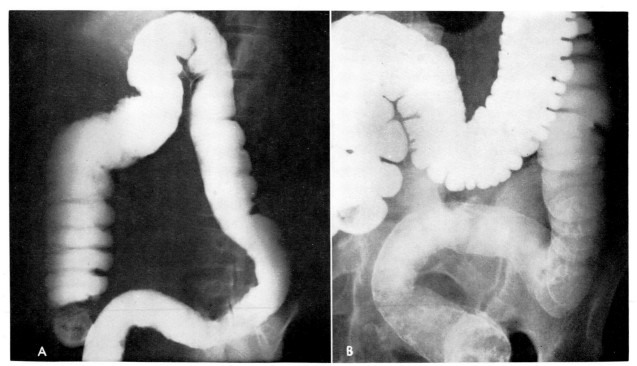

FIG. 620

Fig. 620. Water contrast barium enema in a case of chronic ulcerative colitis affecting the descending and pelvic parts of colon. A: At stage when filled with barium.   The colon is rigid, shortened and has an irregular outline due to chronic ulceration and pseudo-polypi. B: At stage of water contrast.   The sigmoid colon could be passed as normal.   When using the water contrast technique, films of the distal colon must be taken when it is filled with barium as ulcerative colitis might otherwise be overlooked.

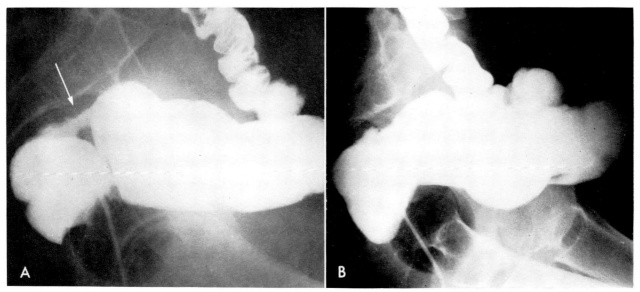

FIG. 621

Fig. 621. Localised distal ulcerative procto-colitis at pelvi-rectal junction. A: True lateral view showing the lesion clearly (arrowed). B: Slightly oblique view. The lesion is obscured by overlying loops of pelvic colon.

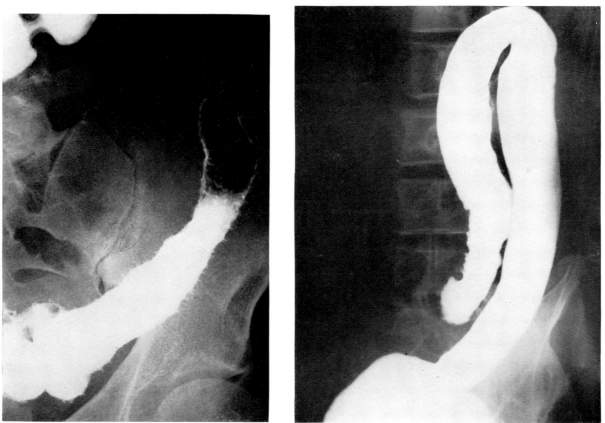

FIG. 622   FIG. 623

Fig. 622. Active distal ulcerative procto-colitis with a large number of ulcer craters. The ulcers are deeper and sharper than usual and initially raised the suspicion of Crohn's disease. **Fig. 623.** Chronic ulcerative colitis with previous history of histologically proven Crohn's disease. Smooth, shortened colon with absence of haustrations. Previous excision of terminal ileum and proximal colon for Crohn's disease. Subsequently the remainder of the colon and the rectum were excised for classical ulcerative colitis with histological confirmation.

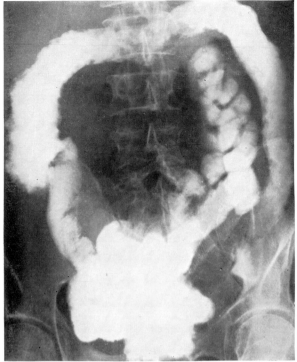

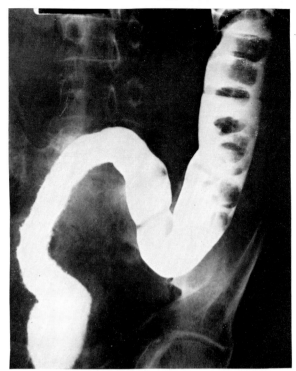

FIG. 624

FIG. 625

Fig. 624. Chronic ulcerative colitis with acute exacerbation. The colon is short and of the inverted 'U' type with lack of haustrations. Large numbers of pseudo-polypi present. Barium passed readily into the ileum which shows some dilatation. At operation the ileum was normal. **Fig. 625.** Acute exacerbation of a chronic ulcerative colitis affecting lower pelvic colon and rectum. Extensive ulceration with narrowing and shortening. Proximal to this the colon is smooth due to chronic, relatively inactive disease, and it contains numerous smooth, well formed faecal masses—a common finding in chronic ulcerative colitis.

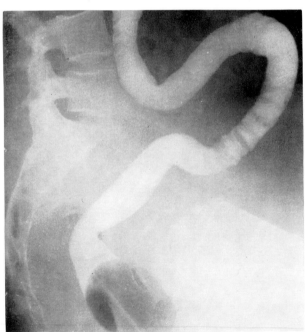

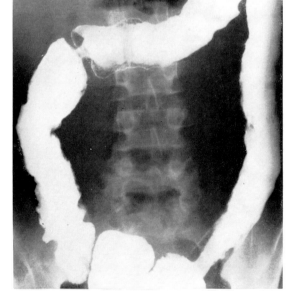

FIG. 626

FIG. 627

Fig. 626. Chronic ulcerative colitis. The pelvic colon and rectum are smooth and contracted and are separated from the sacrum by a large space. The translucency is the bulb of the Foley catheter which must always be inflated with particular care in cases of ulcerative colitis. Chronic disease of many years duration. **Fig. 627.** Chronic ulcerative colitis resulting in a narrow, rigid, shortened colon with smooth outline. 'String' stricture at the hepatic flexure which proved to be simple. Radiologically a carcinoma could not be excluded. Total procto-colectomy performed.

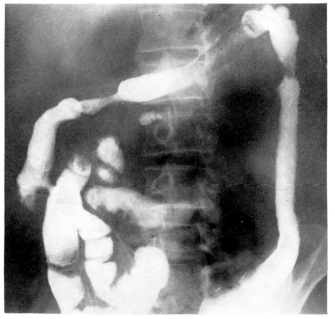

FIG. 628

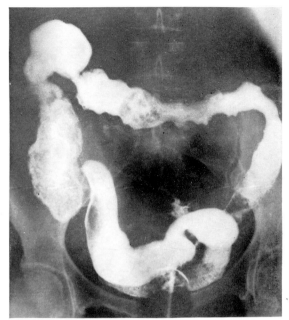

FIG. 629

Fig. 628. Chronic ulcerative colitis resulting in a rigid, diffusely contracted (hose-pipe) colon with several strictures. The ileo-caecal valve is rigid allowing free reflux into the small bowel. **Fig. 629.** Chronic ulcerative colitis of many years duration involving the entire colon with marked shortening, irregularity, and some narrowing. Rigidity of ileo-caecal valve. Dilatation of the terminal ileum. Total procto-colectomy performed. No evidence of disease of the ileum at laparotomy.

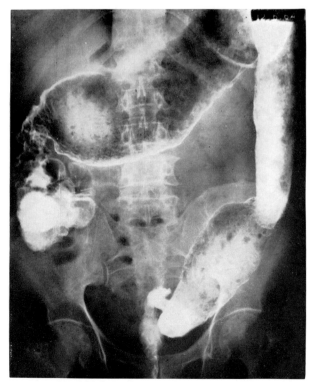

FIG. 630

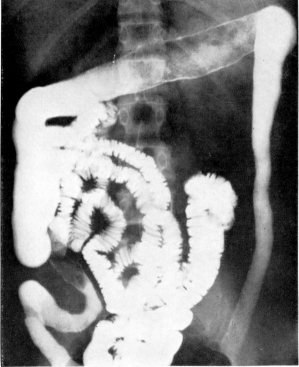

FIG. 631

Fig. 630. Chronic ulcerative colitis with a degree of toxic dilatation. Multiple pseudo-polypi, particularly in the lower descending colon. **Fig. 631.** Chronic ulcerative colitis of many years duration with a shortened, hose-pipe type of colon. The colon filled with great rapidity and is smooth owing to extensive mucosal destruction. Featureless appearance of terminal loop of ileum with lack of mucosal pattern—not necessarily indicating disease on a barium enema. Total procto-colectomy. Ileum carefully examined pathologically and found to be normal.

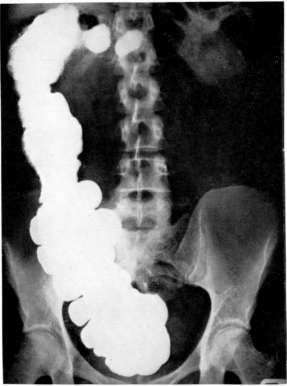

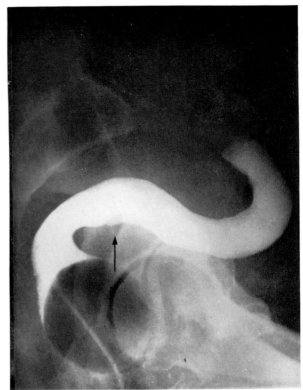

FIG. 632

FIG. 633

Fig. 632. Gross stasis in proximal colon in a case of distal ulcerative procto-colitis. Film six weeks after barium had been given by mouth for barium meal and follow-through. **Fig. 633.** Chronic ulcerative colitis with smooth, shortened and narrowed pelvic colon and with increased retro-rectal space. Early carcinoma (arrowed) on anterior wall.

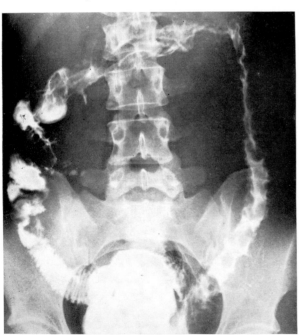

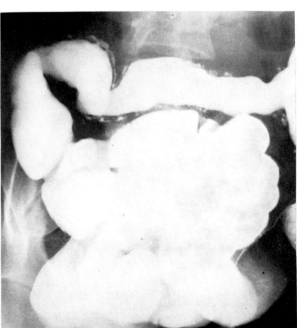

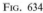

FIG. 634

FIG. 635

Fig. 634. Diffuse ulcerative form of colitis as yet unclassified. The distal colon is particularly affected. Gross mucosal destruction with indentations and thumb-printing due to large pseudo-polypi. Ulceration in descending and sigmoid colon. Clinically and pathologically there were some features of Crohn's disease and some features of ulcerative colitis. **Fig. 635.** Acute severe exacerbation of chronic ulcerative colitis. Multiple, deep, collar-stud type ulcers causing a double contour, especially in the transverse colon.

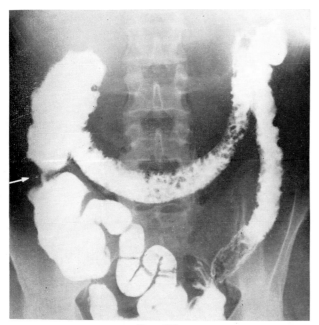

FIG. 636

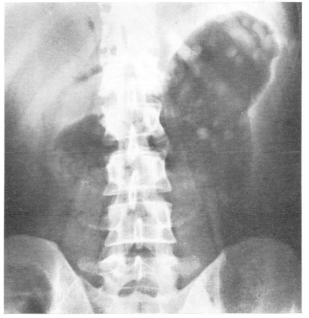

FIG. 637

Fig. 636. Chronic ulcerative colitis of many years duration with carcinoma (arrowed) supervening in ascending colon. The transverse and descending parts of colon are shortened and have a cobble-stone appearance due to ulceration, granulations and pseudo-polypi.

Fig. 637. Toxic dilatation of colon. Case of ulcerative colitis. Pseudo-polypi also present. Increased distance between body of stomach (containing a streak of gas) and transverse colon owing to greater omentum wrapped round the latter. The clinical features suggested Crohn's disease rather than ulcerative colitis.

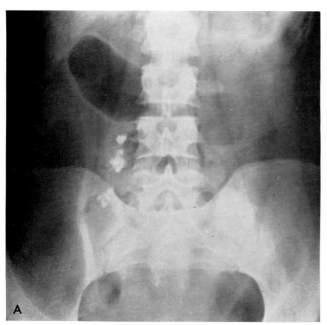

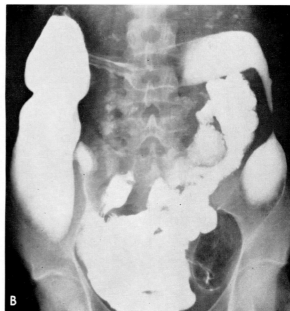

FIG. 638

Fig. 638. Crohn's disease affecting the entire colon and to a lesser extent the small bowel. A: Plain film. Distension of the ascending and proximal part of transverse colon with gas with smooth outline and absence of haustrations. B: Follow-through of barium meal. Smooth rigid shortened colon with lack of haustrations and extensive mucosal destruction. The terminal ileum is also narrowed with mucosal destruction. Organic strictures in transverse and descending colon. Well marked steatorrhoea and malabsorption of vitamin B_{12}.

P

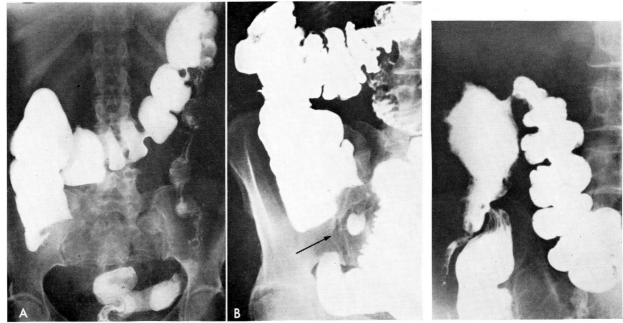

FIG. 639   FIG. 640

Fig. 639. Crohn's disease of ileo-caecal region with a large inflammatory mass. A: Barium enema. Filling defect of caecum causing complete obstruction to the flow of barium. B: Follow-through of barium meal. Large ulcer crater (arrowed) in an otherwise unfilled segment of terminal ileum ('skip' lesion). The inflammatory mass displaces the caecum and terminal ileum.
Fig. 640. Right-sided colitis of the Crohn type with caecal contraction, shortening of ascending colon and a stricture at hepatic flexure. An acute intestinal obstruction subsequently occurred from a date stone. Gross dilatation of terminal ileum.

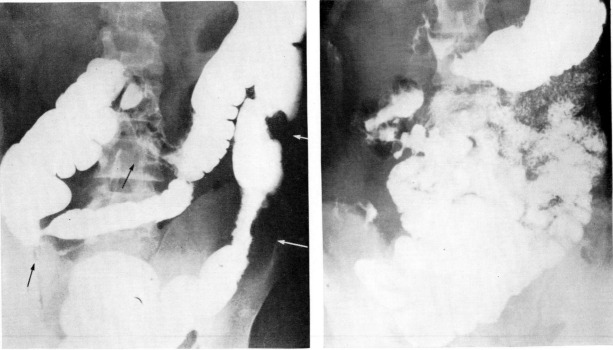

FIG. 641   FIG. 642

Fig. 641. Crohn's disease of colon with a segmental distribution—the common finding. Several areas (arrowed) are involved— the caecum and commencement of ascending colon, the transverse colon and two areas of the descending colon. Ulceration present, particularly obvious in the most distal lesion. Intervening normal colon. **Fig. 642.** Crohn's disease of terminal ileum, caecum and ascending colon. Incomplete filling of affected segments and large, soft tissue mass in right iliac fossa. Three-hour barium follow-through. Because of obstruction, resection carried out and pathological confirmation of Crohn's disease obtained. Subsequently the patient developed a form of colitis which pathologically looked more like ulcerative colitis than Crohn's disease.

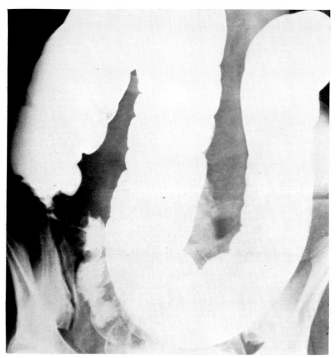

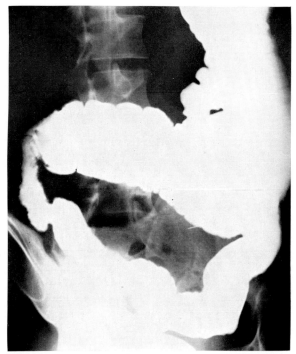

FIG. 643   FIG. 644

Fig. 643. Crohn's disease of ileo-caecal region. Barium enema reveals an irregular filling defect with a grossly narrowed lumen. Macroscopically at laparotomy this looked like a tumour. No other lesion in the small or large bowel. History of constipation for one year, with lower abdominal pain. **Fig. 644.** Right-sided colitis of the Crohn type. Gross shortening with narrowing and superficial irregularity of caecum, ascending colon and hepatic flexure. The distal colon is normal. Rigid and patent ileo-caecal valve allowing gross reflux into terminal ileum which is dilated. Follow-through of barium meal subsequently showed some mucosal destruction in the ileum.

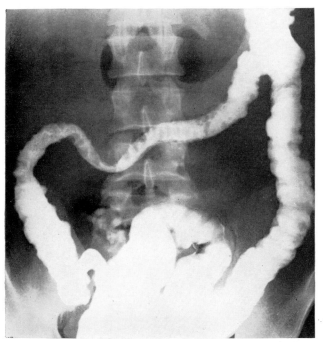

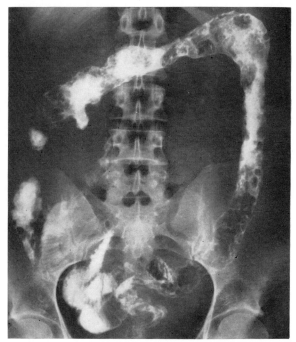

FIG. 645   FIG. 646

Fig. 645. Crohn's disease affecting in particular the proximal half of colon with narrowing, shortening and mucosal destruction. A peri-anal fistula was also present. Only minimal disease in the small bowel on barium follow-through. **Fig. 646.** Extensive Crohn's disease of colon. Marked shortening with mucosal destruction and numerous pseudo-polypi, especially in descending colon. Considerable faecal residue as great difficulty was encountered in clearing the colon. Previous right hemi-colectomy with ileo-colic anastomosis.

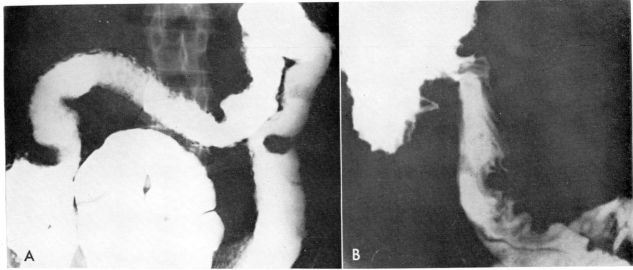

Fig. 647

Fig. 647. Severe Crohn's disease restricted to the colon with histological confirmation. A: Multiple collar-stud ulcers causing a double contour. Barium enema. B: 'Spot' film showing normal appearance of terminal ileum on follow-through of barium meal. The rest of the small bowel was also normal.

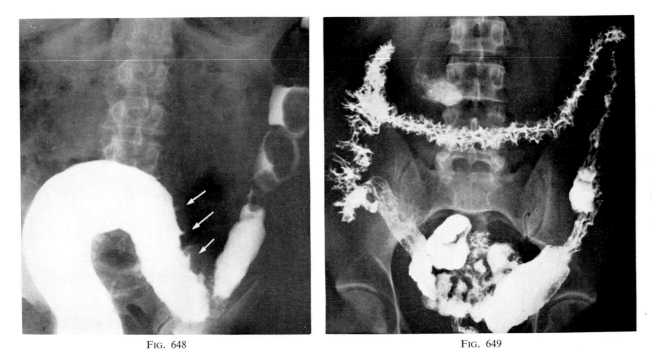

Fig. 648   Fig. 649

Fig. 648. Severe Crohn's disease of pelvic colon with narrowing rigidity and deep fissure-like ulcers (some arrowed). Resection performed because of increasing obstruction.

Fig. 649. Three-hour barium follow-through demonstrating extensive Crohn's disease of colon with shortening, spasticity and a coarse mucosal pattern. The terminal ileum is also involved, the mucosal destruction being well demonstrated. Marked intestinal hurry in the colon. At first sight the appearances suggest the post-evacuation film of a barium enema.

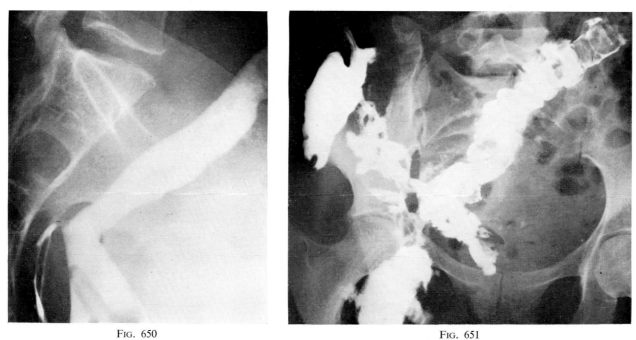

Fig. 650   Fig. 651

Fig. 650. Crohn's disease of pelvic colon and rectum with narrowing, shortening and increased retro-rectal and retro-colic space. Fistula present posteriorly.

Fig. 651. Crohn's disease arising from a short segment of terminal ileum causing extensive fistulous tracts in abdominal wall and retro-peritoneally. The fistulae have been outlined by Gastrografin and there is a connection also with the transverse colon.

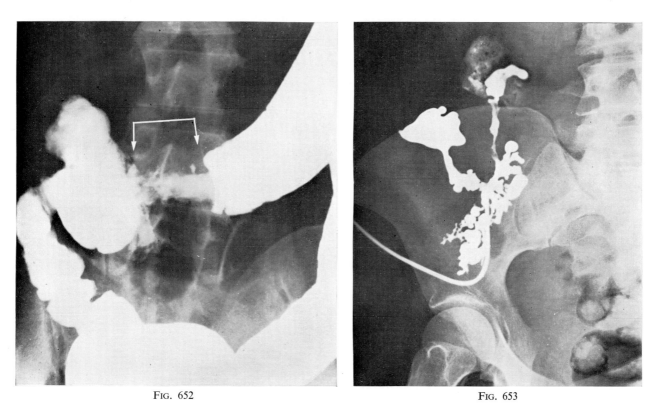

Fig. 652   Fig. 653

Fig. 652. Recurrence of Crohn's disease in transverse colon adjacent to an ileo-transverse colostomy. Irregular filling defect (arrowed) with mucosal destruction.

Fig. 653. Crohn's disease with multiple sinuses and fistulae to the skin, outlined by Gastrografin.

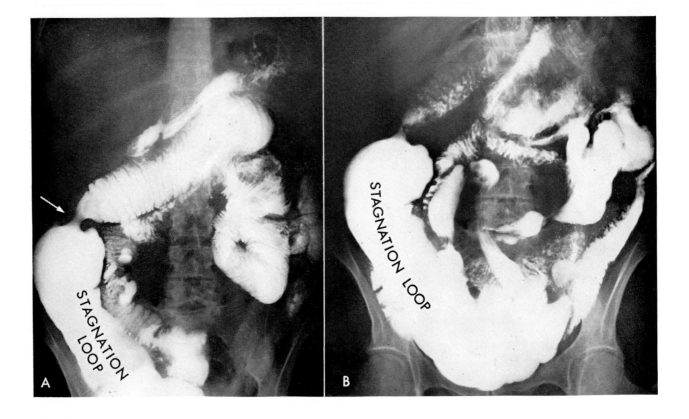

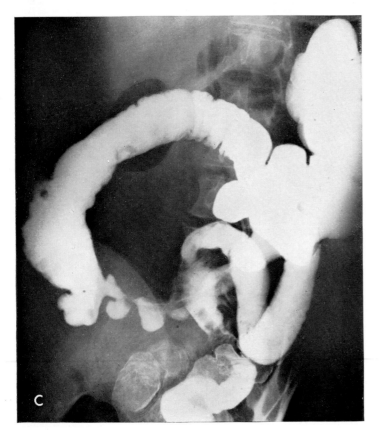

FIG. 654.

Fig. 654. Diffuse Crohn's disease of small bowel and proximal colon. A: Stricture (arrowed) in upper jejunum. Distal to this there is a dilated stagnation loop. One-hour barium follow-through film. B: Three-hour barium follow-through film. The stagnation loop is still obvious. Long segments of jejunum and ileum with smooth outline due to mucosal destruction and with several strictures. C: Barium enema. Diffuse Crohn's disease of caecum and proximal colon with marked contraction particularly of caecum. Strictures and sacculations demonstrated in terminal ileum. Gross malabsorption present.

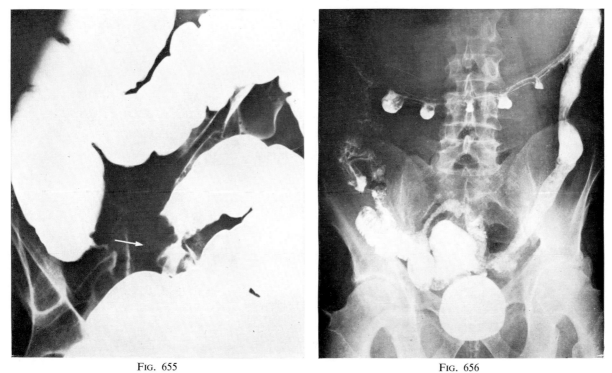

FIG. 655   FIG. 656

Fig. 655. Segment of Crohn's disease (arrowed) in upper pelvic colon due to direct extension from terminal ileum causing a filling defect simulating a carcinoma. Some involvement also of the caecum. Large inflammatory mass present. No filling of terminal ileum. Examination by barium enema. **Fig. 656.** Chronic amoebic colitis. Smooth contraction of colon with lack of haustrations and well-marked sacculations in the transverse colon. Post-evacuation film of barium enema. The patient, a native of south-west Scotland had never been abroad or even to England. A chronic amoebic abscess was also present in the liver.

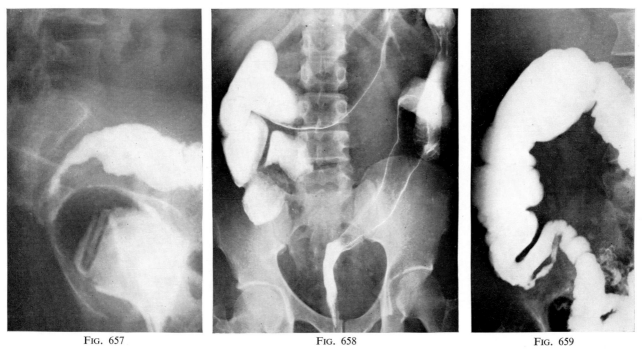

FIG. 657   FIG. 658   FIG. 659

Fig. 657. Chronic amoebiasis affecting the pelvi-rectal junction causing an irregular stricture with mucosal destruction. The radiological appearances are indistinguishable from chronic ulcerative colitis or Crohn's disease. **Fig. 658.** Chronic amoebic colitis affecting the whole colon. Narrowed, shortened, rigid colon with lack of haustrations, and smooth mucosal pattern. **Fig. 659.** Amoebic colitis affecting the caecum, ascending colon and probably also the appendix. Gross caecal contraction—a common finding. Disease still active with many amoebae in the stools. Native of Edinburgh who had had only one short holiday abroad.

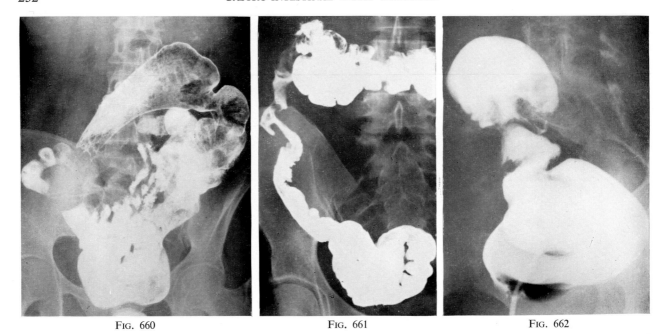

FIG. 660   FIG. 661   FIG. 662

Fig. 660. Actinomycosis of colon with underlying Crohn's disease. Gross distortion with strictures especially in proximal colon. Laparotomy performed because of obstruction when the diagnosis of actinomycosis was established. **Fig. 661.** Tuberculosis of caecum and ascending colon with irregularity, gross contraction and mucosal destruction. Minimal narrowing of terminal 2 to 3 cm. of ileum. Initially considered to be a form of Crohn's disease. Laparotomy performed because of increasing obstruction when the diagnosis of tuberculosis was established. **Fig. 662.** Tuberculosis of pelvic colon with gross irregularity and narrowing. The right ovary was also affected—possibly the initial source of infection in the abdomen.

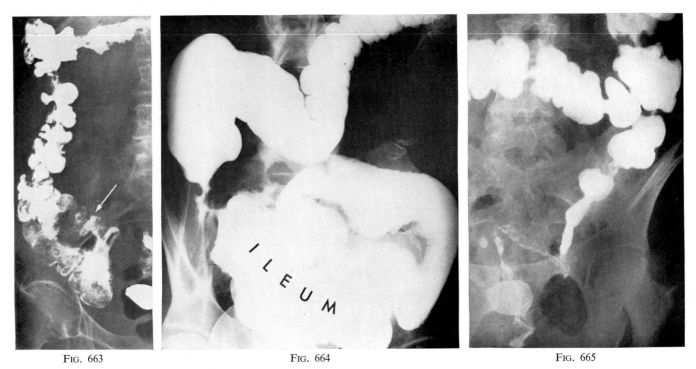

FIG. 663   FIG. 664   FIG. 665

Fig. 663. Chronic inflammatory fibro-fatty mass affecting the lips of the ileo-caecal valve and causing a lobulated filling defect (arrowed). Laparotomy performed with resection of the mass as a carcinoma could not be excluded. **Fig. 664.** Chronic tuberculosis affecting the caecum, the adjacent part of ascending colon and last 5 cm. or so of terminal ileum. Marked irregular narrowing with mucosal destruction. Examination by barium enema. The barium refluxed into the ileum which is grossly dilated. **Fig. 665.** X-irradiation colitis and proctitis. Marked contraction and distortion of pelvic colon and rectum. Treatment twenty years previously by radiotherapy for carcinoma of cervix. Examination of the resected specimen showed that superficial malignancy had developed.

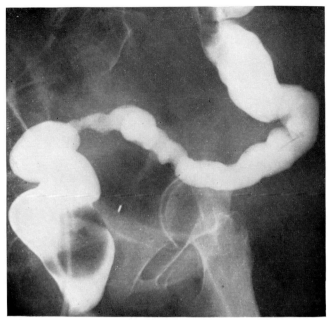

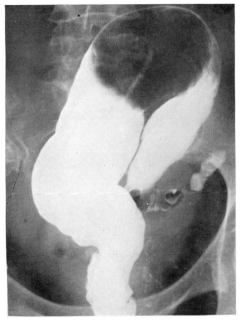

FIG. 666

FIG. 667

Fig. 666. X-irradiation procto-colitis following treatment for carcinoma of cervix. The pelvic colon and rectum, in particular the pelvi-rectal junction, are smooth, narrowed and shortened. **Fig. 667.** X-irradiation procto-colitis following radiotherapy for carcinoma of cervix. Gross narrowing, irregularity and superficial ulceration in lower rectum and proximally in pelvic colon loop where it dips down into the pelvis and lies adjacent to the rectum. The Foley catheter doubled back on itself during insertion so that the tip pointed distally. The balloon thus ascended high up into the pelvic colon and caused the large translucency. At fluoroscopy this could be mistaken for a bulky tumour.

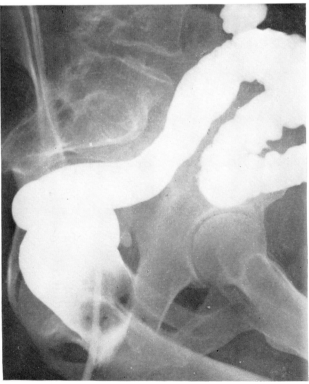

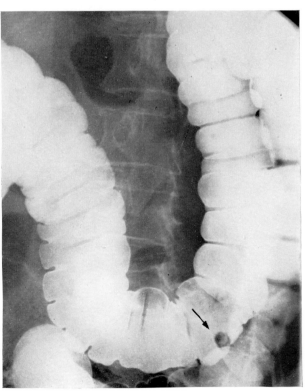

FIG. 668

FIG. 669

Fig. 668. Mild X-irradiation colitis of pelvic colon. The affected area is smooth and shortened, but no actual ulceration noted. Previous radiotherapy for carcinoma of cervix. **Fig. 669.** Polyp (arrowed) in transverse colon. Water contrast phase of barium enema.

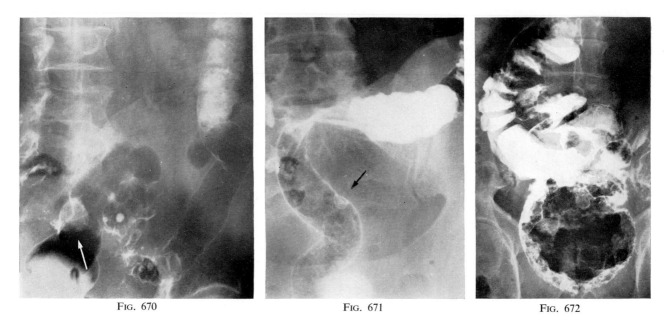

FIG. 670   FIG. 671   FIG. 672

Fig. 670. Polyp (arrowed) in pelvic colon. Localised area of diverticular disease at a higher level. Double contrast barium enema.

Fig. 671. Sessile polyp (arrowed) in pelvic colon. Double contrast barium enema.

Fig. 672. Villous papillomatosis of rectum causing bulky filling defects down to anal margin. The tumours secreted 4 to 5 litres of fluid per day containing a large amount of potassium.

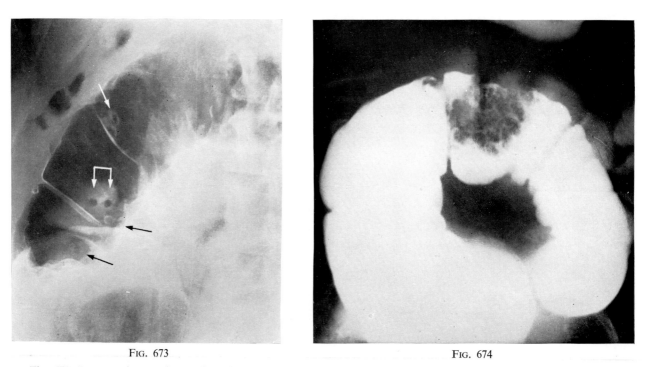

FIG. 673   FIG. 674

Fig. 673. Large carcinoma of ascending colon causing obstruction. Numerous small polypi (arrowed) in ascending colon and at hepatic flexure distal to tumour. Two polypi in a shallow pool of barium cause smooth filling defects (double arrow). Supine film. Double contrast barium enema. Case of familial polyposis.

Fig. 674. Large villous papilloma in mid-pelvic colon shown clearly as an irregular lobulated filling defect.

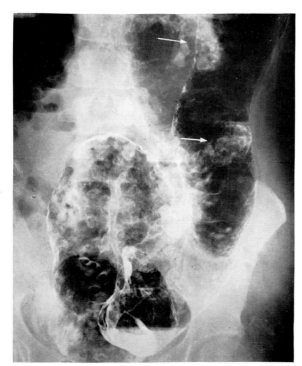

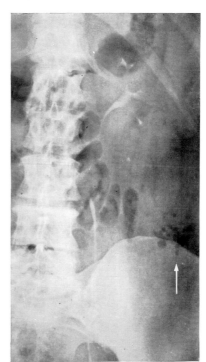

FIG. 675

FIG. 676

Fig. 675. Multiple polyposis with a vast number of polypi. At laparotomy the two bunches of polypi (arrowed) in the descending colon could not be palpated through the intact bowel wall. Double contrast barium enema. Erect film. The small polypi in the pelvic colon are easily distinguished from diverticula as they do not contain fluid levels. **Fig. 676.** Localised abscess with multiple bubbles of gas (arrowed) due to perforation of a carcinoma of descending colon. Mass present, clinically considered to be an enlarged left kidney. Abscess discovered during an I.V.P. examination.

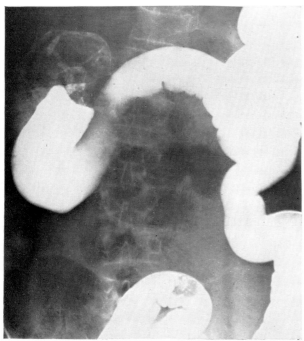

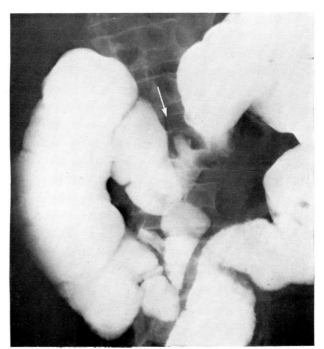

FIG. 677

FIG. 678

Fig. 677. Carcinoma of hepatic flexure causing an almost complete obstruction. The filling defect in the pelvic colon was not persistent and was due to faeces. **Fig. 678.** Lymphosarcoma of middle of transverse colon causing a filling defect with a large ulcer (arrowed). This ulcer subsequently perforated into the jejunum causing bacterial colonisation and gross malabsorption.

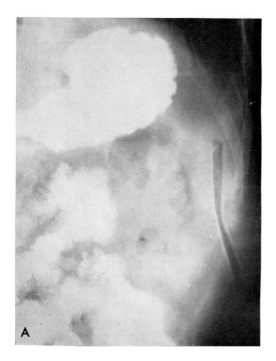
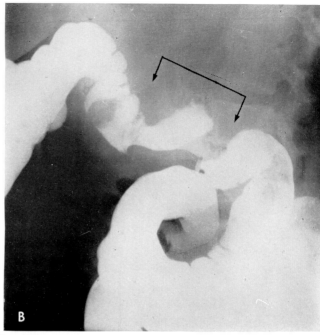

Fig. 679

Fig. 679. Large sub-phrenic abscess on left side due to local perforation of a carcinoma of splenic flexure. A: Follow-through of barium meal shows displacement of the jejunum and to a lesser extent the stomach by a large soft-tissue shadow. Bulging of the left flank. Drainage tube (containing air in its lumen) in situ. B: The large irregular tumour (arrowed) is clearly shown by barium enema. The fistula is not demonstrated. The filling defect proximal to the tumour is due to faeces.

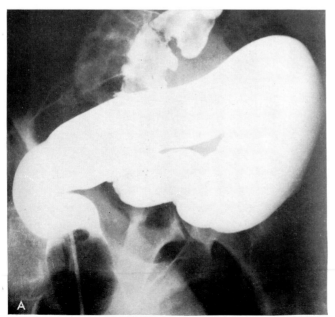
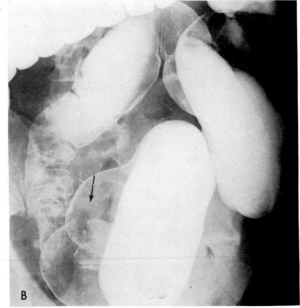

Fig. 680

Fig. 680. Carcinoma high up in pelvic colon obscured by overlying loops of sigmoid colon filled with barium at the beginning of the barium enema examination. A: Early stage with barium alone. No abnormality detected. B: Water contrast stage. The tumour (arrowed) is clearly depicted even although two loops of colon overlie it.

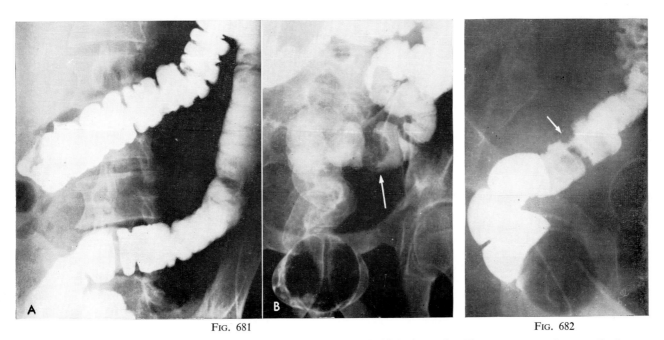

FIG. 681   FIG. 682

Fig. 681. Carcinoma of pelvic colon. A: At the early stage when filled with barium only. The tumour cannot be seen. B: At water contrast stage. The tumour (arrowed) is clearly demonstrated.

Fig. 682. Carcinoma of pelvic colon (arrowed) of string stricture type. It is readily detected on the lateral view but was not seen on the P.A. view.

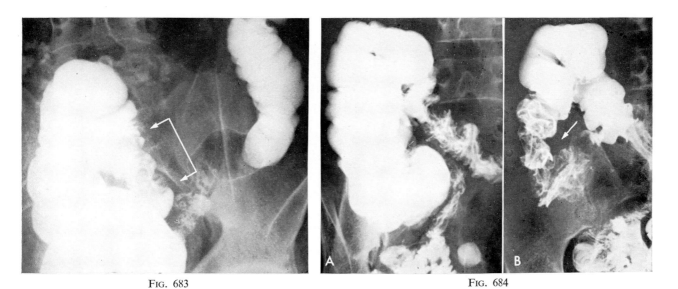

FIG. 683   FIG. 684

Fig. 683. Carcinoma of pelvic colon. Large, irregular filling defect (arrowed) typical of a carcinoma. This tumour could not be detected on the post-evacuation film.

Fig. 684. Carcinoma of ascending colon. A: The carcinoma is obscured on the filled film as the affected segment contains too much barium. B: After most of the barium has been evacuated into the can during fluoroscopy, the tumour (arrowed) is demonstrated and causes a filling defect with mucosal destruction.

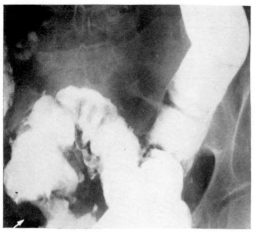

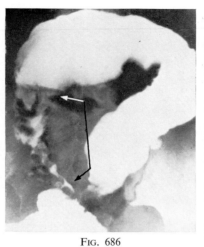

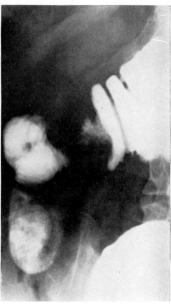

Fig. 685

Fig. 686

Fig. 685. Napkin-ring type of carcinoma (arrowed) in pelvic colon. Proximal to the tumour there is an area of diverticular disease but the tumour is at the point of greatest narrowing.

Fig. 686. Carcinoma of pelvic colon (arrowed) causing irregularity with narrowing and mucosal destruction over a large area. The tumour has spread and involved the pelvic colon proximally where it dips down into the pelvis.

Fig. 687

Fig. 687. Recurrence of carcinoma of colon at the anastomosis near hepatic flexure. Previous right hemi-colectomy for carcinoma. The filling defect is so large that it cannot be mistaken for a fibrous stricture.

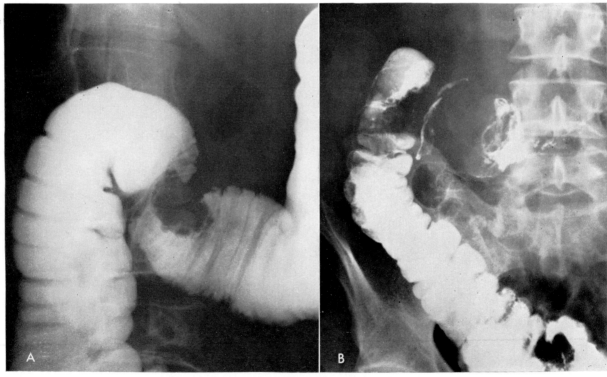

Fig. 688

Fig. 688. Malignant papilloma immediately distal to hepatic flexure. A: Characteristic filling defect with short stalk shown at stage of filling by barium enema. B: Post-evacuation film. The filling defect is confirmed and there is indication of partial intussusception, namely coating of entering loop with widening. Complaint of bleeding per rectum for several months with intermittent colicky abdominal pain presumably coinciding with partial intussusception.

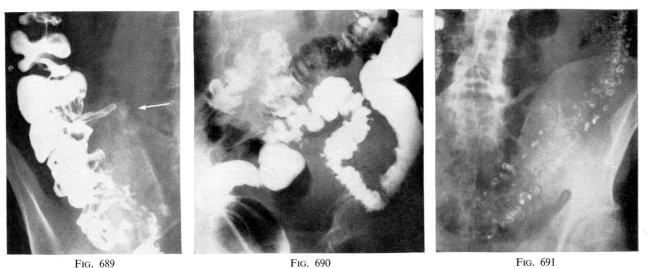

FIG. 689   FIG. 690   FIG. 691

Fig. 689. Traction diverticulum of ascending colon caused by an adhesion to a calcified mesenteric node (arrowed).

Fig. 690. Diverticular disease of sigmoid colon showing distally a zig-zag appearance and proximally transverse ridging due to muscular thickening and with the presence of a few diverticula between the ridges.

Fig. 691. Extensive diverticular disease of distal colon. The diverticula are disposed in a regular fashion indicating that the primary abnormality is unlikely to be inflammatory. Post-evacuation film of barium enema.

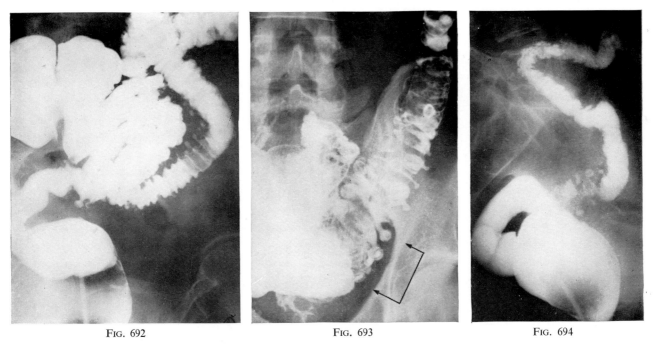

FIG. 692   FIG. 693   FIG. 694

Fig. 692. Diverticular disease of sigmoid colon. The uniformly disposed transverse bars due to thickened circular muscle are clearly seen. The diverticula arise uniformly from between these bars, and thus also have a regular distribution.

Fig. 693. Diverticular disease. Note residual barium forming a nucleus in several colonic diverticula (arrowed) from a follow-through one week previously. The diverticula are also disposed in a regular fashion.

Fig. 694. Segment of diverticular disease of pelvic colon with superadded infection, i.e. diverticulitis causing irregularity with distortion and narrowing. Tender mass in the left iliac fossa. Patient complained of pain with diarrhoea. Local excision performed. In addition to the well marked muscular hypertrophy there was fibrosis and evidence of chronic inflammation—a true diverticulitis.

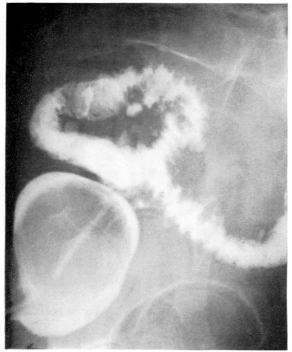

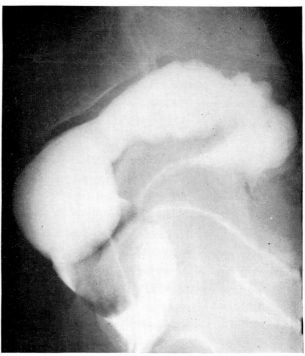

FIG. 695   FIG. 696

Fig. 695. Severe diverticular disease with distortion and irregularity and the presence of many diverticula. Peri-diverticulitis also present causing the upper loop of pelvic colon to be adherent to the pelvi-rectal junction.

Fig. 696. Obstruction of upper pelvic colon by a para-colic abscess—proved at laparotomy to have resulted from diverticulitis. The diverticulitis could not be detected radiologically as it was not possible to fill the affected segment by barium enema.

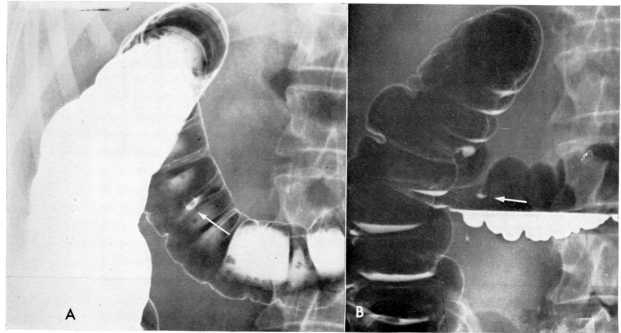

FIG. 697

Fig. 697. Diverticulum (arrowed) in transverse colon. Double contrast barium enema. A: Supine view. The diverticulum simulates a polyp. B: Erect. The diverticulum contains a fluid level confirming the diagnosis and definitely excluding a polyp.

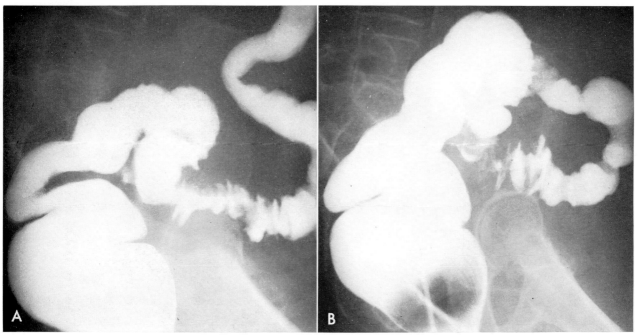

Fig. 698

Fig. 698. Localised diverticular disease with peri-diverticulitis of upper pelvic colon. Patient complained of abdominal pain. Tender mass in left iliac fossa. A: Irregular narrowing over a considerable length of upper sigmoid colon with marked spasticity. B: One month later. Palpable mass even larger. The radiological changes are more obvious.

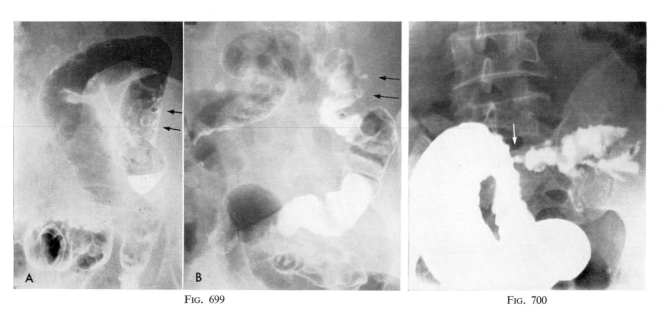

Fig. 699   Fig. 700

Fig. 699. Diverticula simulating polypi in one view on double contrast barium enema. A: Ring structures (arrowed) near splenic flexure. B: Oblique view shows that these definitely extend beyond the lumen and are thus diverticula (arrowed) and not polypi.

Fig. 700. Short segment of diverticulitis with fistula (arrowed) to the ileum.

Q

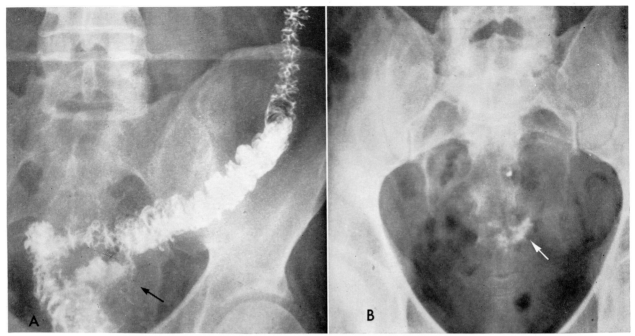

FIG. 701

Fig. 701. Diverticulitis with fistula. A: Deformity of pelvic colon due to diverticulitis. An amorphous mass of barium (arrowed) outwith the colon indicating the presence of a fistula. B: Plain film one week later. Still residual barium (arrowed) in the loculation.

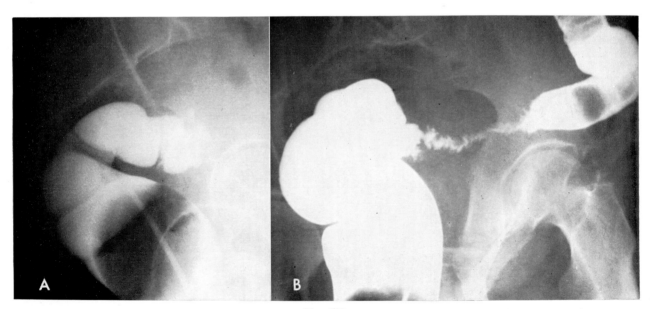

FIG. 702

Fig. 702. Obstruction of upper pelvic colon due to a markedly active diverticular disease. A: Even with the use of a Foley catheter the patient could not retain the enema and a complete obstruction was encountered. As two or three diverticula are indistinctly seen the diagnosis of diverticulitis rather than a carcinoma was suggested. B. Second barium enema following 30 mg. Buscopan intravenously. The spasm was partially relieved and a long narrowed segment of diverticulitis revealed.

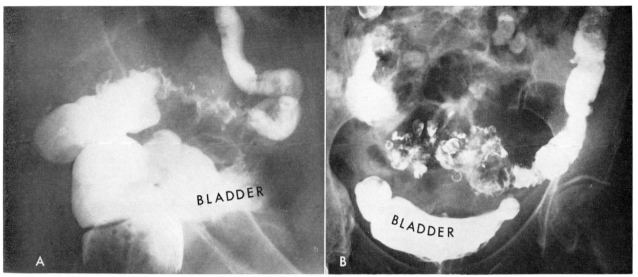

FIG. 703

Fig. 703. Vesico-colic fistula from diverticulitis. A: Severe diverticulitis of pelvic colon demonstrated by barium enema. The bladder contains a large amount of barium and some gas. B: Post-evacuation film. Residual barium in the bladder. The segment of well marked diverticulitis in the pelvic colon is also clearly seen. The actual fistula is not demonstrated.

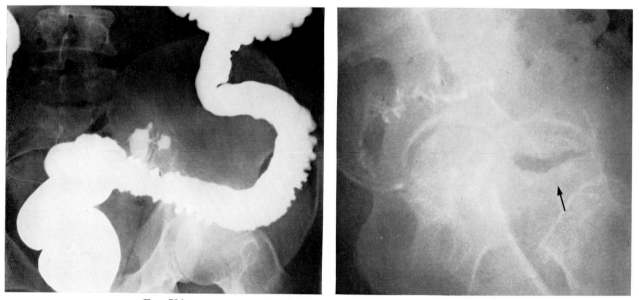

FIG. 704   FIG. 705

Fig. 704. Short segment of diverticulitis in upper pelvic colon with a fistula into an abscess cavity. The changes of diverticular disease in the colon are minimal.

Fig. 705. Vesico-colic fistula. Gas in bladder (arrowed) (post-evacuation film of barium enema). No barium on this occasion entered the bladder.

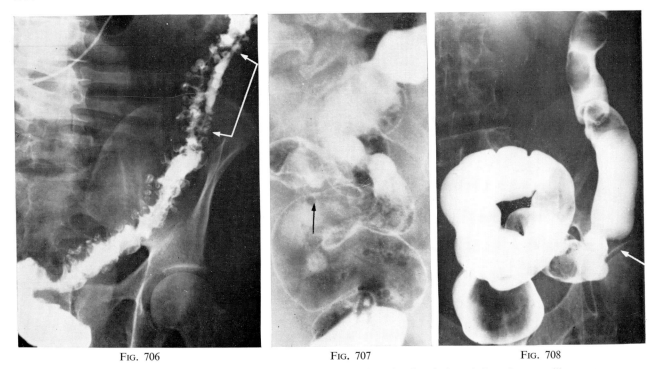

FIG. 706   FIG. 707   FIG. 708

Fig. 706. Severe diverticular disease after long myotomy (arrowed). The diverticula and distortion are still present.

Fig. 707. Endometriosis involving the pelvic colon. Filling defect with central ulcer (arrowed). History of intermittent colonic obstruction with bleeding per rectum coinciding with menstruation. Double contrast barium enema.

Fig. 708. Stricture of descending colon (arrowed) from a healed localised ischaemic colitis.

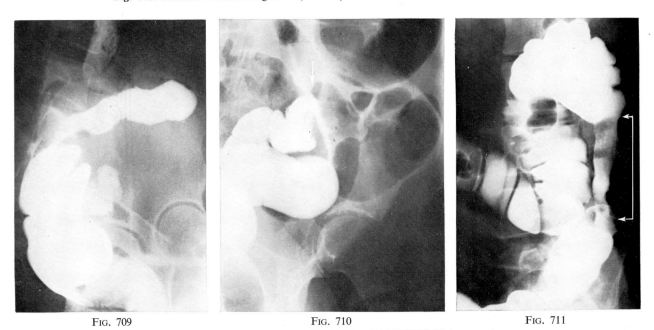

FIG. 709   FIG. 710   FIG. 711

Fig. 709. Endometriosis. Large mass in pelvis displacing the pelvic colon—indistinguishable radiologically from an ovarian cyst. Known case of endometriosis.

Fig. 710. Ischaemia of descending colon. Barium enema demonstrates a complete obstruction (arrowed) simulating a carcinoma high up in pelvic colon. At operation the obstruction coincided with the lower end of an almost gangrenous loop resulting from an inferior mesenteric thrombosis. Patient presented with intestinal obstruction.

Fig. 711. Localised subacute ischaemic colitis. Barium enema shows narrowed area (arrowed) at upper end of descending colon. Complaint of attacks of abdominal pain with diarrhoea and blood in the stool. This segment was resected.

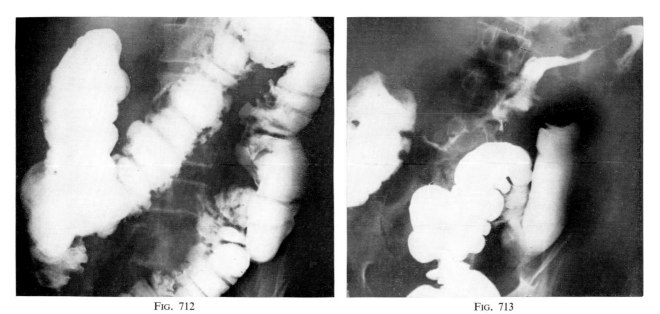

FIG. 712   FIG. 713

Fig. 712. Chronic ischaemic colitis in a case of mitral stenosis. Irregular diverticula-like sacculations in a dilated inert colon which was impossible to clear satisfactorily of faeces.

Fig. 713. Extensive contraction and irregularity of transverse colon, splenic flexure and upper part of descending colon from ischaemia. Previous gastrectomy for carcinoma of stomach. At laparotomy diffuse metastatic deposits were present in the transverse meso-colon causing vascular obstruction and thrombosis.

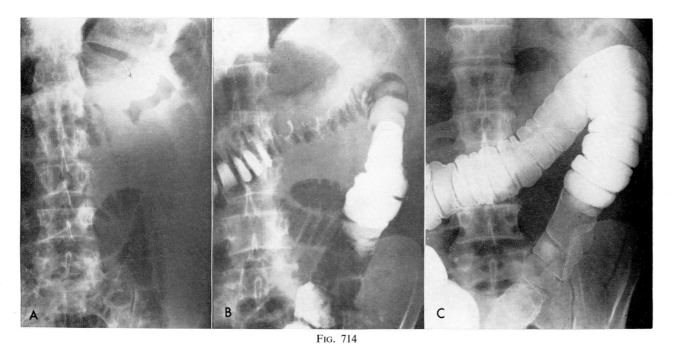

FIG. 714

Fig. 714. Acute ischaemic colitis affecting the splenic flexure area of the colon. Patient presented as an abdominal emergency with abdominal pain, shock, diarrhoea and the passage of a large amount of blood. A: Plain film shows narrowing of splenic flexure with a soft-tissue shadow due to oedema of bowel wall. The lumen of the bowel is depicted by gas and is narrowed. Some dilatation of the bowel proximally. B: Barium enema a fortnight later. Narrowing in the region of the splenic flexure with thumb-printing, transverse ridging and a large soft-tissue shadow. Considerable clinical improvement at this stage. C: Barium enema two months later. The colon is now normal.

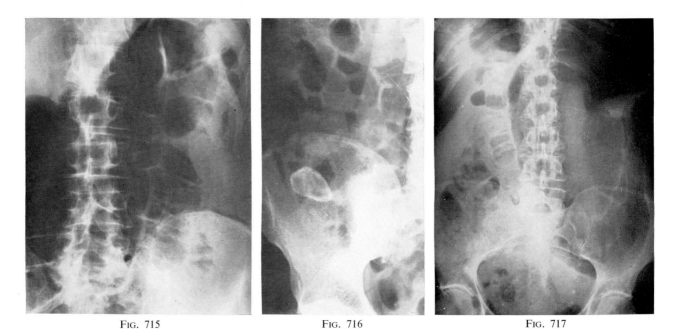

FIG. 715   FIG. 716   FIG. 717

Fig. 715. Vascular occlusion of inferior mesenteric artery with gangrene of descending colon which was distended with fluid—operative confirmation. Plain film shows almost complete absence of gas in descending colon. Dilatation of proximal colon and small bowel. At operation the proximal colon was distended but was otherwise normal.

Fig. 716. Calcified faecolith in caecum confirmed subsequently by barium enema.

Fig. 717. Herpes zoster causing gross ileus of distal colon. Patient presented with abdominal pain and increasing distension. Plain film shows marked dilatation of distal half of colon. Laparotomy performed but no obstruction found. The following day the patient developed herpes zoster.

(By courtesy of Mr. E. L. Farquharson and Dr. W. Macleod.)

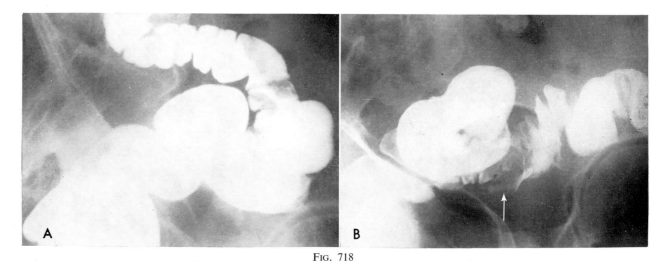

FIG. 718

Fig. 718. Faecolith in pelvic colon adherent to bowel wall—operative proof. A: Initial stage when outlined solely by barium. No abnormality detected. B: At water contrast stage. Moderately large filling defect (arrowed) simulating a carcinoma.

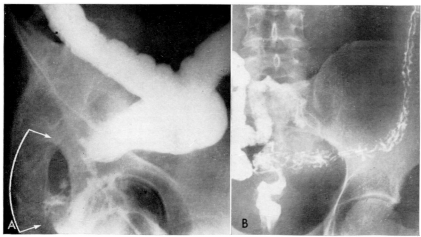
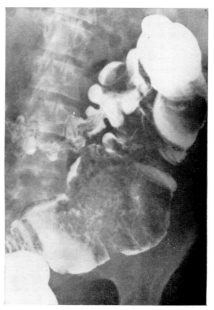

Fig. 719

Fig. 719. Large faecal mass in pelvic colon. A: Filling defect in pelvi-rectal region (arrowed) seen on initial lateral view of pelvic colon. A carcinoma is a possibility. B: Post-evacuation film. This area is clearly normal. The bowel is reduced to its normal narrow calibre excluding a bulky tumour.

Fig. 720

Fig. 720. Faecal impaction. Gross distension of upper pelvic colon which contains large faecal masses. Considerable obstruction encountered on barium enema.

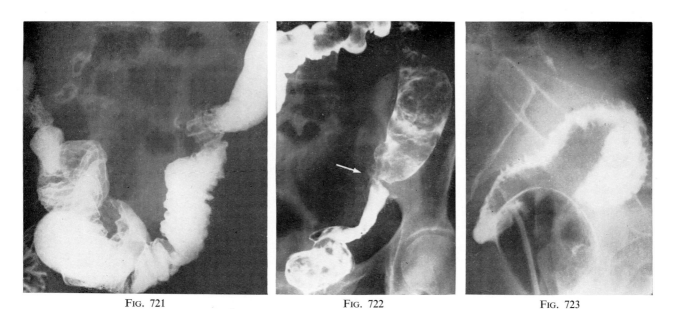

Fig. 721   Fig. 722   Fig. 723

Fig. 721. Gross oedema of pelvic colon and rectum with coarse thickened mucosal folds. Case of cirrhosis of the liver with gastric and oesophageal varices. Gross ascites was also present.

Fig. 722. Smooth simple stricture (arrowed) at site of previous resection for a carcinoma. Faecal impaction in the colon proximally.

Fig. 723. Gross oedema of pelvic colon and rectum causing diffuse narrowing with an extremely coarse mucosal pattern—confirmed at sigmoidoscopy. Case of carcinoma of the descending colon with enlarged lymph nodes in the mesentery causing lymphatic obstruction.

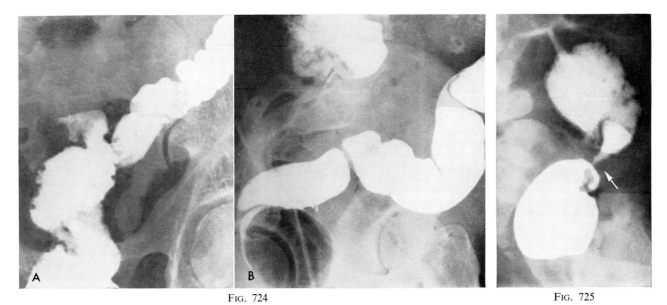

FIG. 724   FIG. 725

Fig. 724. Demonstration of healing following local resection of a tumour. A: Pocket of barium with a short sinus leading from the suture line. Barium enema three weeks after resection. B: Two years later. Only a little narrowing at the site of the previous anastomosis.

Fig. 725. Hirschsprung's disease. Characteristic narrowed segment in pelvic colon (arrowed) with dilatation proximally.

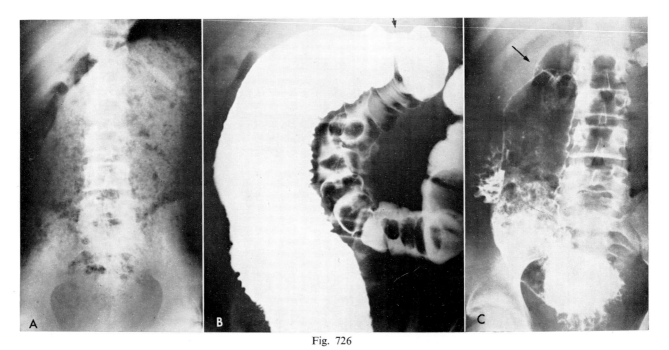

Fig. 726

Fig. 726. Idiopathic megacolon. Ganglion cells present on rectal biopsy. A: Plain film. Large, soft-tissue shadow extending from the pelvis to the epigastrium and presenting a mottled appearance due to faeces and gas. B: Barium enema. Gross distension of pelvic colon and rectum with atony. There is a sharp demarcation point (arrowed) between the normal pelvic colon proximally and the abnormal bowel distally. C: Post-evacuation film. The distal pelvic colon and rectum are still grossly distended. The point of demarcation (arrowed) between normal and abnormal bowel is even more clearly seen.

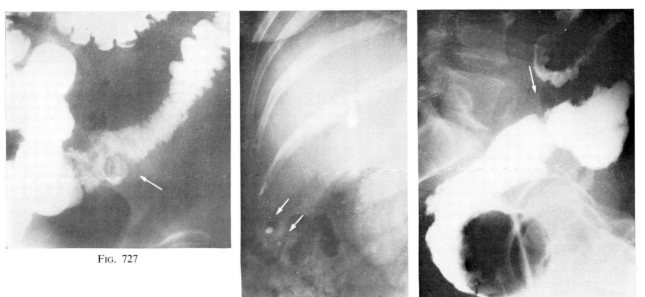

Fig. 727

Fig. 728

Fig. 729

Fig. 727. Granuloma (arrowed) at site of anastomosis causing a filling defect indistinguishable from malignant recurrence. It is coated with barium at the water contrast stage of a barium enema. Resection for carcinoma six months previously. **Fig. 728.** Calcification of two appendices epiploicae (arrowed) at hepatic flexure of colon. Incidental finding. Calcified gall stone also present at a higher level. **Fig. 729.** Torsion of an appendix epiploica in the pelvic colon causing subacute obstruction. Narrowing (arrowed) with typical signet-ring appearance. Operative confirmation.

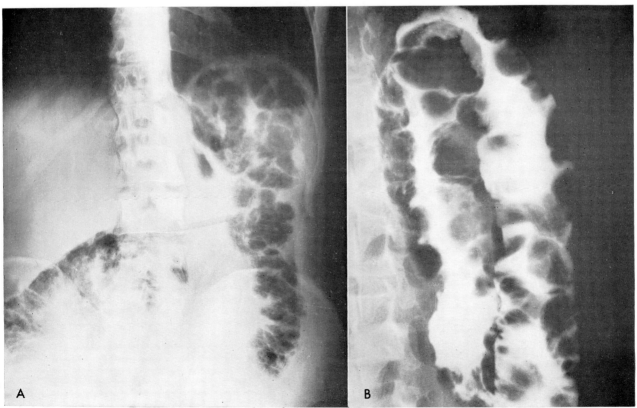

Fig. 730

Fig. 730. Pneumatosis cystoides intestinalis. A: Plain film shows gas-containing cysts in colon, particularly in descending colon and at splenic flexure. B: Barium enema shows large gas-containing cysts with a broad base causing a markedly irregular and narrowed lumen. Obvious marginal thumb-printing. Typical history of bloody diarrhoea for years, simulating ulcerative colitis. The barium enema was performed with great difficulty because of intense colonic spasm.

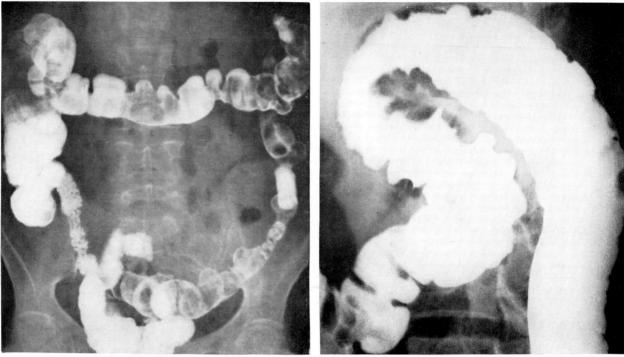

FIG. 731   FIG. 732

Fig. 731. Diffuse systemic sclerosis (scleroderma). Typical sacculations in transverse and sigmoid colon. The wall of the bowel opposite the sacculations is smooth with absence of normal haustrations. **Fig. 732.** Pneumatosis cystoides intestinalis. Characteristic gas translucencies causing marginal thumb-printing in region of splenic flexure. There is also some emphysema of the wall of the colon presumably due to rupture of a cyst. Case of gross obstructive airways disease with clinical features suggesting ulcerative colitis.

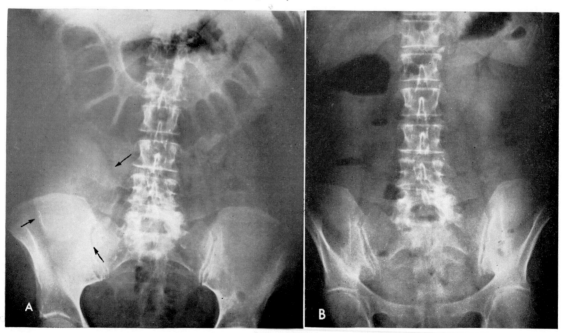

FIG. 733

Fig. 733. Obstruction of distal colon by a carcinoma causing gross dilatation of proximal colon. A: Plain film. Supine. Gross distension of caecum causing a large soft-tissue shadow (arrowed) in the right iliac fossa. There is a small amount of gas in the caecum floating on the surface of a large amount of fluid. B: Erect film. Air-fluid level at hepatic flexure—the caecum and ascending colon being filled with a large amount of fluid and relatively little gas. The one or two tiny fluid levels represent gas trapped in colonic haustrations. The ileo-caecal valve in this case did not permit reflux of gas or fluid colonic content into the ileum, i.e. it was competent—contributing to the caecal distension.

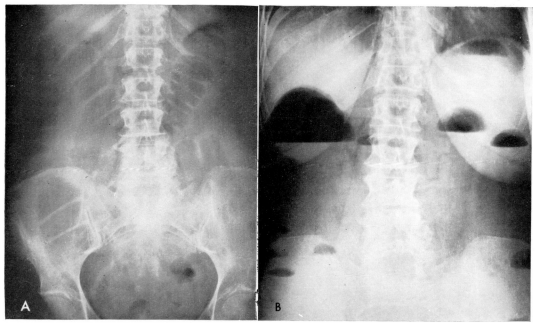

Fig. 734

Fig. 734. Obstruction in descending colon by a carcinoma. A: Supine film. There is a large amount of fluid in the proximal colon, in particular the caecum and ascending and transverse colon. There is a small amount of gas floating on this fluid. The colon is thus wider than would appear from the gaseous translucencies. B: Erect. A large air-fluid level is at hepatic flexure. The caecum and ascending colon are dilated and filled with fluid up to the air-fluid level except for a few small pockets trapped in haustrations.

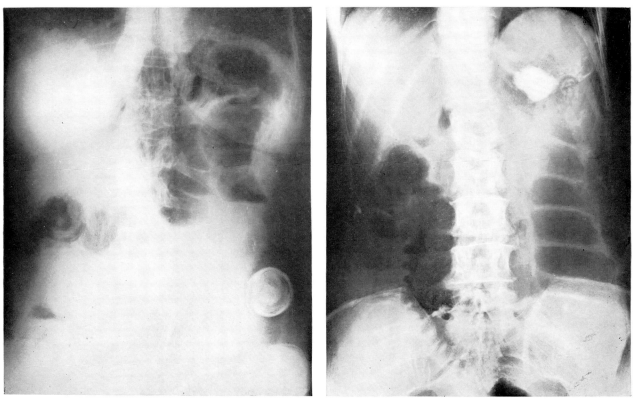

Fig. 735   Fig. 736

Fig. 735. Obstruction of descending colon by a large faecolith which had presumably originated in the caecum. Erect film. There is a considerable column of fluid between the faecolith and the air-fluid level in the descending colon. **Fig. 736.** Obstruction at splenic flexure by a carcinoma. Mass of bismuth (given because of history of indigestion) impacted at the site of the tumour. Marked dilatation of the proximal colon which contains a large amount of fluid and gas. The dilated transverse colon dips down into the pelvis.

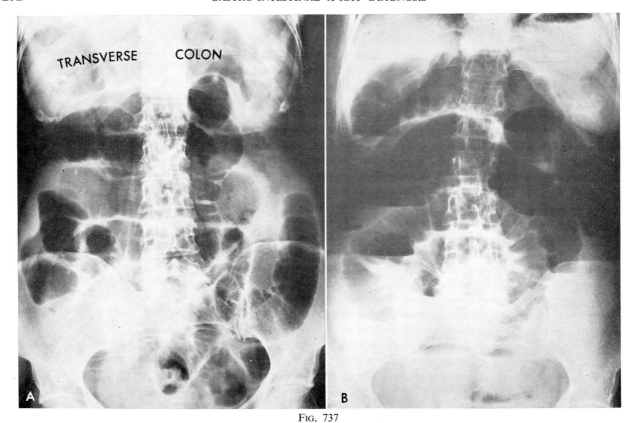

Fig. 737

Fig. 737. Colonic obstruction due to a carcinoma at splenic flexure. A: Supine film. Some distension of proximal colon but no gas distal to splenic flexure. The small bowel is considerably dilated indicating incompetence of the ileo-caecal valve which acts as a safety valve—the more usual finding. B: Erect. Multiple fluid levels especially in small bowel. The site of the obstruction is not so obvious on the erect film.

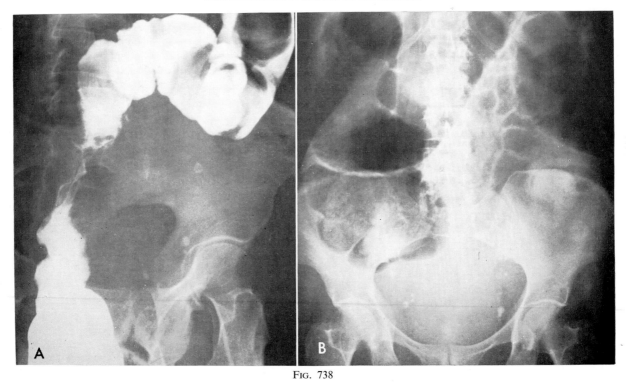

Fig. 738

Fig. 738. Obstruction of pelvic colon by a large ovarian carcinoma. A: Barium enema shows compression and infiltration of pelvic colon by a large extra-colonic tumour. B: Plain film one month later. Patient admitted with intestinal obstruction. Gross distension of proximal colon and caecum. No reflux of gas into the small bowel as the ileo-caecal valve was competent. Dangerous degree of caecal distension.

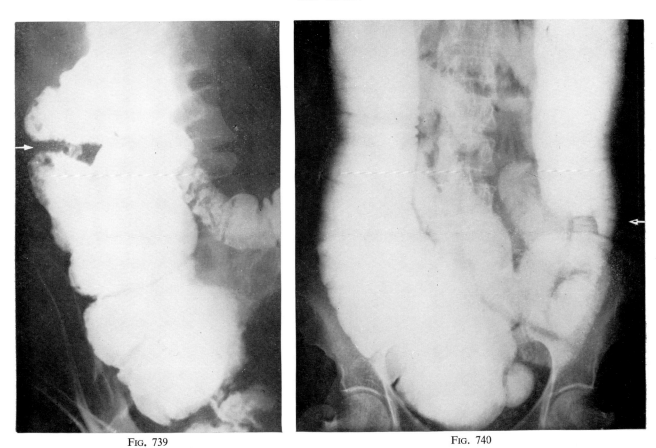

FIG. 739   FIG. 740

Fig. 739. Obstruction of ascending colon by a congenital band (arrowed). Operative confirmation. The narrow constriction looks remarkably like a carcinoma. **Fig. 740.** Obstruction of descending colon (arrowed) by a carcinoma. Plain film five weeks after a barium meal for a doubtful haematemesis. Gross dilatation of small and large bowel which are uniformly opacified by the barium. The even distribution of the barium with absence of clumping is due to atony of the small and large bowel. This degree of intestinal obstruction was not suspected clinically.

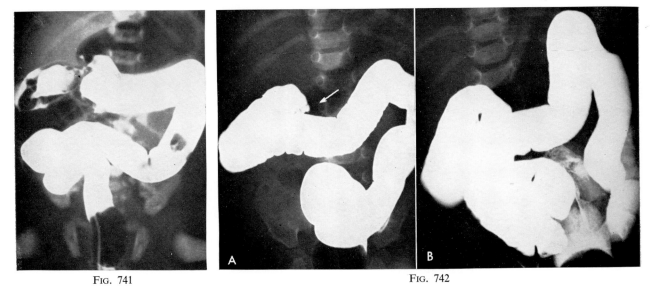

FIG. 741   FIG. 742

Fig. 741. Obstruction in transverse colon in a newborn by a meconium plug. The baby evacuated a long worm-like plug of inspissated meconium with the Gastrografin resulting in cure. Gastrografin (diluted 50 per cent) enema. **Fig. 742.** Intussusception in a baby reduced by a barium enema. A: Obstruction (arrowed) encountered at hepatic flexure. B: With a little persistence the obstruction was overcome and the proximal colon and ileum were filled, with reduction of the intussusception.

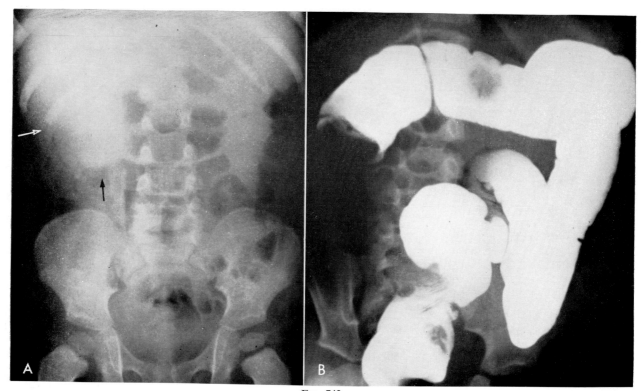

FIG. 743

Fig. 743. Intussusception in a child. A: Plain film. Intussusception causing a round, soft-tissue shadow (arrowed) in right hypochondrium. B: Barium enema. Obstruction at hepatic flexure by the intussusception which could not be reduced.

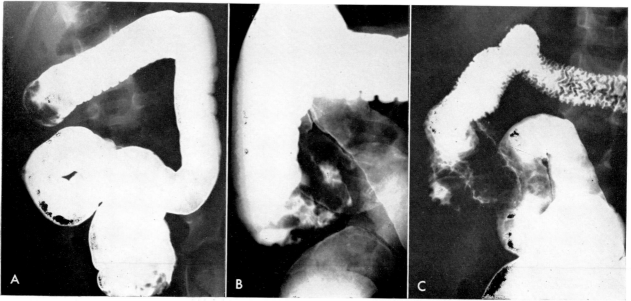

FIG. 744

Fig. 744. Intussusception reduced by barium enema. A: Obstruction in transverse colon near hepatic flexure with a little coating of the entering loop. B: The intussusception is almost completely reduced. C: Complete reduction with filling of terminal ileum. Narrowing of caecum and ascending colon due to residual spasm and oedema.

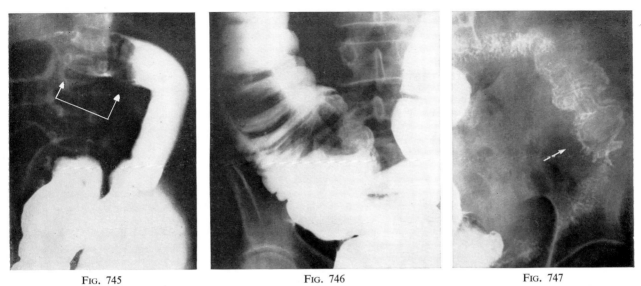

FIG. 745   FIG. 746   FIG. 747

Fig. 745. Classical intussusception in a baby causing a defect (arrowed) coated by barium in transverse colon and a complete obstruction. The intussusception could not be reduced.

Fig. 746. Ileo-colic intussusception. The ileum is clearly seen within the lumen of the ascending colon. Barium enema.

Fig. 747. Intussusception caused by a large polyp (arrowed) on a long stalk. Post-evacuation film of barium enema.

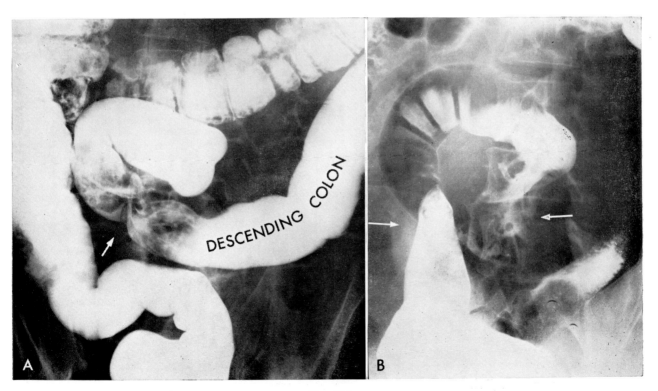

FIG. 748

Fig. 748. Volvulus of sigmoid colon demonstrated by barium enema. A: Postero-anterior view. The twist (arrowed) is clearly seen. B: Oblique view. The twist and main loop of the sigmoid colon are clearly shown. The extremities (arrowed) are also approximated.

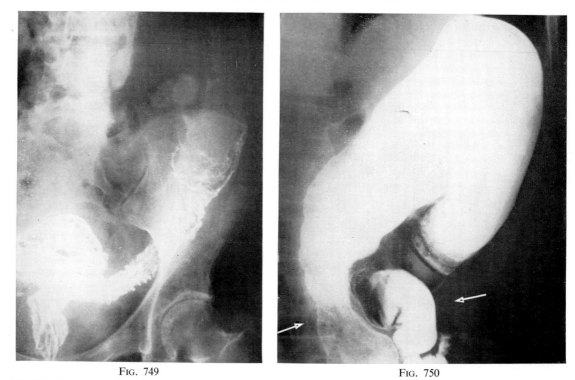

FIG. 749   FIG. 750

Fig. 749. Intussusception of descending colon due to a carcinoma. The entering loop is coated with barium and causes bulging of the receiving loop. Post-evacuation film. **Fig. 750.** Subacute volvulus of sigmoid colon. Barium enema clearly shows approximation of the extremities (arrowed) of the volvulus. Some redundancy and dilatation of sigmoid colon.

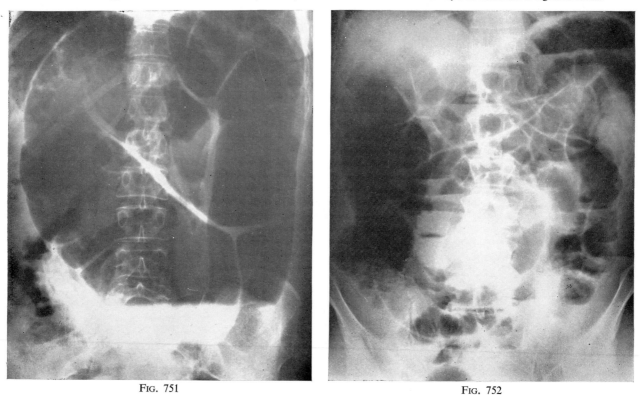

FIG. 751   FIG. 752

Fig. 751. Volvulus of sigmoid colon. Erect film shows a grossly distended sigmoid colon extending up into the epigastrium. The degree of distension suggests that the volvulus developed over a number of days. Fluid level present. **Fig. 752.** Acute volvulus of pelvic colon. The soft-tissue shadow in the centre of the abdomen is due to the affected loop being filled with fluid. Its distension is not marked because of the rapidity of onset and development. Dilatation of proximal colon and small bowel.

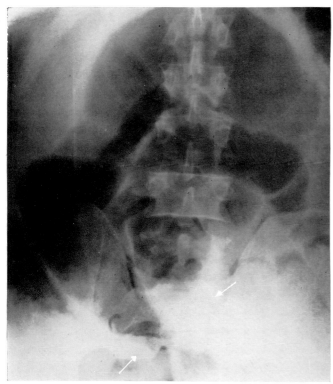

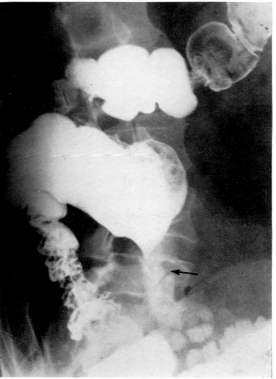

Fig. 753   Fig. 754

Fig. 753. Subacute volvulus of pelvic colon. Plain film shows considerable distension with approximation and tapering of the extremities (arrowed) of the volvulus. **Fig. 754.** Adhesion of transverse colon to a calcified node (arrowed). The right half of the transverse colon is drawn downwards causing considerable deformity.

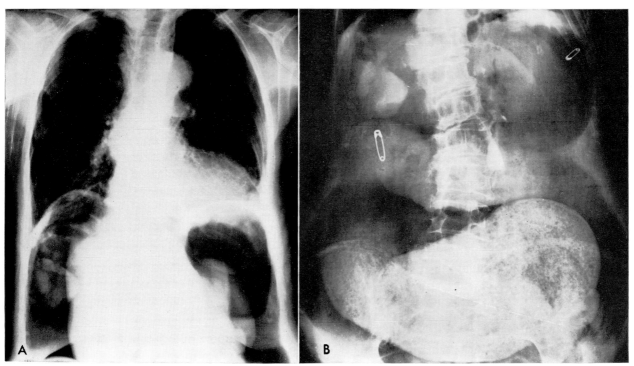

Fig. 755

Fig. 755. Rupture of caecum due to an obstruction in distal colon. A: Erect. Large pneumo-peritoneum with intra-peritoneal filling defects, especially on the right side, due to faecal material. B: Supine film. The grossly distended caecum loaded with faeces and extending to the left iliac fossa is clearly seen as it is surrounded by gas. The faecal material in the peritoneal cavity is again obvious opposite the liver.

R

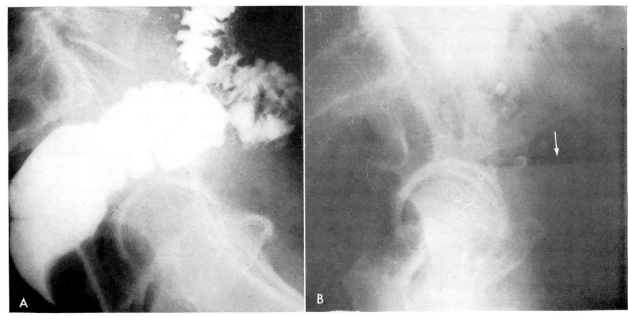

FIG. 756

Fig. 756. Diverticulitis of pelvic colon with fistula to urinary bladder. Lateral views. A: Barium enema showing gross diverticulitis of pelvic colon but no fistula. B: Following insufflation of air at sigmoidoscopy. Erect film. Air-fluid level (arrowed) clearly seen in the bladder.

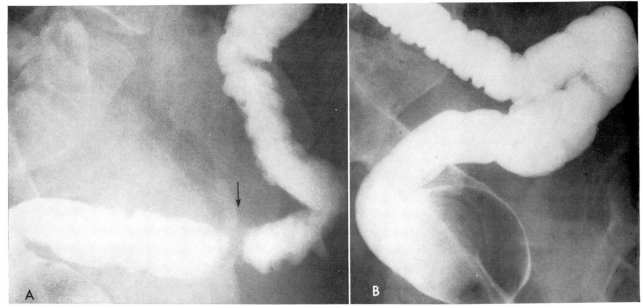

FIG. 757

Fig. 757. Spasm of upper pelvic colon initially suggesting a carcinoma. A: First barium enema. The area of spasm (arrowed) could be mistaken for a carcinoma. B: Second barium enema following intravenous injection of Buscopan. The narrowed area is no longer seen.

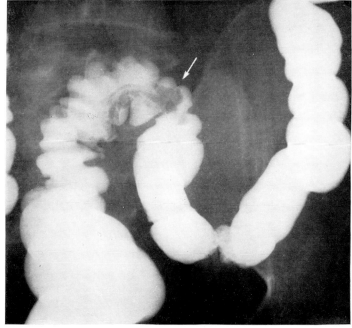

FIG. 758

Fig. 758. Polyp (arrowed) with a long stalk arising from pelvic colon. Water contrast barium enema.

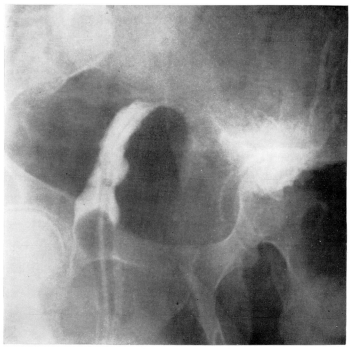

FIG. 759

Fig. 759. Recurrence of carcinoma in rectal stump. Colectomy for ulcerative colitis 15 years previously. Gastrografin enema shows a narrowed irregular rectum with fistula to abdominal wall. The amorphous opacity is Gastrografin on abdominal wall.

CHAPTER VIII

THE BILIARY TRACT

RADIOLOGICAL METHODS OF INVESTIGATION AND CLINICAL RADIOLOGY

THERE are numerous radiological methods of investigation of the biliary tract. In most instances plain films followed by oral cholecystography and intravenous cholangiography provide adequate information.

PLAIN FILMS

For most purposes the film is taken in the prone position with the right side slightly elevated. This view is also of particular value in cases of acute cholecystitis for demonstrating gas in a persistently distended duodenal bulb. The erect view is also helpful in these cases but it must be remembered that a fluid level in the duodenal bulb is present in some normal cases. To show traces of gas in the ducts the erect view is preferable.

The normal gall-bladder can occasionally be seen as a faint soft-tissue shadow below the liver margin.

ORAL CHOLECYSTOGRAPHY

This is the most important single method of investigation. It has the great merit of being simple and practically without side-effects—a mild diarrhoea being the most frequent. Many media are used but Telepaque* (each tablet containing 500 mg. iopanoic acid) is satisfactory. Some Telepaque is not absorbed and thus the colon is usually speckled with tiny radio-opaque particles. This rarely causes confusion and has the advantage of confirming that the patient has actually taken the Telepaque.

Six tablets of Telepaque, i.e. 3 g., are taken after a light supper, following which only sips of water are permitted. Using fluoroscopy for positioning, films are taken erect the following morning 12 to 14 hours later. In the female a pendulous right breast should be held up by the patient. Spot films with compression and graduated rotation are of great help. If the gall-bladder overlies the pelvis an attempt should be made to displace it upwards clear of the iliac crest when the films are taken. In cases of poor concentration television equipment is of great value in identifying the gall-bladder. Sometimes its position can be determined by giving a little barium to outline the first and second parts of the duodenum. A supine film is useful particularly to show the neck of the gall-bladder.

In many centres the examination is completed by a fatty meal—its main purpose being to estimate the ability of the gall-bladder to contract. In most cases, however, a fatty meal is superfluous because if the gall-bladder is well opacified it must have been empty beforehand. Occasionally in the contracted gall-bladder Rokitansky-Aschoff sinuses, compartmental disease, or tiny stones are more clearly demonstrated. In all cases the ducts are better and more consistently shown by intravenous Biligrafin†.

Normal Appearances

The gall-bladder is opacified 12 to 14 hours after Telepaque has been taken. The shadow of a normal gall-bladder can be clearly identified and is denser than the liver shadow. In the erect position the density is greatest at the fundus and gradually decreases towards the neck due to admixture with pre-existing non-opaque bile and mucus. Sometimes the common bile duct is faintly opacified.

Contraction occurs within half an hour following a

---

* Manufactured by The Bayer Products Company, Surbiton on Thames, England.
† Manufactured by Schering A. G., Berlin. Called Cholegrafin in the U.S.A.

fatty meal or Prosparol * and within a few minutes after injection of Pancreozymin† or cholecystokinin.

The gall-bladder may be opacified for three or more days due to re-absorption from the intestine of a proportion of the medium and its re-excretion by the liver.

Significance of the Normally Concentrating Gall-bladder

If the gall-bladder concentrates well and has a dense easily identified shadow and shows no stones or other abnormality, it is presumed to be normal.

Significance of the Poorly or Non-concentrating Gall-bladder

Concentration by the gall-bladder is considered to be poor if its shadow is faint, and at most only slightly more dense than the liver shadow.

In the great majority of cases with poor or absent concentration, certainly over 90 per cent., the gall-bladder is diseased and this is confirmed if gall-stones are present. Furthermore, if the common bile duct is opacified this indicates adequate absorption of Telepaque from the alimentary tract and satis-factory excretion by the liver and provides additional evidence of gall-bladder disease.

In the remainder, 10 per cent. or less, the gall-bladder is normal. The faint or absent shadow is then due to one of the following causes:

1. *Inadequate absorption* from (*a*) vomiting, diar-rhoea, the malabsorption syndrome, or (*b*) retention of Telepaque in duodenal or intestinal diverticula or in the stomach, e.g. from a duodenal ulcer with stenosis. In these cases the Telepaque usually forms a clump and is obvious on the films. In the stomach it causes an opaque meniscus in the erect position.

2. *Inadequate excretion* by the liver, e.g. from cirrhosis, metastases, hepatitis, most cases with jaundice. In most instances the cause is obvious from the history and/or clinical data.

ORAL CHOLANGIOGRAPHY

The medium used is Solu-Biloptin‡ (2 sachets, i.e. 6 g.). This investigation is employed in the rare instances when intravenous Biligrafin is considered

unsuitable or unsafe, e.g. history of severe sensitivity reactions. Films are taken as for an intravenous Biligrafin investigation (see below), but starting approximately three hours after the medium has been swallowed.

Normal Appearances

Solu-Biloptin is absorbed and excreted rapidly so that the ducts are outlined after three hours. The opacification however is not so dense or so consistent as that which follows intravenous Biligrafin. The gall-bladder subsequently opacifies even if its con-centrating power is lost, provided that there is no obstruction of the cystic duct or at the neck of the gall-bladder.

INTRAVENOUS CHOLANGIOGRAPHY

Forty millilitres of 50 per cent. Biligrafin are injected intravenously, the patient having been questioned and tested for sensitivity. The injection is given slowly taking 5 to 10 minutes—with a pause of approximately one minute following the injection of the first millilitre. If an allergic reaction occurs the injection is immediately stopped. Following a mild reaction, e.g. nausea or vomiting, there should be a short pause following which the injection is given very slowly.

Three films are taken half an hour after injection with the patient supine and the left side slightly elevated and with slightly differing degrees of obliquity. After inspection further films may be required until the lower end of the common bile duct is clearly shown and in many instances tomograms are necessary.

The examination is complete if adequate films of the gall-bladder opacified with Telepaque have been previously obtained. Failing this, films are taken between one and two hours after injection in the erect and supine positions. At this time the gall-bladder should be opacified provided there is no obstruction in the cystic duct or at the neck of the gall-bladder.

Contra-indications

(*a*) Known sensitivity to Biligrafin. If an intra-venous cholangiogram is considered necessary, the medium should be given under steroid cover, e.g.

* Manufactured by Duncan, Flockhart & Evans Ltd., London, England.
† Manufactured by Messrs. Boots Pure Drug Company Ltd., Nottingham, England.
‡ Manufactured by Schering A. G., Berlin.

prior injection of 100 mg. hydrocortisone intramuscularly.

(b) Severe disease of the liver, in particular hepatitis, and of the kidneys.

At the onset of jaundice from any cause, excretion of Biligrafin may be adequate for diagnostic purposes even with a serum bilirubin level up to 4 mg. per cent. When jaundice has been present for a week or so excretion is inadequate, and thus a cholangiogram should be delayed as long as possible and at least until the serum bilirubin level falls below 2 mg. per cent. Excretion is also impaired to a greater or lesser degree in certain chronic liver diseases, e.g. cirrhosis, but even so, in some cases the examination is helpful.

Normal Appearances

The ducts are well opacified half an hour after injection and after a further half-hour or so the opacification gradually diminishes. The calibre is variable but a measurement of 10 mm. in the widest part of the common bile duct is the upper limit of normal. This is at the junction of the common hepatic and common bile ducts and there is usually uniform tapering from that point to the ampulla of Vater.

Half an hour after injection a trace of Biligrafin is noted in the duodenum and the gall-bladder begins to fill. In the erect position the dense bile containing Biligrafin sinks to the fundus of the gall-bladder causing a translucent layer which may be 1 cm. thick in the middle of the gall-bladder due to pre-existing non-opaque bile and mucus.

A variable amount of Biligrafin is excreted in the urine. Care must be taken not to mistake a calyx of the right kidney or the right ureter for the common bile duct.

The appearance of the lower end of the common bile duct may change—sometimes it is sharply cut off, sometimes conical.

When Biligrafin enters the duodenum some refluxes into the bulb which can look remarkably like the gall-bladder. Careful scrutiny of the films should prevent such an error. If doubt still remains, the duodenum can be identified after the patient has swallowed a mouthful of barium.

BARIUM MEAL

This is usually performed in the investigation of cases with obstructive jaundice. Hypotonic duodeno-

graphy following intubation is sometimes helpful. Particular attention is paid to the junction of the first and second parts of the duodenum and to the shape of the duodenal loop for evidence of a tumour of the head of the pancreas. Spot films are also taken of the ampullary region to detect a carcinoma or finely calcified stone at the lower end of the common bile duct. The duodenal bulb should be carefully palpated and films taken for evidence of a penetrating posterior wall duodenal ulcer or for finger-printing indicating a carcinoma of the head of the pancreas extending up behind the duodenum.

An additional purpose of the barium meal is to detect or exclude a lesion in the oesophagus, stomach or duodenum. If gas is present in the biliary tract a search is made for a fistula.

GASTROGRAFIN MEAL

This investigation is normally carried out in suspected cases of acute cholecystitis. The prone view is of particular value.

BARIUM ENEMA

This is rarely necessary. Its main purpose is the investigation of a mass in the right hypochondrium or a suspected fistula to the colon.

PERCUTANEOUS TRANSHEPATIC CHOLANGIOGRAPHY

This procedure is carried out in the X-ray Department under television control*. The most common indication is obstructive jaundice when other methods have failed to provide adequate pre-operative information. Because of the dangers of haemorrhage or biliary peritonitis it should be performed immediately prior to surgical intervention. Furthermore, any deficiency in coagulation factors must have been rectified.

In a successful examination the exact site of the obstruction, in particular whether it is intra- or extra-hepatic can be demonstrated. A tumour of the liver near the porta hepatis displaces and narrows the ducts. Non-opaque stones show as translucencies in the ducts. An intraductal carcinoma or papilloma causes an irregular obstruction which is sometimes difficult or impossible to differentiate from a sclerosing cholangitis. In carcinoma of head of the pancreas

* See Recommended Reading, p. 267.

the obstruction is usually immediately distal to the junction of the cystic duct and common hepatic duct.

Following previous operations on the biliary tract this procedure is helpful in determining the position and calibre of the ducts and the presence or absence of stones.

OPERATIVE CHOLANGIOGRAPHY

This is performed during the course of an operation when it is considered necessary to examine the ducts further for stones or an obstruction. The injection is made into the common bile duct or the cystic duct at the discretion of the surgeon. It is an advantage to inject 1/100 gr. (0·6 mg.) atropine intravenously immediately beforehand in order to relieve any spasm of the sphincter of Oddi. The patient should be slightly rotated raising his left side. It is usually necessary to take serial films including one following removal of stones to verify that none remain.

POST-OPERATIVE CHOLANGIOGRAPHY

This examination is usually carried out on the ninth or tenth post-operative day for the purpose of excluding residual stones and to demonstrate patency of the ampulla of Vater. It is preferably performed under television control and care must be taken not to inject air bubbles. Five to ten millilitres 25 per cent. Hypaque* are injected through the T tube and two or three films taken as considered necessary. The right hepatic duct has numerous branches and is readily detected. However, the main left hepatic duct is smaller, its branches are fewer and absence of filling, e.g. from obstruction by a stone, can easily be overlooked without careful scrutiny.

Normally the ducts should not be dilated and the appearance of the lower end of the common bile duct should be as already described and no stones should be present. Medium enters the duodenum readily. Occasionally translucencies due to air bubbles are present, and should there be any difficulty in interpretation an erect film is helpful.

In 5 to 10 per cent. of cases medium enters the lower end of the pancreatic duct. Some medium may also reflux along the side of the tube into the gall-bladder bed, where bubbles of gas may also be present for several days after cholecystectomy.

Following the removal of a stone from the lower end of the common bile duct, some irregularity of the ampullary region may persist.

CONGENITAL ANOMALIES OF THE GALL-BLADDER

A *septum* may be present and is unimportant unless stasis occurs in the distal pouch causing compartmental disease (p. 265).

In *Phrygian cap deformity* the fundus is bent over the body causing a form of septum. It is of no significance.

CONGENITAL ANOMALIES OF THE DUCTS

A *choledochal cyst* is a rare abnormality and usually arises from the common bile duct. The cyst may be large requiring surgical intervention. Intravenous cholangiography is necessary for its demonstration.

An *accessory right hepatic duct* is a common anomaly and its recognition is important as it could be mistaken at operation for the cystic duct.

Occasionally the junction between the cystic duct and common bile duct is low down near the ampulla of Vater in the head of the pancreas. In some cases the cystic duct passes behind the common hepatic duct entering it from the left side.

The common bile duct may enter a duodenal diverticulum. If infection or fibrosis occurs in this diverticulum, obstructive jaundice may follow.

DISEASES AND ABNORMALITIES
Gall-stones

Stones are the most common abnormality found in the biliary tract.

Calcified Gall-stones. Approximately 40 per cent. of gall-stones are calcified and can be seen on a plain film. They may be single or multiple. When multiple they are commonly of approximately the same size but occasionally there may be one or two large stones and several smaller ones indicating that they have been produced at different periods. A large stone usually has concentric rings of calcification and sometimes a calcified dot in the centre. In other cases the stones contain gas-filled clefts which cause fine stellate translucencies. When films are taken

---

* Manufactured by The Bayer Products Company, Surbiton on Thames, England.

in the erect and supine positions the relative position of the stones may vary. When multiple and large they may be faceted. Care should always be taken to look for stones in the common bile duct.

Calcified costal cartilages, calcification in an appendix epiploica or stones in the right kidney may cause confusion. Oblique views are helpful but usually it is necessary and desirable to carry out an oral cholecystogram and an intravenous cholangiogram.

In cases of jaundice a finely calcified stone may be demonstrated at the lower end of the common bile duct on a barium meal. This stone may escape detection on a plain film but can be located accurately by an unchanging position in relation to the second part of the duodenum.

Occasionally a calcified stone in the gall-bladder may be masked on a cholecystogram because of similar density to the contrast medium. Thus plain films beforehand are of the utmost importance. If the density of the medium in the gall-bladder is altered by taking a film in the supine position and thereby mixing the dense and translucent gall-bladder content the stone may then be demonstrated.

Non-opaque Stones. Occasionally a non-opaque stone can be seen on a plain film because it contains gas-filled clefts (the Mercedes star appearance). Even more rarely a large cholesterol stone may be detected by being slightly more translucent than the neighbouring soft tissues.

Translucent stones in the gall-bladder can be demonstrated by an oral cholecystogram provided that the concentration is adequate. They tend to congregate together and sink to the fundus of the gall-bladder in the erect position. In some cases the stones float causing a translucent band in the middle of the gall-bladder while in others floating and sinking stones co-exist.

Translucent stones in the gall-bladder may be demonstrated following intravenous Biligrafin when an oral cholecystogram has failed to opacify the gall-bladder. This is because the Biligrafin excreted by the liver is sufficiently dense and does not require concentration by the gall-bladder to demonstrate such stones as filling defects. In these cases erect films with compression several hours after the injection, when the medium has been allowed to settle, are helpful.

By giving Telepaque over a period of several days

a non-opaque stone may occasionally be rendered opaque by the adsorption of opaque medium on its surface. This is an inconsistent finding and not a procedure to be recommended as a routine.

To detect non-opaque stones in the ducts an intravenous cholangiogram is necessary. When the excretion is adequate they show as translucent filling defects and dilatation of the ducts is usually, though not always, present. Failure of opacification of the gall-bladder when the ducts are shown is definite evidence of cystic duct obstruction or obstruction of the neck of the gall-bladder, usually by a stone.

Care must be taken not to mistake bubbles of gas caught up in the mucosal folds of the duodenum and overlying the duct for translucent stones. In cases of doubt tomograms are most helpful. Very occasionally stones, in particular non-opaque stones, disappear from the gall-bladder or ducts. The most likely explanation is that they have been passed.

Residual Stones. In a few instances stones are left behind in the ducts following operation. On a post-operative cholangiogram they show as persistent translucencies. Care must be taken to scrutinise the ducts proximal to the T tube, in particular the left hepatic duct.

Calcified Sludge (Limey Bile)

This causes a granular opacity which gravitates to the fundus in the erect position. It may pass into the cystic duct and common bile duct and thence into the duodenum. It may be present in association with stones.

Calcification of the Gall-bladder (Porcelain Gall-bladder)

This usually has a characteristic egg-shell appearance but in some cases on a plain film may simulate a large gall-stone. Following intravenous Biligrafin the gall-bladder fills with medium unless the cystic duct is blocked by a stone.

Gas in the Biliary Tract

An erect film of the abdomen is of particular value in the demonstration of gas.

CAUSES:

1. (*a*) Previous sphincterotomy of the sphincter of Oddi. (*b*) A functioning anastomosis between the

gall-bladder or common bile duct and the duodenum or jejunum. Following such operations disappearance of the gas indicates blockage of the stoma usually by a stone or stricture and is associated with jaundice, fever, pain, etc.

2. Incompetence of the sphincter of Oddi from the recent passage of a stone.

3. Perforation of an empyema of the gall-bladder into the bowel causing a fistula.

4. Gall-stone ileus—the gall-stone having ulcerated into the duodenum or jejunum.

5. In rare instances the gas is due to intestinal obstruction from other causes—the gas having been forced up by the high intra-duodenal pressure alone.

6. Distortion of the ampulla of Vater from a second part duodenal ulcer or carcinoma.

7. Infection of the gall-bladder by gas-forming organisms.

The gas is usually restricted to the larger ducts and the gall-bladder. Thus, the differentiation from gas in the portal circulation is relatively easy since in the latter instance the gas extends almost to the periphery of the liver.

In most cases when gas is present, barium refluxes into the biliary tract at a barium meal. A barium enema is usually necessary to demonstrate a fistula to the colon.

Infection of the Gall-bladder and Ducts

Acute Cholecystitis. Plain films may show (a) a soft-tissue shadow below the liver; and/or (b) gall-stones, especially one in the region of the neck of the gall-bladder; and/or (c) persistent distension of the duodenal bulb with gas in the prone position and with a fluid level in the erect position. It must be remembered that in some cases especially in long thin individuals a fluid level may normally be present in the duodenal bulb in the erect position.

It is recommended that the next stage in investigation is a Gastrografin meal since this, in addition to giving additional evidence of an acute cholecystitis, helps to exclude a perforated peptic ulcer and an acute pancreatitis (pp. 95 and 309). Furthermore an immediate diagnosis can usually be made.

Following a Gastrografin meal the main radiological features of acute cholecystitis are (a) persistent narrowing immediately distal to the bulb due to oedema or spasm from the adjacent inflamed gall-bladder, (b) persistent distension of the bulb, and

(c) sometimes an unusually patent pylorus. The prone position in particular is of value in demonstrating these features. Sometimes the gall-bladder lies more laterally in which case the narrowing affects the upper part of the second part of the duodenum. More rarely the distended gall-bladder overlies the antrum causing a filling defect simulating a carcinoma.

In some cases an intravenous Biligrafin examination may be performed. This has the disadvantage of being time-consuming, requiring an ill patient to be in the X-ray Department for more than two hours. In addition, excretion of Biligrafin in these cases is commonly poor. Films are taken in the usual manner, but particular attention should be paid to the film two hours after injection. A common finding then is non-opacification of the gall-bladder due to obstruction of the cystic duct. Less commonly the gall-bladder slowly fills with Biligrafin demonstrating numerous translucent stones.

If untreated an acute cholecystitis may progress to a frank empyema with increasing size of the soft-tissue shadow and elevation of the right dome of diaphragm. The empyema may rupture into the bowel causing gas in the gall-bladder.

Mucocoele of the Gall-bladder. In some instances where the infection is less severe a mucocoele develops. It causes a soft-tissue shadow below the liver and a stone may be seen at the neck of the gall-bladder.

Subacute and Chronic Cholecystitis. These are associated with poor or absent concentration on oral cholecystography. Stones may also be present.

Following intravenous Biligrafin, the following appearances may be noted:

1. The gall-bladder fills with Biligrafin but there is little or no increase in the density of the shadow.

2. Non-opaque gall-stones may be demonstrated in the gall-bladder.

3. The gall-bladder does not become opacified. When the ducts are opacified this always indicates an obstruction of the cystic duct or of the neck of the gall-bladder, usually by a stone.

A barium meal occasionally shows some distortion and narrowing of the duodenal bulb or post-bulbar region, caused by adhesions.

Compartmental Disease. In this condition there is a septum present with infection in the distal pouch which usually contains stones. This compartment does not opacify if the communication with the main body of the gall-bladder is blocked, e.g. by a stone, and the erroneous diagnosis of a normal gall-bladder might be made. Sometimes the blockage is intermittent. Usually, however, the distal pouch opacifies rendering non-opaque stones obvious.

Cholesterosis (*'Strawberry' Gall-bladder*). Doubt exists as to whether this is an infection or a metabolic disorder but it is convenient to discuss it at this point. The gall-bladder concentrates well on oral cholecystography. The marginal translucent filling defects caused by the localised swellings in the gall-bladder wall are seen on spot films with compression of good quality. Stones may also be present.

Rokitansky-Aschoff Sinuses (*Cholecystitis Glandularis Proliferans*). The gall-bladder usually concentrates well on oral cholecystography and a variable number of small diverticula are present especially at the fundus. These cause a double contour usually more clearly shown following a fatty meal.

Cholangitis. Radiology plays little part in diagnosis in the acute stage. In the subacute stage an intravenous cholangiogram sometimes shows spasm or irregularity of the common bile duct. Rarely part of the wall sloughs off causing a filling defect simulating a stone.

Strictures of the Common Bile Duct

The most common form is at the extreme lower end in association with stones or following the removal of stones. The most likely cause is mild chronic infection.

Intravenous cholangiography shows obvious stasis in the ducts so that they are well opacified even after four hours. The stricture may involve a short segment or a considerable length of the common bile duct. Tomograms are of great value in demonstrating the stricture and differentiating it from stones or non-opaque debris. Sometimes a stricture reforms after sphincterotomy in which case there is an absence of gas in the biliary tract. In all cases a search should be made for gall-stones which are commonly present proximal to the stricture.

A stone or a stricture may be present at the origin of the left hepatic duct causing obstruction with dilatation proximally. If the obstruction is complete there is absence of filling and this can easily be missed without careful scrutiny.

The common bile duct is narrowed often markedly so by a carcinoma of the head of the pancreas and sometimes by chronic pancreatitis (pp. 310 and 311), in particular calcific pancreatitis.

Sclerosing Cholangitis

In this condition there is a progressive fibrosis with narrowing of the ducts, both extra- and intrahepatic, with dilatation proximally. It is difficult or impossible to differentiate from diffuse malignant papillomatosis. The fibrosis may start at the lower end of the common bile duct or at the porta hepatis. Only in early cases is an intravenous cholangiogram of help because of the subsequent development of obstructive jaundice. The stenosis can later be shown by a percutaneous or an operative or postoperative cholangiogram.

Cystic Duct Remnant

Only rarely does this cause symptoms. When excretion of Biligrafin is adequate the remnant can be outlined but tomograms are usually necessary to show dilatation or residual stones.

Adhesions

In chronic cholecystitis, adhesions sometimes form around the gall-bladder. These may cause deformity of the gall-bladder, especially at the fundus—demonstrated by intravenous Biligrafin. In some cases a barium meal shows distortion and narrowing of the duodenum especially distal to the bulb.

Fistulae

A fistula may form by rupture of an acutely inflamed gall-bladder or empyema of the gall-bladder into the bowel, usually the duodenum or the hepatic flexure of the colon. Gas is present in the biliary tract. The gall-bladder and ducts may be outlined by a barium meal when a fistula to the duodenum is present, but to demonstrate a cholecysto-colic fistula a barium enema is usually necessary.

Fistulae to other organs are rare.

Post-cholecystectomy Syndrome

The symptoms in many cases labelled as such are due to previously unrecognised disease such as hiatus hernia, diverticulitis, duodenal ulcer. In some cases, however, there is a stricture at the lower end of the common bile duct with or without recent or residual stones. Only rarely is a stone in a cystic duct remnant found.

An intravenous cholangiogram is the diagnostic method of choice in the first instance. For further investigation a barium meal or barium enema may be necessary.

Vagotomy and Post-gastrectomy Sequelae

Following these operations some dilatation of the gall-bladder with stasis commonly occurs. It is this which presumably predisposes to the development of gall-stones and acute or chronic cholecystitis—complications which are now being more frequently recognised.

Tumours

Polypi in the Gall-bladder. On oral cholecystography these show as smooth persistent filling defects in a well concentrating gall-bladder. A stone adherent to the gall-bladder wall has a similar appearance.

An adenomyoma usually occurs at the fundus of the gall-bladder. Characteristically it causes a smooth filling defect with a dimple in the middle simulating an ulcer.

Papillomatosis of the Ducts. This condition is of very low malignancy and causes irregular obstruction with dilatation proximally. It is difficult or impossible to differentiate from sclerosing cholangitis.

Carcinoma of the Gall-bladder. Usually the gall-bladder can be opacified only following intravenous Biligrafin because of co-existing chronic cholecystitis. The tumour causes an irregular filling defect in the gall-bladder. Stones are commonly present and sometimes the gall-bladder wall is calcified. When the gall-bladder is enlarged a barium meal shows deformity and displacement of the adjacent part of the duodenum.

Carcinoma of the Common Bile Duct. This generally occurs at the extreme lower end and less commonly at a higher level. Because of the presence of jaundice an intravenous cholangiogram is pointless except at a very early stage. A barium meal is performed in the first instance and spot films of the ampullary region should always be taken. These may show the presence of a filling defect or mucosal destruction. A percutaneous transhepatic cholangiogram will demonstrate an obstruction at the site of the tumour.

RECOMMENDED READING

SHALDON, S., BARBER, K. M. and YOUNG, W. B. (1962). Percutaneous transhepatic cholangiography. A modified technique. *Gastroenterology*, **42**, 371-379.

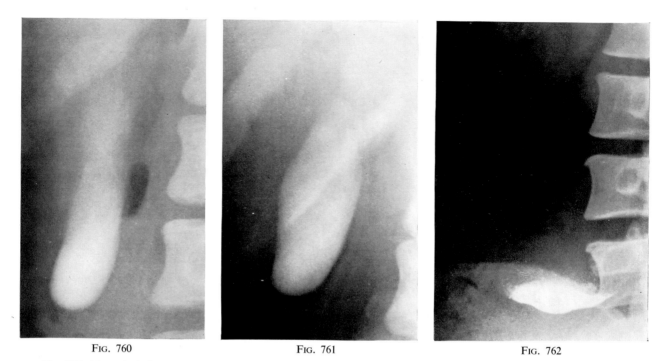

FIG. 760   FIG. 761   FIG. 762

Fig. 760. Normal cholecystogram 13 hours after Telepaque. Erect film positioned with fluoroscopic control. Dense gall-bladder shadow easily identifiable and becoming fainter towards its neck. **Fig. 761.** Normal cholecystogram 13 hours after Telepaque. Erect film positioned with fluoroscopic control. Gall-bladder shadow getting less dense near the neck. Common bile duct of normal calibre and faintly opacified even without a fatty meal. It is situated immediately medial to the gall-bladder. **Fig. 762.** Non-opacification of gall-bladder due to retention of Telepaque in the stomach. Erect film 14 hours after Telepaque which has formed a dense meniscus in the pyloric antrum. Previous vagotomy and pyloroplasty with gastric stasis.

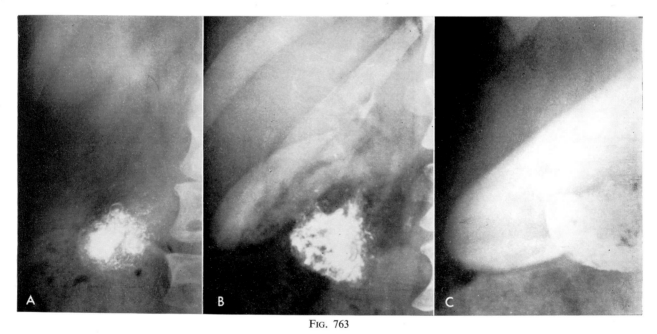

FIG. 763

Fig. 763. Absence of opacification of gall-bladder due to non-absorption of Telepaque—initially suggesting gall-bladder disease. A: Film 14 hours after Telepaque. The gall-bladder is not shown. Dense granular opacity due to retained Telepaque in the stomach. Subsequent barium meal showed a chronic duodenal ulcer with stenosis and a large gastric residue. B: One hour after injection of Biligrafin. Supine film. Excretion good. Ducts of normal calibre. Gall-bladder partially filled and presents a normal appearance. C: One hour after injection of Biligrafin. Erect film. Gall-bladder partially filled. Normal translucent zone near the fundus due to pre-existing non-opaque bile and mucus.

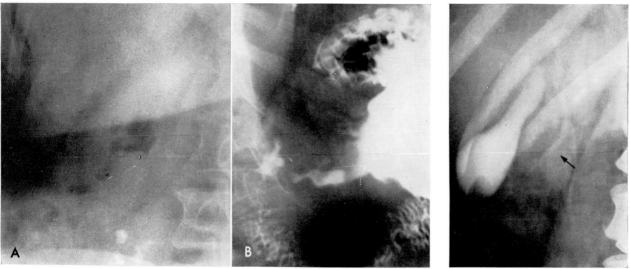

Fig. 764   Fig. 765

Fig. 764. Non-opacification of gall-bladder due to the patient having vomited the Telepaque. A: Plain film 14 hours after Telepaque. The gall-bladder is not shown. No obvious Telepaque in stomach or colon. Calcified lymph nodes in lower abdomen. B: Barium meal the following day. Large ulcerated filling defect in the antrum with gross narrowing due to a carcinoma. Prone film. (Print reversed.)

Fig. 765. Normal intravenous cholangiogram half an hour after injection of Biligrafin and 14 hours after Telepaque by mouth. Supine film. Normal common bile duct (arrowed). Some excretion by the right kidney—a common finding. Care must be taken not to mistake a calyx of the right kidney or the right ureter (which is faintly opacified) for the common bile duct.

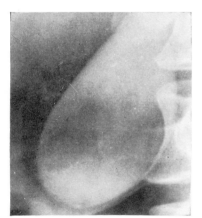

Fig. 766

Fig. 766. Normal intravenous cholangiogram. Erect film of gall-bladder 1½ hours after injection. Translucent area in the middle of the gall-bladder due to pre-existing non-opaque bile and mucus.

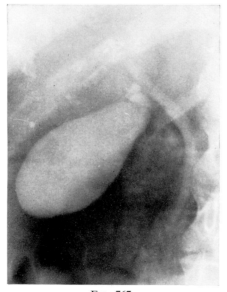

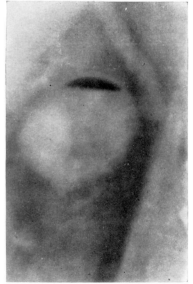

Fig. 767   Fig. 768

Fig. 767. Normal intravenous cholangiogram. Two-hour supine film. Normal gall-bladder and ducts. Faint opacification of duodenal loop by Biligrafin.

Fig. 768. Opacification of duodenal bulb with Biligrafin. Two hours after injection. Erect film. Normal common bile duct. The duodenal bulb contains an air-fluid level making its identification certain. On the supine film the duodenal bulb mimicked the gall-bladder.

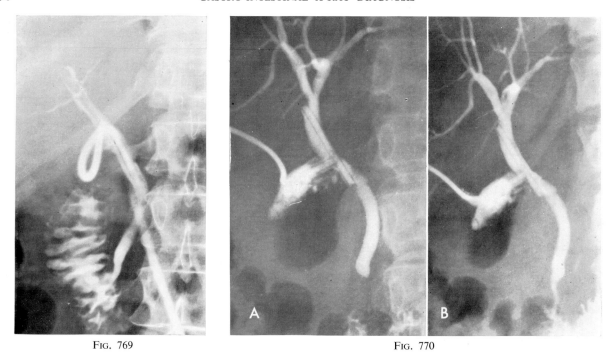

FIG. 769   FIG. 770

Fig. 769. Normal tapered lower end of common bile duct. Post-operative cholangiogram. Medium enters the duodenum satisfactorily. Only minimal filling proximal to the tube—an occasional finding. **Fig. 770.** Changing appearances of lower end of common bile duct. A: Post-operative cholangiogram. The lower end is sharply cut off. This is a common transient finding. B: A few seconds later. Tapering lower extremity—within normal limits. Reflux of medium along the side of the T tube into the gall-bladder bed—a relatively common finding.

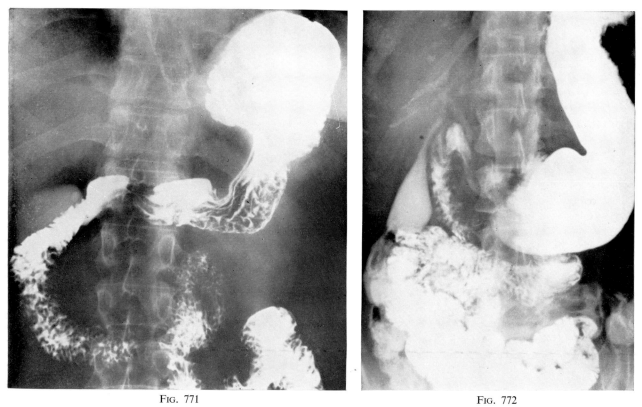

FIG. 771   FIG. 772

Fig. 771. Cholecystogram and barium meal. Supine film showing position of gall-bladder in relation to duodenum. Small calcified stone present at neck of gall-bladder. Normal stomach and duodenum. **Fig. 772.** Gall-bladder still opacified 72 hours after Telepaque. Supine film. Contraction of the gall-bladder had occurred immediately prior to the film causing opacification of the common bile duct.

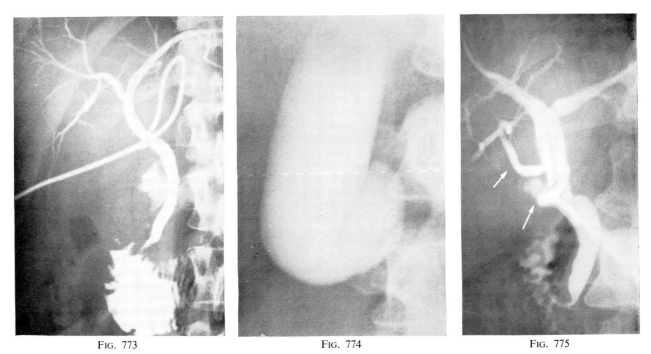

FIG. 773   FIG. 774   FIG. 775

Fig. 773. Post-operative cholangiogram. Normal. Medium enters the duodenum satisfactorily and some has refluxed into the duodenal bulb. **Fig. 774.** Phrygian cap deformity of gall-bladder—of no significance. The fundus of the gall-bladder is bent over causing a form of septum. 14 hours after Telepaque. **Fig. 775.** Accessory right hepatic duct (top arrow). Cystic duct remnant also present (lower arrow). Post-operative cholangiogram. A little dilatation of the ducts. Medium enters the duodenum satisfactorily. No calculi seen.

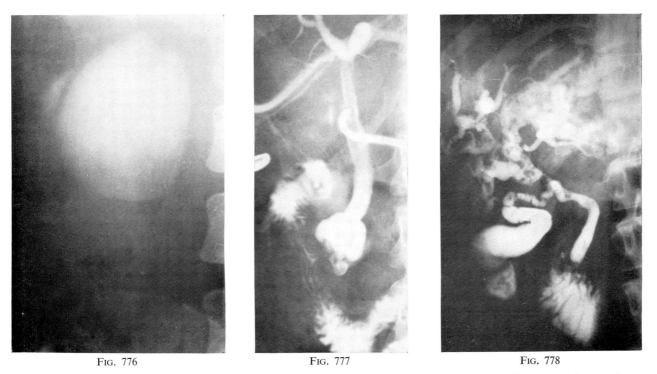

FIG. 776   FIG. 777   FIG. 778

Fig. 776. Choledochal cyst. Four hours after injection of Biligrafin. The large cyst is well opacified. Operative proof. **Fig. 777.** Common bile duct entering duodenal diverticulum. Post-operative cholangiogram. **Fig. 778.** Congenital anomaly of intrahepatic ducts with dilatation, tortuosity and irregularity. Patient subsequently developed gross cirrhosis of the liver with oesophageal and gastric varices. Post-operative cholangiogram.

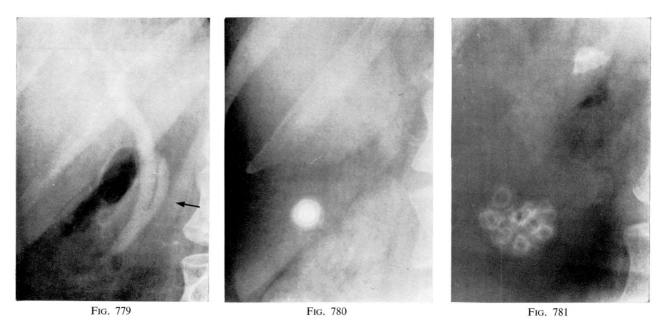

FIG. 779   FIG. 780   FIG. 781

Fig. 779. Low insertion of cystic duct into common bile duct. Half an hour after injection of intravenous Biligrafin. The cystic duct (arrowed) enters the common bile duct on its medial aspect having passed behind the common hepatic duct.

Fig. 780. Calcified gall-stone in gall-bladder with characteristic concentric rings.

Fig. 781. Numerous stones in fundus of gall-bladder and one at its neck. Oral cholecystogram 14 hours after Telepaque. The gall-bladder is not opacified due partly to co-existing chronic cholecystitis but mainly to obstruction at its neck.

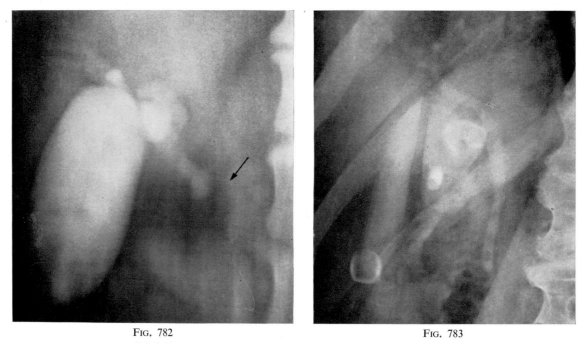

FIG. 782   FIG. 783

Fig. 782. Anomalous position of cystic artery causing indentation of common bile duct. Operative proof. Tomographic cut 2 hours after injection of Biligrafin and 14 hours after Telepaque. Curious obstruction (arrowed) in common bile duct the nature of which radiologically was not certain. Numerous translucent gall-stones in gall-bladder.

Fig. 783. Calcified stones in gall-bladder which did not concentrate Telepaque or opacify with Biligrafin. Film 14 hours after Telepaque and half an hour after Biligrafin injection. The common bile duct is of normal calibre. The translucencies opposite the common bile duct are due to bubbles of gas trapped in mucosal folds in the duodenum and do not represent non-opaque stones. The long vertical translucency is due to a skin fold. Good nephrogram of right kidney.

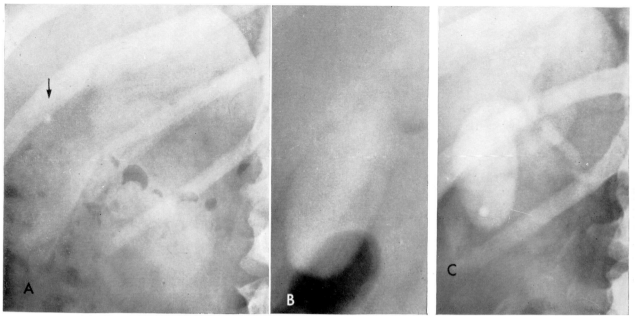

FIG. 784

Fig. 784. Small calcified stone in gall-bladder. ' A: Plain film. The stone (arrowed) could readily be mistaken for calcification in a costal cartilage. B: Oral cholecystogram. Erect film. The stone is not seen as it is obscured by opaque medium of approximately the same density. C: Supine film half an hour after injection of Biligrafin and immediately following the oral cholecystogram. The stone is seen in the gall-bladder due to mixing of the gall-bladder content resulting in a change in its opacification. Normal ducts.

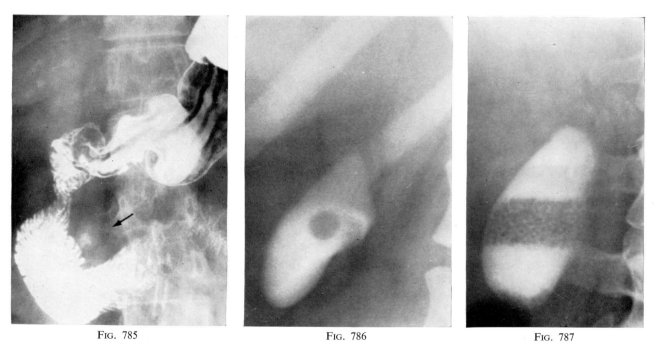

FIG. 785   FIG. 786   FIG. 787

Fig. 785. Gall-stone (arrowed) at lower end of common bile duct—located by barium meal. Case of deep jaundice and thus cholecystography and cholangiography were contra-indicated.

Fig. 786. Solitary non-opaque translucent floating stone. Oral cholecystogram with good concentration. Erect film. The decreased translucency near the neck of the gall-bladder is clearly seen—the characteristic finding in normally concentrating gall-bladders.

Fig. 787. Co-existing floating and sinking stones in gall-bladder. Oral cholecystogram 14 hours after Telepaque. Erect.

S

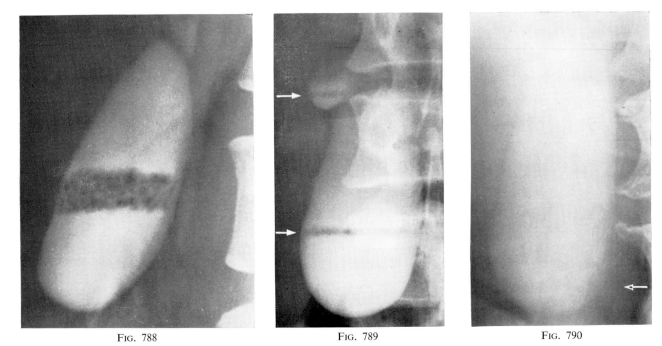

FIG. 788   FIG. 789   FIG. 790

Fig. 788. Non-opaque floating stones demonstrated by oral cholecystogram. Erect film shows a large number of non-opaque stones causing an irregular translucent band in the middle of the gall-bladder.

Fig. 789. Cholecystogram showing floating gall-stones (arrowed) in gall-bladder and in Hartmann's pouch. Erect film 14 hours after Telepaque.

Fig. 790. Dilatation with stasis in gall-bladder with stones, following partial gastrectomy and vagotomy. Erect film 14 hours after Telepaque. Enlarged gall-bladder with poor opacification and layer of floating stones (arrowed) just visible near the fundus.

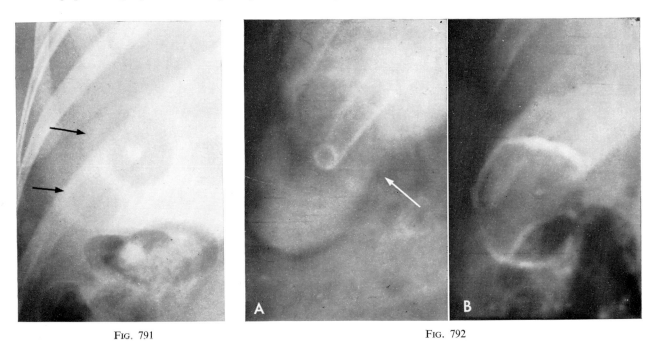

FIG. 791   FIG. 792

Fig. 791. Non-opaque cholesterol stones (arrowed). Oral cholecystogram with poor concentration. On a plain film of gall-bladder area they were just able to be detected because of their increased translucency (similar to fat). One of the stones has a calcified central nucleus making its identification easy

Fig. 792. Gall-stone opacified following Telepaque given for four days. A: 14 hours after first dose of Telepaque, the gall-bladder is faintly opacified and shows a large non-opaque stone (arrowed). B: After four administrations of Telepaque. The rim of the gall-stone is opacified due to adsorption of the medium.

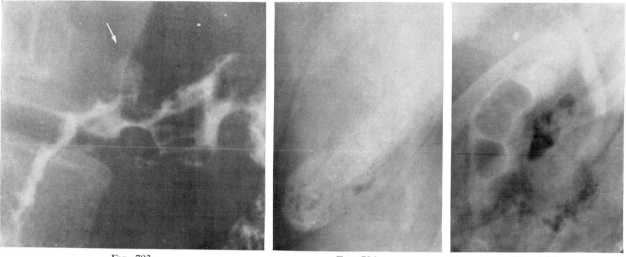

FIG. 793   FIG. 794   FIG. 795

Fig. 793. Barium meal showing deformity of duodenal bulb due to adhesions from the gall-bladder. Case of chronic chole-cystitis with gall-stone (arrowed) in gall-bladder.

Fig. 794. Multiple non-opaque stones in gall-bladder. Erect film 14 hours after Telepaque. The gall-bladder concentrates poorly suggesting that it is pathological. Two years prior to this examination a solitary stone had been removed from the gall-bladder. Because the gall-bladder appeared healthy cholecystectomy at that time was not performed.

Fig. 795. Five or six large non-opaque stones in gall-bladder demonstrated by intravenous Biligrafin. Two-hour film. On a previous occasion the gall-bladder did not concentrate Telepaque suggesting it was pathological. Thus the diagnosis suspected on oral cholecystography was confirmed by an intravenous cholangiogram. Normal common bile duct.

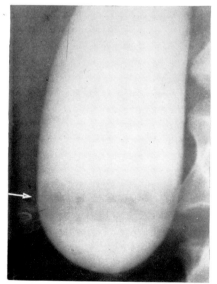

FIG. 796

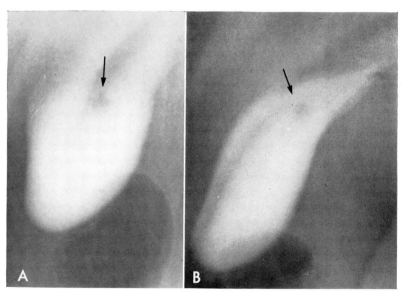

FIG. 797

Fig. 796. Translucent stones in gall-bladder. Erect film two hours after intravenous Biligrafin. Translucent band near fundus due to pre-existing non-opaque bile and mucus and partially opacified by mixture with Biligrafin. There are a number of trans-lucent stones (arrowed) in this band. Operative confirmation.

Fig. 797. Small floating stone in gall-bladder. Previous pyloroplasty and vagotomy for duodenal ulcer. A: Erect film 14 hours after Telepaque. Translucency (arrowed) seen near the interface between opacified bile and pre-existing non-opaque bile and mucus. B: As a polyp could not be excluded the patient was turned on her back to mix the bile and mucus then returned to the erect position. The translucency (arrowed) due to the stone is in a different position.

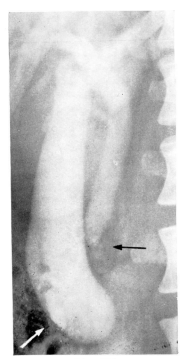

Fig. 798

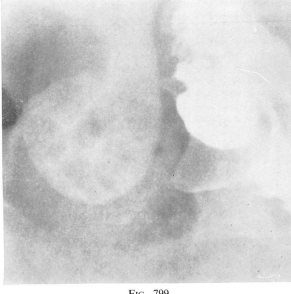

Fig. 799

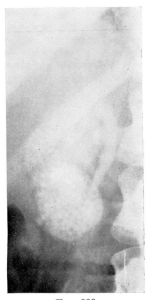

Fig. 800

Fig. 798. Calcified stone (arrowed) at lower end of common bile duct causing some dilatation. Calcified debris (arrowed) in gall-bladder. Two-hour film following Biligrafin. **Fig. 799.** Poorly functioning gall-bladder with multiple non-opaque stones. Erect film 13 hours after Telepaque. The gall-bladder could not be identified on fluoroscopy but its position was localised by giving a little barium and outlining the duodenal bulb. In addition, firm compression had to be applied to displace the gall-bladder out of the pelvis. If possible the films of the gall-bladder should be obtained clear of the ilium. **Fig. 800.** Multiple stones in gall-bladder shown by intravenous Biligrafin. The mottled appearance in the supine position is characteristic but the stones were even more clearly seen when erect. Normal common bile duct.

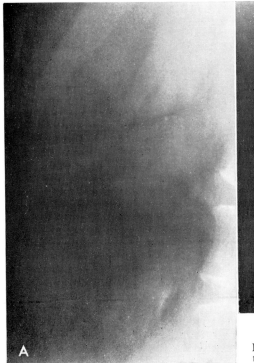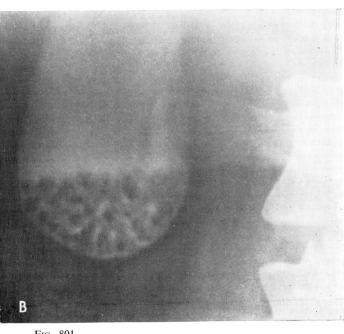

Fig. 801

Fig. 801. A: Cholecystogram. Non-functioning gall-bladder suggesting that it is pathological. B: Two-hour film following intravenous Biligrafin. The gall-bladder has been outlined by Biligrafin and shows a number of non-opaque stones in the fundus of the gall-bladder—confirming disease. Erect film positioned by fluoroscopy.

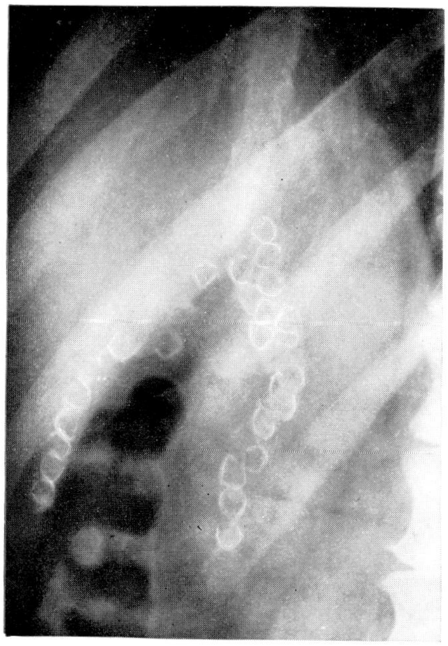

FIG. 802

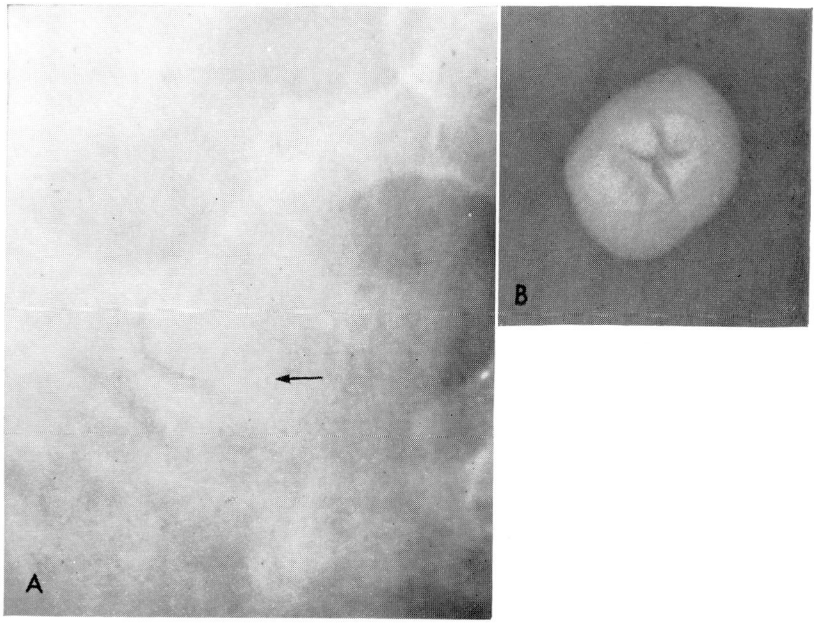

FIG. 803

Fig. 802. Numerous calcified and faceted gall-stones in common bile duct, common hepatic duct, cystic duct and gall-bladder.

Fig. 803. Gall-stone showing Mercedes star appearance due to gas-filled clefts. A: Plain film. Magnified print. The stone (arrowed) containing gas-filled clefts is clearly seen. B: X-ray of stone after removal.

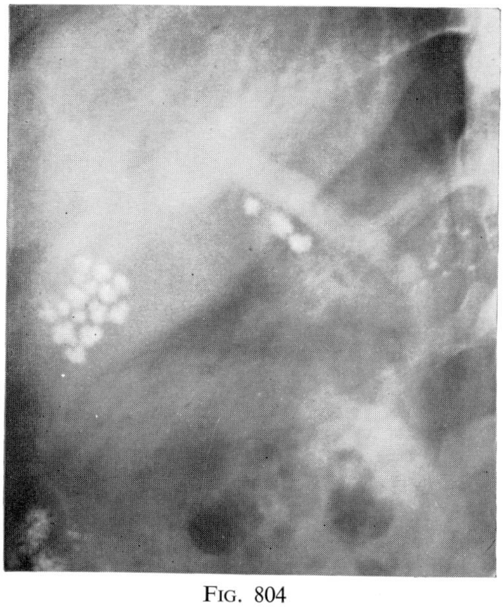

FIG. 804

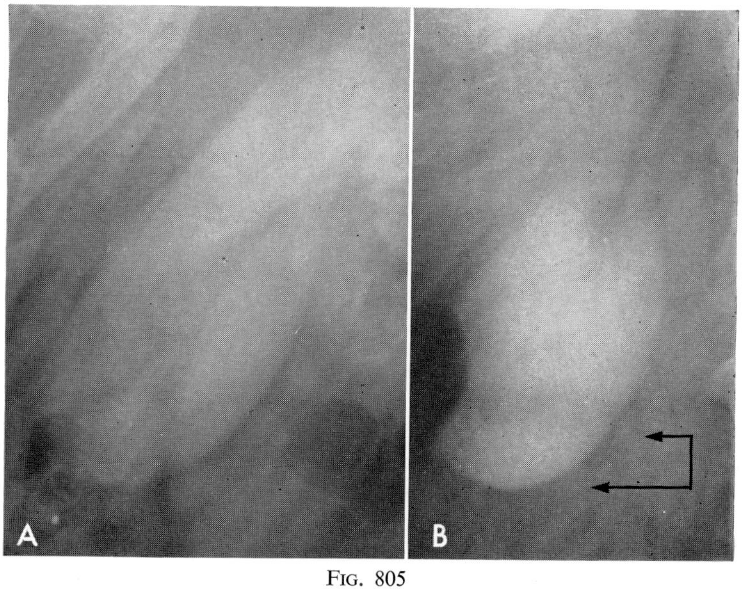

FIG. 805

Fig. 804. Calcified gall-stones in gall-bladder and in cystic duct—the latter causing obstruction, and preventing Telepaque and Biligrafin from entering the gall-bladder. Two-hour film following injection of intravenous Biligrafin, and 14 hours after Telepaque. The common bile and common hepatic ducts are of normal calibre and contain no stones. Particles of unabsorbed Telepaque in the colon (normal).

Fig. 805. Multiple finely calcified stones in gall-bladder. A: Supine view. The stones are invisible. Two hours after injection of Biligrafin. B: Erect. The stones (arrowed) are faintly seen having collected in the fundus of the gall-bladder. The gall-bladder did not concentrate Telepaque on a previous oral cholecystogram.

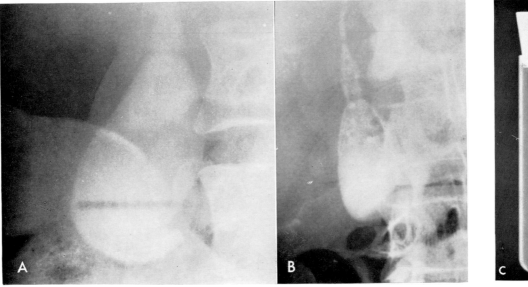

FIG. 806

Fig. 806. Multiple non-opaque stones in gall-bladder. A: Oral cholecystogram 13 hours after Telepaque. Erect. Translucent band due to multiple non-opaque stones. B: Plain film, supine, 3½ months after Telepaque and intravenous Biligrafin. Persistent opacification of gall-bladder with numerous translucent stones near its neck. Cholecystectomy performed with removal of stones. The gall-bladder content was of a tarry consistency and this material had also blocked the cystic duct. This blockage must have occurred immediately following the Telepaque and Biligrafin and thus the stones had been bathed in these media for 3½ months. C: X-ray of stones surrounded by water in a test tube. The stones are not seen and although surrounded by Telepaque and Biligrafin for 3½ months, no medium had become adsorbed on their surfaces.

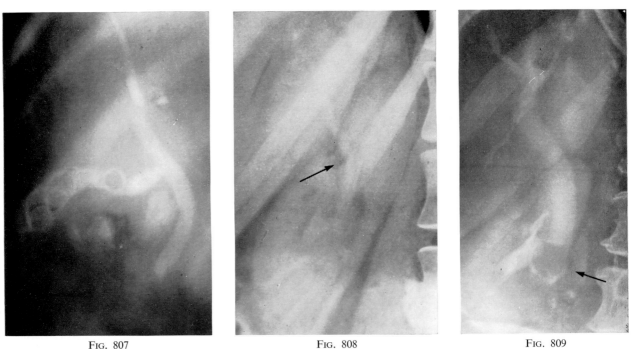

FIG. 807   FIG. 808   FIG. 809

Fig. 807. Non-opaque stones in gall-bladder without cystic duct obstruction. Tomogram two hours after injection of intravenous Biligrafin. Ducts and gall-bladder well opacified. **Fig. 808.** Oral cholecystogram showing non-functioning gall-bladder suggesting that it is pathological. Faint opacification of common bile and common hepatic ducts (arrowed) proving that the Telepaque has been absorbed and excreted in adequate amounts. This indicates an obstruction of the cystic duct (proved at operation to be due to a stone). **Fig. 809.** Dilated common bile duct with non-opaque stone (arrowed) near its lower end. Two-hour film after injection of Biligrafin. The gall-bladder did not fill due to obstruction of the neck of the gall-bladder by another non-opaque stone. Good excretion of Biligrafin by the right kidney. (Care must always be taken not to mistake a calyx or the ureter for the common bile duct.)

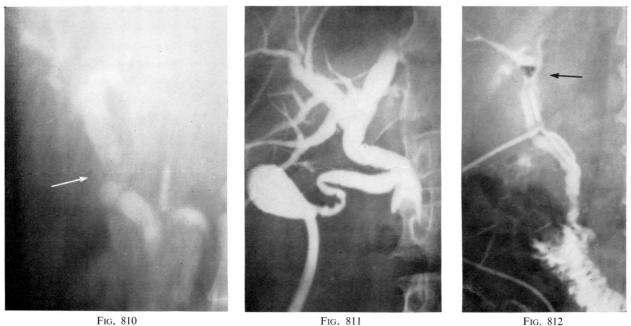

FIG. 810   FIG. 811   FIG. 812

Fig. 810. Residual non-opaque stone (arrowed) in common bile duct with a little dilatation of ducts and slight narrowing at lower end of common bile duct. Tomogram one hour after injection of intravenous Biligrafin. The stone was obscured by overlying bowel shadows on the ordinary film without tomography. Previous cholecystectomy. **Fig. 811.** Non-opaque stone obstructing the common bile duct with dilatation proximally. Operative cholangiogram. Patient presented with deepening jaundice. **Fig. 812.** Residual faceted non-opaque stone (arrowed) in common hepatic duct proximal to the T tube. Medium enters the duodenum satisfactorily. Post-operative cholangiogram. In all cases the ducts proximal to the T tube must be carefully scrutinised.

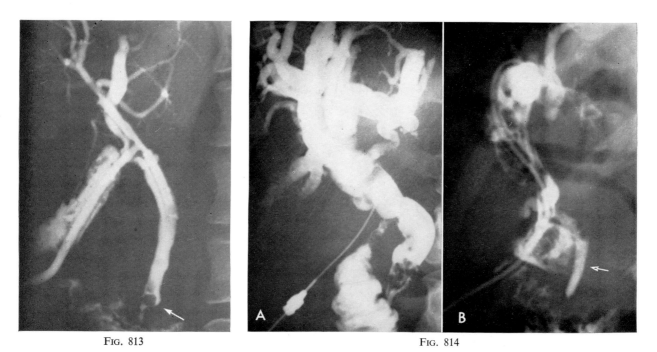

FIG. 813   FIG. 814

Fig. 813. Residual stone (arrowed) at lower end of common bile duct. The two translucencies slightly proximal to this are air bubbles—proved by their later disappearance. Some dilatation of left hepatic duct. Medium has leaked into the gall-bladder bed along the side of the tube—a not uncommon finding. Post-operative cholangiogram. **Fig. 814.** Gross dilatation of bile and hepatic ducts which contain calculi and debris. A: Percutaneous transhepatic cholangiogram. Stones near lower end of common bile duct and in the ducts within the liver. B: Post-operative cholangiogram one month later following removal of stones, sphincterotomy of the sphincter of Oddi, and choledocho-duodenostomy. Unusually marked reduction in calibre of the ducts, in particular of the common bile duct (arrowed).

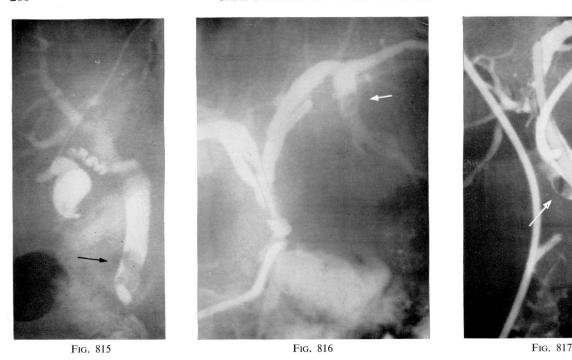

FIG. 815   FIG. 816   FIG. 817

Fig. 815. Large non-opaque stone (arrowed) at lower end of common bile duct. Some dilatation of common bile duct. At previous laparotomy for obstructive jaundice, the gall-bladder was drained. A trace of medium has entered the lower end of the pancreatic duct. Post-operative cholangiogram. **Fig. 816.** Residual non-opaque stone (arrowed) in left hepatic duct. Post-operative cholangiogram. A number of stones had been removed at operation and this stone ultimately passed into the common bile duct from where it was subsequently removed. **Fig. 817.** Residual stone (arrowed) in cystic duct remnant. Post-operative cholangiogram. Some narrowing of common bile duct due to co-existing chronic pancreatitis.

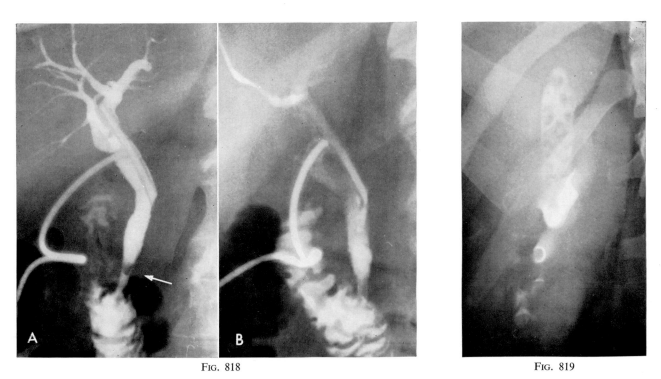

FIG. 818   FIG. 819

Fig. 818. Residual stone at lower end of common bile duct. A: Post-operative cholangiogram shows non-opaque stone (arrowed). B: After treatment with ether and Renacidin* the stone has disappeared. **Fig. 819.** Calcified debris in gall-bladder together with a number of non-opaque stones—discovered during the course of an intravenous pyelogram. Supine film.

* Manufactured by The Gaurdian Chemical Corporation, New York.

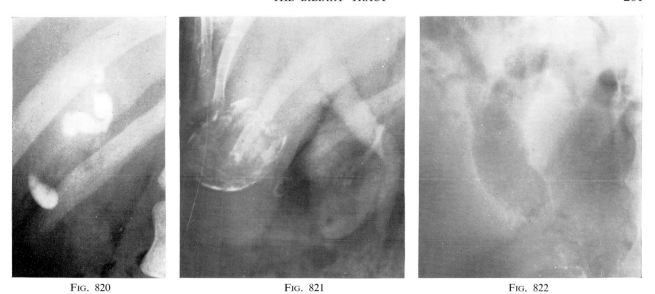

FIG. 820   FIG. 821   FIG. 822

Fig. 820. Plain film (prone) showing calcified debris in gall-bladder and cystic duct. **Fig. 821.** Calcification in gall-bladder wall (porcelain gall-bladder). Supine film one hour after injection of Biligrafin. No medium has entered the gall-bladder owing to obstruction of cystic duct by a non-opaque stone. A moderate pyelogram has also been obtained. Some dilatation of common bile and hepatic ducts. **Fig. 822.** Gas in the biliary tract. Previous sphincterotomy for stenosis at ampulla of Vater with removal of numerous stones from common bile duct. Gross residual dilatation of ducts. The presence of gas indicates patency of the lower end of the common bile duct.

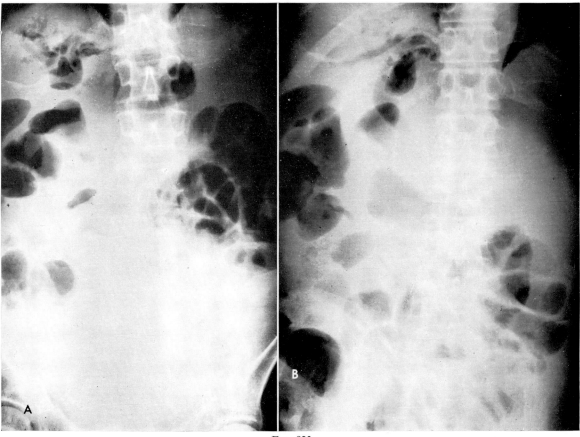

FIG. 823

Fig. 823. Gas in the biliary tract more clearly seen erect than supine. Previous Whipple's operation for carcinoma of pancreas. Gross ascites and some small bowel obstruction from peritoneal metastases. The gas-filled loops are more clearly seen than usual as they are thrown into relief by the ascitic fluid. A: Erect. The gas in the biliary tract is very clearly seen. Most of the loops of bowel have floated on the fluid and are displaced out of the pelvis. B: Supine. The gas in the biliary tract is not so obvious. The distended loops of bowel are again clearly depicted.

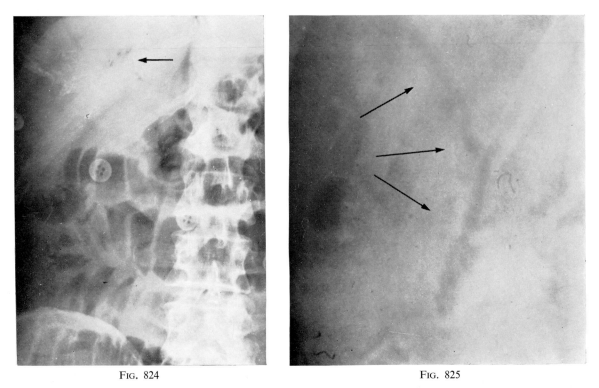

FIG. 824   FIG. 825

Fig. 824. Gas in the biliary tract (arrowed) from a high intestinal obstruction (due to adhesions from a previous operation). The gas was forced up the common bile duct by the high intra-duodenal pressure. No previous operation on the biliary tract itself. **Fig. 825.** Gas in the common bile and common hepatic ducts (arrowed) from recent passage of a stone. Some dilatation and irregularity—subsequently proved to be due to the presence of multiple small gall-stones. History of recent pain, jaundice and fever. Magnified print.

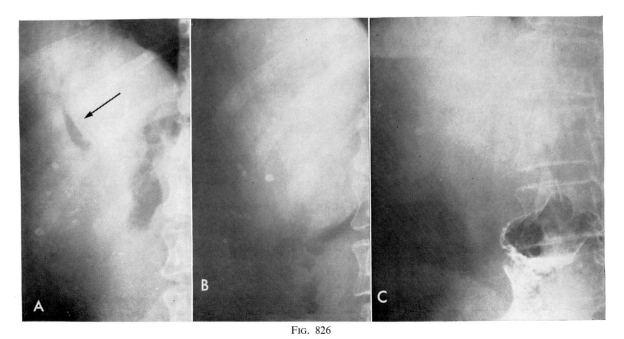

FIG. 826

Fig. 826. Intermittently functioning cholecyst-duodenostomy performed for stricture of common bile duct. Patient complained of attacks of pain with transient jaundice coinciding with absence of gas in the biliary tract. A: Patient well. No pain or jaundice. Gas in the intrahepatic ducts (arrowed) causing branching translucencies. B: Plain film at time of attack of pain with jaundice. No gas in the biliary tract. C: Barium meal same day. No gas in the biliary tract. No reflux of barium into the biliary tract. At operation a gall-stone was present on the suture line producing a ball-valve action at the anastomosis.

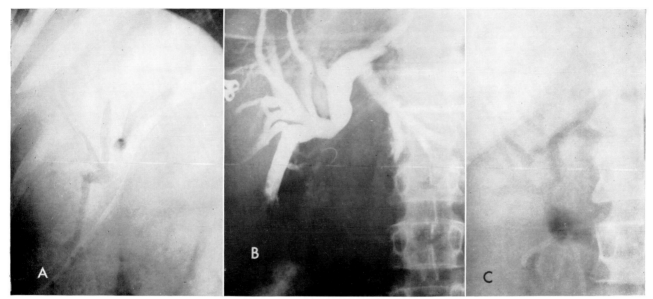

FIG. 827

Fig. 827. Recurrence of stricture of common hepatic duct. A: Gas in the biliary tract indicating a well-functioning anastomosis between the common hepatic duct and the jejunum (carried out for stricture of common bile duct following removal of stones). Patient well and free from jaundice. B: Two years later. Recurrence of pain, jaundice, fever, and absence of gas in the biliary tract on a plain film. Operative cholangiogram shows dilatation of the intra-hepatic ducts but absence of gas. Complete obstruction at origin of common hepatic duct—found to be due to a stricture. Anastomosis refashioned. C: One month later. Plain film shows obvious gas in the biliary tract and a patent anastomosis. Patient now well with absence of jaundice and fever.

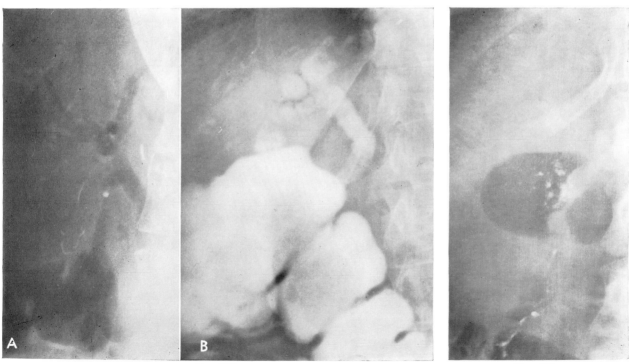

FIG. 828   FIG. 829

Fig. 828. Cholecysto-colic fistula due to an acute cholecystitis seven years previously with perforation of gall-bladder into hepatic flexure of colon. A: Plain film shows gas in biliary tract. B: Barium enema. The gall-bladder and ducts are outlined by barium. The fistula was not outlined on follow-through of a barium meal. **Fig. 829.** Acute cholecystitis. Marked distension of duodenal bulb with gas and a patent pylorus. Prone view. (Print reversed.)

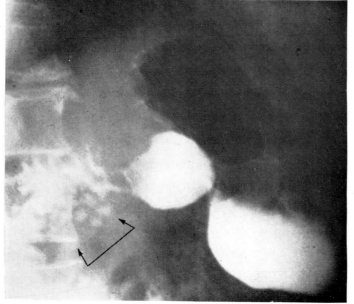

FIG. 830

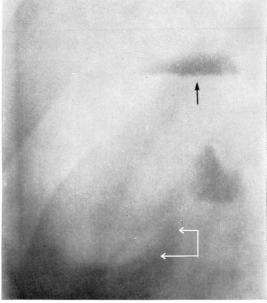

FIG. 831

Fig. 830. Acute cholecystitis. Gastrografin meal shows dilated duodenal bulb with narrowing at its apex—due to indentation and spasm from the adjacent infected gall-bladder. Four or five small calcified gall-stones (arrowed) are also present in the fundus of the gall-bladder. Prone position. (Print reversed.)

Fig. 831. Acute cholecystitis. Erect film following Telepaque. No concentration of Telepaque suggesting a pathological gall-bladder. Granular opacity at the fundus due to a collection of finely calcified stones (arrowed). Persistent distension of the duodenal bulb with a fluid level (top single arrow).

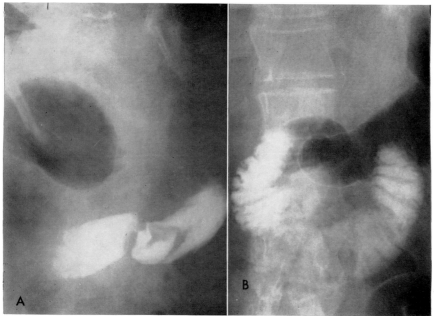

FIG. 832

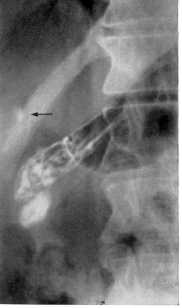

FIG. 833

Fig. 832. Acute cholecystitis. A: Gastrografin meal. Obstruction at the apex of the duodenal bulb due to the adjacent in-flamed gall-bladder. Prone film, (Print reversed.) The large collection of gas is in the fundus of the stomach. B: Two hours later. Some of the Gastrografin has passed onwards. Still obvious distension of the duodenal bulb with a patent pylorus. Duodenal diverticulum arising from the second part. Supine film. Operative confirmation.

Fig. 833. Acute cholecystitis. Gastrografin meal shows temporary hold-up in the upper part of the second part of the duodenum. Small gall-stone (arrowed) in the neck of gall-bladder. At operation the gall-bladder was situated more laterally than usual.

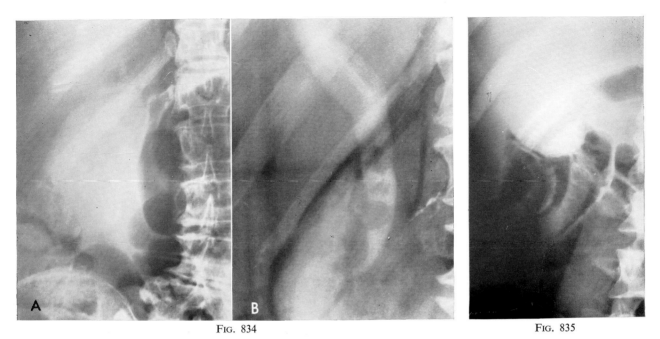

Fig. 834   Fig. 835

Fig. 834. Acute cholecystitis. A: Large soft-tissue swelling in right hypochondrium due to the distended gall-bladder with a surrounding inflammatory mass. B: Two hours after injection of Biligrafin. Excretion good. The common bile and hepatic ducts are dilated and contain numerous non-opaque stones. No medium has entered the gall-bladder indicating an obstruction of the cystic duct or at the neck of the gall-bladder, presumably by a stone. This supports the diagnosis of an acute cholecystitis.

Fig. 835. Acute cholecystitis. Soft-tissue shadow in right hypochondrium projecting from below the liver margin caused by an enlarged inflamed gall-bladder. Local ileus of jejunum.

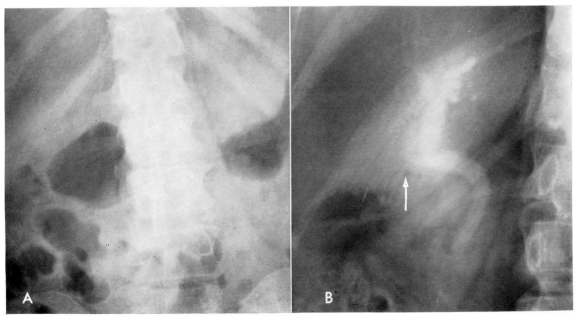

Fig. 836

Fig. 836. Acute cholecystitis. A: Supine film. Marked distension of duodenal bulb with gas. B: Two hours after injection of Biligrafin. Excretion good. The gall-bladder did not opacify due to an obstruction of the cystic duct (arrowed). At laparotomy this was found to be caused by a stone. Some dilatation of common hepatic duct and common bile duct with a little narrowing at its lower end.

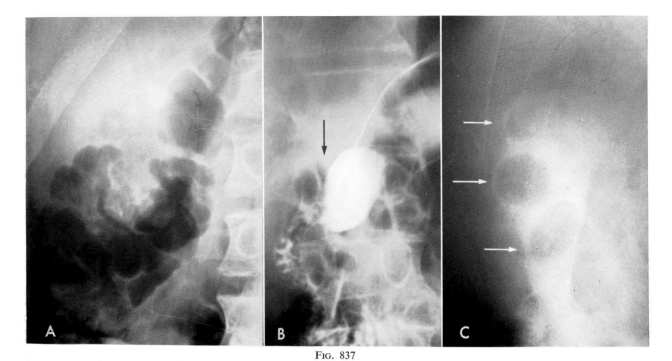

FIG. 837

Fig. 837. Acute cholecystitis. A: Plain film shows soft-tissue shadow in right hypochondrium displacing transverse colon and hepatic flexure. B: Gastrografin meal. Characteristic narrowing (arrowed) at apex of duodenal bulb due to indentation by the inflamed gall-bladder. C: Two hours after injection of intravenous Biligrafin. Enough Biligrafin has entered the gall-bladder to demonstrate at least three large non-opaque stones (arrowed).

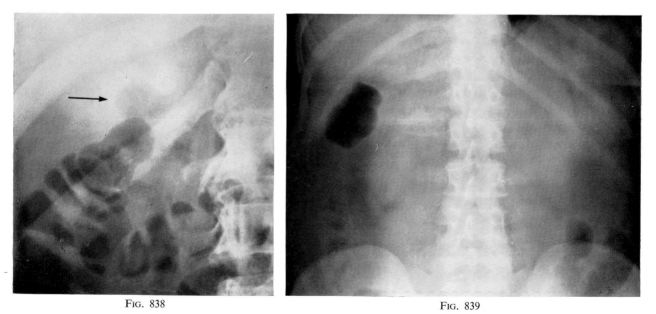

FIG. 838   FIG. 839

Fig. 838. Empyema of gall-bladder with perforation into hepatic flexure of colon. The gall-bladder is outlined by gas (arrowed) and is situated in the middle of a large soft-tissue shadow caused by an inflammatory mass.

Fig. 839. Acute cholecystitis. Operative confirmation. Dilatation with atony of hepatic flexure of the colon—persistent on other films. This is an appearance more commonly seen in association with acute pancreatitis.

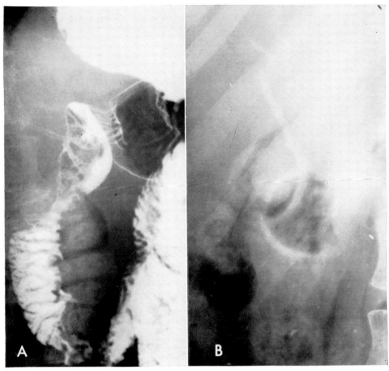

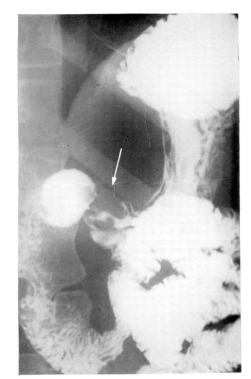

Fɪɢ. 840

Fɪɢ. 841

Fig. 840. Empyema of gall-bladder. A: Barium meal showing deformity with narrowing of first and second parts of duodenum due to indentation by the enlarged gall-bladder. B: Intravenous Biligrafin two hours after injection. The common bile duct is faintly opacified but no medium has entered the gall-bladder due to an obstruction at its neck—a common appearance. This was found to be due to a stone. **Fig. 841.** Chronic empyema of gall-bladder. Clinically a mass was palpable. Barium meal shows deformity of the antrum (arrowed) indistinguishable radiologically from a carcinoma. At operation the gall-bladder was situated more medially than usual, overlying the antrum and causing the above deformity.

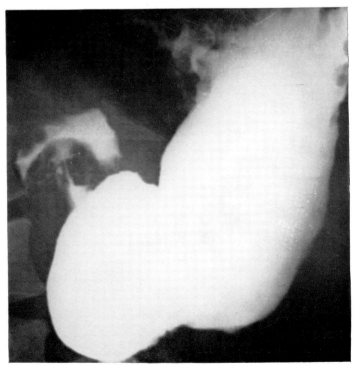

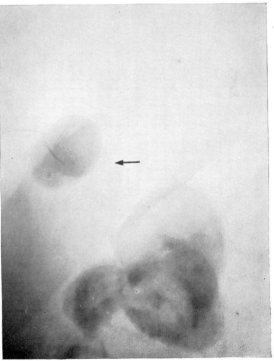

Fɪɢ. 842

Fɪɢ. 843

Fig. 842. Chronic empyema of gall-bladder causing a filling defect in pyloric antrum considered radiologically to be a carcinoma. Some indentation also of base of duodenal bulb. Prone view. (Print reversed.) Operative proof. **Fig. 843.** Acute cholecystitis with perforation into hepatic flexure of colon. Operative confirmation. The gall-bladder is filled with gas (arrowed) and is in the middle of a large soft-tissue shadow due to an inflammatory mass.

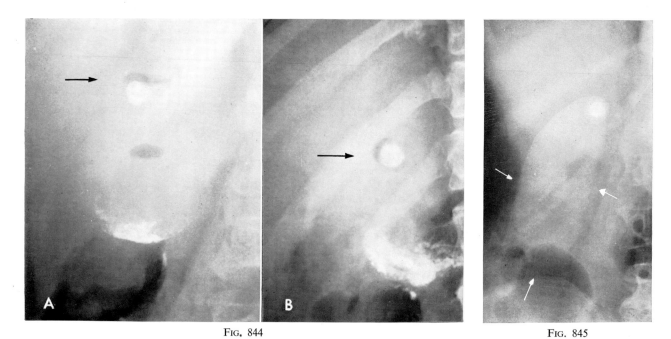

FIG. 844   FIG. 845

Fig. 844. Empyema of gall-bladder containing gas due to infection by gas-forming organisms. Stone in Hartmann's pouch. Operative confirmation. No fistula found. Films 14 hours after Telepaque some of which has been retained in the stomach. No concentration by the gall-bladder. A. Erect. Calcified gall-stone and gas (arrowed) in gall-bladder. The lower fluid level is in the duodenal bulb. Opaque meniscus of Telepaque in stomach. B. Supine. Gall-stone and gas (arrowed) in gall-bladder.
Fig. 845. Mucocoele of gall-bladder causing a large soft-tissue shadow (arrowed) remarkably like the right kidney. Calcified stone impacted in neck of gall-bladder. Operative confirmation.

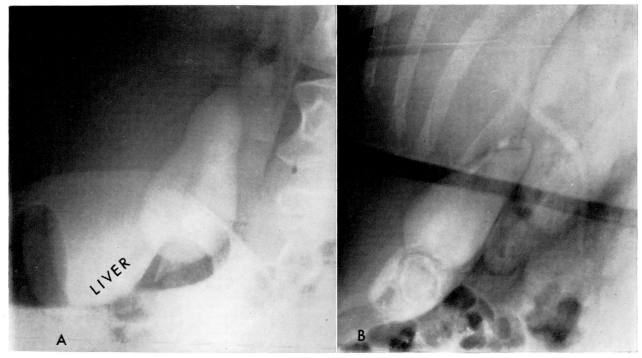

FIG. 846

Fig. 846. A: Cholecystogram. Fourteen-hour film. Apparently normally functioning gall-bladder without evidence of stones and failing to show the existing compartmental disease. B: Intravenous cholangiogram two hours after injection (and sixteen hours after Telepaque). The distal pouch has now filled and it contains two large gall-stones. Supine film. The transverse linear translucency is due to air trapped between skin folds in a very stout patient. Normal ducts.

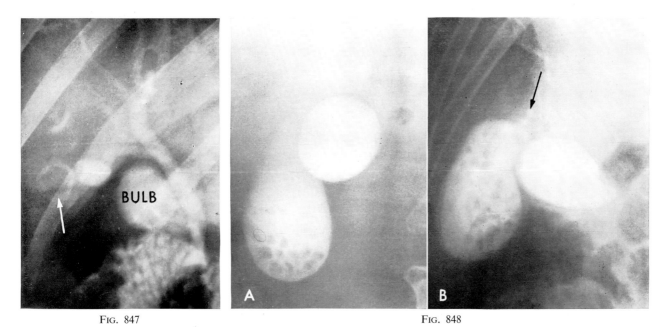

FIG. 847   FIG. 848

Fig. 847. Compartmental disease. Supine film two hours after injection of intravenous Biligrafin. The gall-bladder has filled showing a proximal and distal pouch with a stricture between. The distal pouch contains a large non-opaque stone (arrowed). The ducts are normal and medium has entered the duodenum. The duodenal bulb is well filled and must not be mistaken for the gall-bladder.

Fig. 848. Compartmental disease. Oral cholecystogram. A: Erect. The proximal compartment looks like a dilated Hartmann's pouch. Stones clearly seen in distal compartment. B: Supine film. Obstruction (arrowed) in middle of gall-bladder. Stones clearly seen.

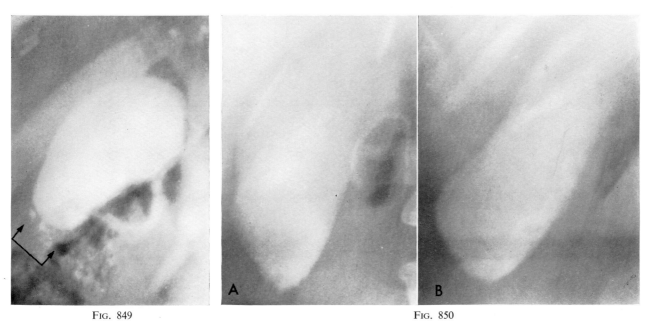

FIG. 849   FIG. 850

Fig. 849. Rokitansky-Aschoff sinuses. Typical double contour of fundus of gall-bladder (arrowed). The gall-bladder and ducts are otherwise normal. Supine film. Fourteen hours after Telepaque and half an hour after injection of intravenous Biligrafin.

Fig. 850. 'Strawberry' gall-bladder causing multiple small filling defects which are only faintly seen in the gall-bladder wall. Oral cholecystogram with good concentration. A: The defects are seen most clearly along the margin near the fundus. B: The defects cause a faintly mottled appearance of the gall-bladder with a scalloped border of fundus and medial aspect of body.

T

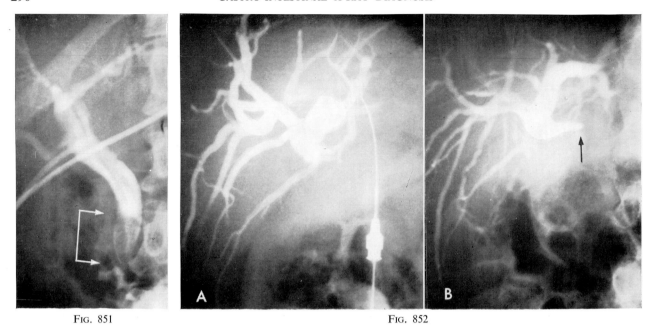

Fig. 851   Fig. 852

Fig. 851. Severe cholangitis. Part of the mucous membrane lining the common bile duct has sloughed off causing a conical filling defect (arrowed) at the lower end of the common bile duct. Operative proof. Post-operative cholangiogram. The defect was considered radiologically to represent a stone.

Fig. 852. Obstruction at porta hepatis—proved at laparotomy to be due to a subhepatic abscess secondary to an empyema of the gall-bladder. Patient presented with deepening jaundice and a mass in the right hypochondrium. Percutaneous trans-hepatic cholangiogram under television control. A: Supine film. Considerable dilatation of the intrahepatic ducts. B: Ten minutes later. Erect film. The point of obstruction (arrowed) is more clearly seen and is tapered suggesting an external mass at the porta hepatis.

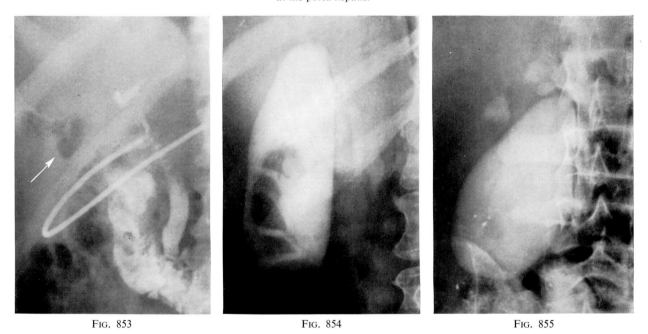

Fig. 853   Fig. 854   Fig. 855

Fig. 853. Infection in gall-bladder bed after cholecystectomy suggested by an excessive amount of gas (arrowed) and a soft-tissue shadow 12 days after operation. The abscess subsequently ruptured externally. Some dilatation of the common bile duct. (Stones were removed from it at cholecystectomy.) Post-operative cholangiogram.

Fig. 854. Distended gall-bladder in a patient who developed herpes zoster the following day. 13 hours after Telepaque and half an hour after injection of Biligrafin. Herpes zoster may also cause adynamic ileus of the bowel.

Fig. 855. Dilatation and atony of the gall-bladder following vagotomy and partial gastrectomy. Several non-opaque stones are also seen as faint translucent filling defects in the middle of the gall-bladder. Supine film 13 hours after Telepaque and half an hour after injection of intravenous Biligrafin.

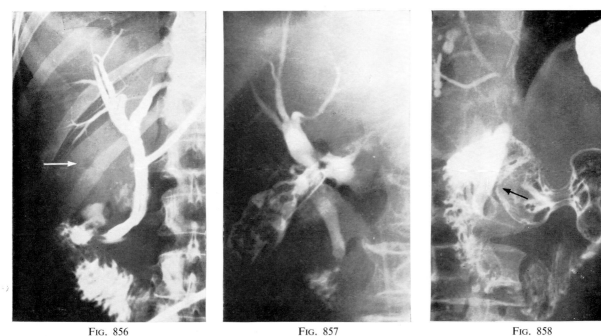

FIG. 856   FIG. 857   FIG. 858

Fig. 856. Normal post-operative cholangiogram ten days after cholecystectomy. Trace of gas (arrowed) in the gall-bladder bed—normal. A little medium has entered the lower end of the pancreatic duct. **Fig. 857.** Rupture of an abscess into common bile duct demonstrated by instillation of Gastrografin through an abdominal sinus. Previous gastrectomy for carcinoma of stomach. **Fig. 858.** Reflux of barium into common bile duct (arrowed) during a barium meal. Previous removal of stones and sphincterotomy for stricture at lower end of common bile duct. Opacities opposite lower dorsal spine are due to Myodil from a previous myelogram.

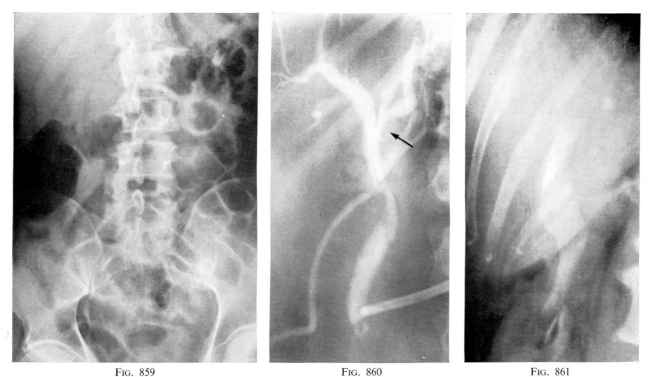

FIG. 859   FIG. 860   FIG. 861

Fig. 859. Adynamic ileus of small and large bowel which are moderately distended with gas to a similar degree in a patient with biliary colic. The cause of the ileus cannot be determined from this film. **Fig. 860.** Stenosis of origin of left hepatic duct (arrowed). Post-operative cholangiogram. Care must always be taken to note that this duct has been outlined following cholangiography as non-filling can easily be overlooked. **Fig. 861.** Re-stenosis of lower end of common bile duct with dilatation proximally and absence of gas in biliary tract. Previous sphincterotomy for stricture. Two-hour film following injection of intravenous Biligrafin. Moderately good pyelogram.

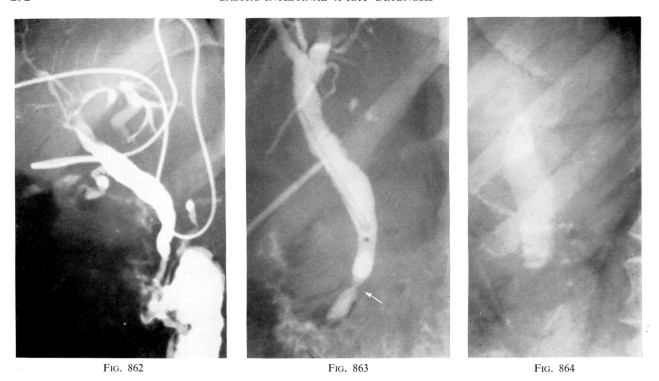

FIG. 862   FIG. 863   FIG. 864

Fig. 862. Sclerosing cholangitis. Gross irregularity with narrowing of ducts at porta hepatis. Dilatation proximally especially of branches of left hepatic duct. This condition is extremely difficult or impossible to differentiate from malignant papillomatosis. Cystic duct remnant also present. Post-operative cholangiogram. **Fig. 863.** Stricture (arrowed) near lower end of common bile duct demonstrated by post-operative cholangiogram. Medium however enters the duodenum satisfactorily. At original operation a stone impacted at lower end of common bile duct was removed. **Fig. 864.** Dilatation of common bile and common hepatic ducts with stricture at lower end. Previous cholecystectomy. Four-hour film after injection of Biligrafin still shows dense opacification of ducts. Very little if any medium in duodenum. (By courtesy of Messrs. Butterworths.)

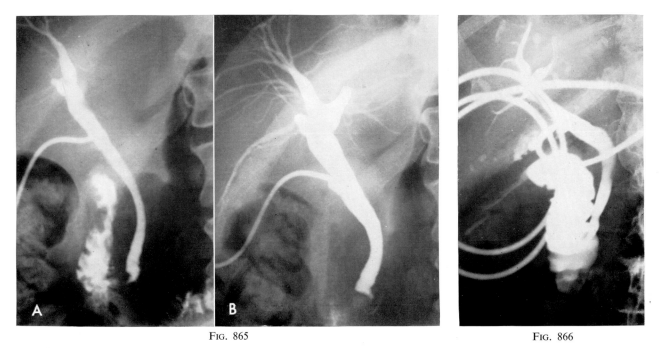

FIG. 865   FIG. 866

Fig. 865. Normal post-operative cholangiogram. A: The common bile duct is of normal calibre. B: A little dilatation of ducts due to spasm of lower end induced by too rapid injection of more medium. **Fig. 866.** Non-filling of left hepatic duct due to obstruction at its junction with right hepatic duct. Without careful scrutiny this can readily be overlooked.

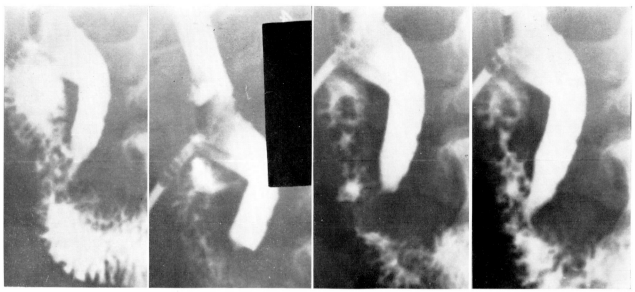

Fig. 867

Fig. 867. Four spot films showing changing appearances of lower end of common bile duct. Post-operative cholangiogram ten days after removal of stones. Note in particular the temporary sharply cut-off appearance in second spot film. Medium enters the duodenum satisfactorily.

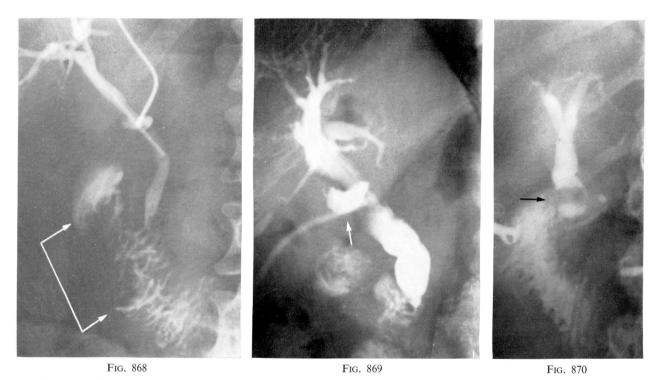

Fig. 868   Fig. 869   Fig. 870

Fig. 868. Deformity of second part of duodenum (arrowed) due to oedema of its wall after incision for sphincterotomy of sphincter of Oddi. Normal ducts. Post-operative cholangiogram.

Fig. 869. Dilated cystic duct remnant (arrowed) immediately above the T tube. Considerable dilatation of ducts also present with stricture at lower end of common bile duct. A little medium has ultimately entered the duodenum. Cholecystectomy ten days previously with removal of stones from common bile duct.

Fig. 870. Displacement of common bile duct (arrowed) by a small circumscribed mass which was found to be an aberrant pancreatic nodule. Operative cholangiogram. A trace of medium has entered the lower end of the pancreatic duct.

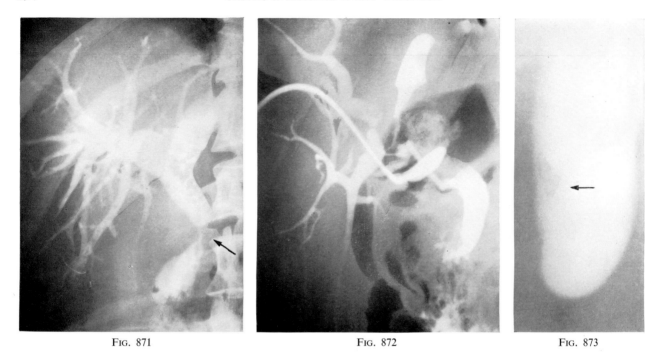

FIG. 871   FIG. 872   FIG. 873

Fig. 871. Choledocho-duodenostomy with development of a stricture (arrowed) at the anastomosis. Dilatation of ducts which contain multiple non-opaque stones showing as a mottled appearance in common hepatic duct. Note absence of gas in hepatic ducts indicating obstruction at the anastomosis. History of pain and intermittent jaundice after the original operation. Percutaneous transhepatic cholangiogram. **Fig. 872.** Papillomatosis of the ducts. Gross irregular narrowing of the ducts with filling defects at porta hepatis and with dilatation proximally. Some dilatation also of the common bile duct from a stricture at its lower end. Post-operative cholangiogram. **Fig. 873.** Polyp in gall-bladder causing a small persistent lobulated filling defect (arrowed). Fourteen hours after Telepaque.

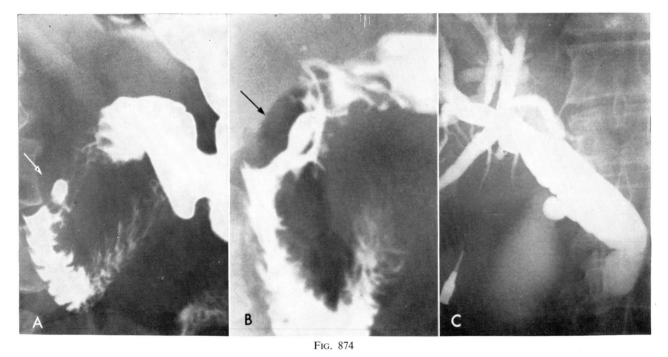

FIG. 874

Fig. 874. Carcinoma of common bile duct with infiltration of pancreas and duodenal wall—indistinguishable from carcinoma of head of pancreas. A: Barium meal prone view. Indentation with narrowing and ulcer (arrowed) at junction of first and second parts of duodenum. B: Supine view. The ulcer (arrowed) is seen in the deformed area. C: Percutaneous transhepatic cholangiogram. Gross dilatation of the ducts with an obstruction at lower end of common bile duct—the common site for a carcinoma. Some medium has entered the gall-bladder causing it to be faintly opacified.

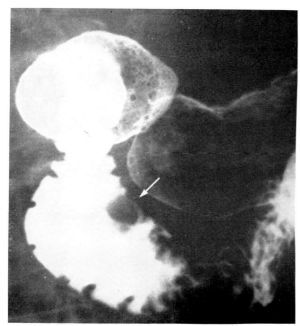

FIG. 875

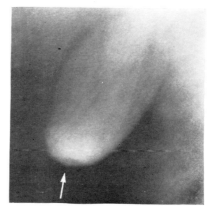

FIG. 876

Fig. 875. Carcinoma of duodenum (arrowed) adjacent to ampulla of Vater causing an irregular filling defect. The patient presented with pain and jaundice.

Fig. 876. Adenomyoma of gall-bladder. Smooth filling defect (arrowed) at the fundus of gall-bladder—the common site. Oral cholecystogram.

Fig. 877. Carcinoma of common bile duct. Operative cholangiogram showing high obstruction (arrowed) with dilatation of ducts proximally. The lower end of the common bile duct is the more common site of a carcinoma.

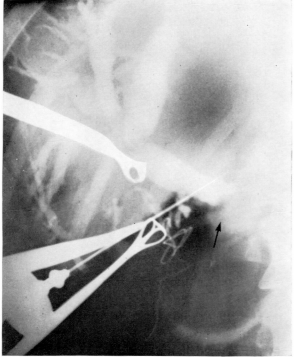

FIG. 877

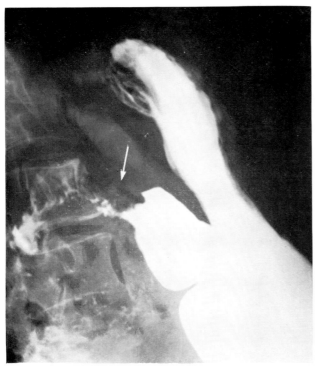

FIG. 878

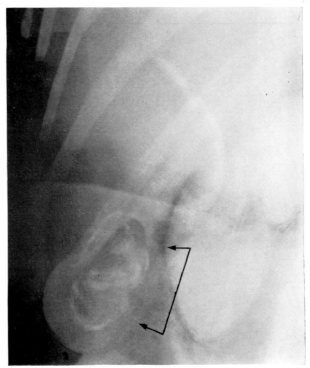

FIG. 879

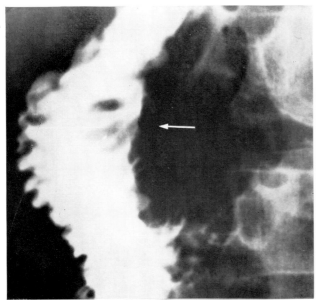

FIG. 880

Fig. 878. Carcinoma of gall-bladder. Persistent irregularity with narrowing (arrowed) at junction of first and second parts of duodenum due to local extension of the tumour. Barium meal. Prone view. (Print reversed.)

Fig. 879. Carcinoma of gall-bladder. Calcification (arrowed) subsequently found to be partially in gall-bladder wall and partially in a large stone. The gall-bladder did not opacify, owing to obstruction by the stone. Intravenous Biligrafin two hours after injection.

Fig. 880. Carcinoma of ampulla of Vater. Spot film of second part of the duodenum shows a filling defect (arrowed) which was persistent. Case of deepening jaundice.

CHAPTER IX

THE LIVER

RADIOLOGICAL METHODS OF INVESTIGATION

THE liver does not lend itself to radiological investigation as readily as other abdominal organs.

Plain Films. A supine film, a P.A. film of the chest and a right lateral view of the upper abdomen to include the diaphragm are necessary. Because of its shelving inferior surface the lower the X-ray beam is centred the smaller is the soft-tissue shadow of the liver when examined in the supine position.

Fluoroscopy is of value in diagnosing infection which causes impaired movement of the right dome of the diaphragm. A very large liver because of its size has a similar effect.

A barium meal and barium enema are carried out to determine the nature of a mass in the upper abdomen and may demonstrate the possible site of a primary tumour. In cirrhosis a barium meal is given to look for oesophageal and gastric varices. A standing left lateral view with the patient bending forwards attempting to touch his toes is valuable in differentiating between deformity of the fundus of the stomach due to an intrinsic lesion and indentation by the liver (or spleen). In the former the deformity persists whereas in the latter it disappears or alters.

Splenic venography may be used in cases of suspected cirrhosis or tumours of the liver and to show the splenic and portal veins and any collateral circulation. It is also of value in demonstrating the patency of a porto-caval anastomosis and in distinguishing between an intra- and extrahepatic portal obstruction.

Aortography and selective coeliac axis angiography are sometimes of value in demonstrating space-occupying lesions in the liver and differentiating a tumour of the liver from a retroperitoneal tumour by its blood supply. Occasionally these methods may be employed in the diagnosis of cirrhosis.

Pneumoperitoneum is sometimes used to define the position of the diaphragm and thus differentiate between a supra- and infradiaphragmatic opacity.

Liver Scanning. Using appropriate radioactive isotopes, the liver can be scanned and its size, shape and function demonstrated. When a tumour or abscess is present there is an area of absent uptake. In cases of multiple tumours several such areas may be demonstrated. In cirrhosis there may be patchy areas of reduced uptake.

CLINICAL RADIOLOGY

Congenital Anomalies

A Riedel's lobe extends downwards often to below the level of the iliac crest. As it is smooth and tongue-like it can usually be differentiated from enlargement of the liver from other causes.

Congenital elevation of the right dome of diaphragm causes the liver to be situated higher than normal.

Congenital herniation of a part of the liver through the right dome of diaphragm is rare. On a plain P.A. and lateral film of the chest a smooth opacity is noted above the right dome of diaphragm. A pneumoperitoneum is diagnostic as the herniated portion of liver is seen to be surrounded by a cap of gas.

Congenital cystic disease of the liver may be associated with a similar condition in the pancreas and kidneys. Occasionally solitary cysts are present. The wall of a cyst may show fine curvilinear plaques of calcification.

Calcifications in the Liver

A hydatid cyst (Echinococcus cyst) may calcify causing an irregular scalloped appearance.

A gumma of the liver is rare and usually the calcification is granular or mottled.

Armillifer armillatus is a rare parasite and causes punctate or crescentic areas of calcification in the peritoneum and pleura in addition to the liver.

An amoebic abscess may occur in an untreated case of amoebiasis. Its wall may ultimately calcify.

Carcinomata, primary or secondary, on rare occasions show fine calcification.

Miscellaneous calcifications, the nature of which cannot be precisely determined, are sometimes noted in the liver. In some cases they probably represent old tuberculous foci or congenital cysts and in others simple tumours, e.g. dermoid cysts.

Other rare causes are brucellosis, old pyaemic abscesses, histoplasmosis and intrahepatic calculi. Flecks of calcification may be seen in the portal vein, especially in cases of cirrhosis, but localisation is difficult without a splenic venogram.

Enlargement of the Liver

There are many causes, e.g. tumours, especially metastases, heart failure, amoebiasis and some cases of cirrhosis. An enlarged right lobe displaces the stomach downwards and to the left. An enlarged left lobe displaces the stomach downwards and backwards and causes an increase in the distance between the fundus of the stomach and the base of the left lung. Occasionally on a barium meal it indents the fundus simulating a gastric carcinoma.

Liver Abscess

The liver is enlarged with elevation of the right dome of the diaphragm and impaired movement on fluoroscopy. There are usually also inflammatory changes at the base of the right lung. In some instances a liver abscess is present without enlargement or impaired diaphragmatic movement. Its detection may be extremely difficult even at laparotomy.

Following drainage of an amoebic abscess, its size, position and rate of healing may be demonstrated by the injection of a water soluble organic iodine contrast medium, e.g. 25 per cent. Hypaque into the abscess cavity. In the late stage calcification may occur. Sometimes a diffuse amoebiasis causes enlargement without a localised abscess.

Cirrhosis

The liver may be either small or large. For further investigation a barium meal followed by a splenic venogram is necessary.

When varices are present in the lower oesophagus they can be demonstrated by a barium meal in the great majority of cases. Gastric varices, however, are more difficult to show and can easily be mistaken for simple coarse mucosal folds. Occasionally a dilated left gastric vein indents the lesser curvature of the stomach (pp. 9 and 43).

A splenic venogram shows patent splenic and portal veins but with diminished rate of flow through the liver. There is narrowing of the intrahepatic veins sometimes with distortion. Flecks of calcification in the portal vein may be seen. Gastric and oesophageal varices are demonstrated with greater accuracy than by barium meal and dilated collateral channels are usually present. It must be remembered, however, that in some normal cases there is an apparent blockage of the splenic vein near the spleen for no obvious reason.

If a porto-caval anastomosis becomes blocked, no medium passes into the inferior vena cava from the portal vein and the gastric and oesophageal varices return.

Gas in the Portal Circulation

Gas may be present in the portal circulation in gangrene of the small intestine and necrotising enteritis, and is a grave sign. The gas shows as branching translucencies extending far out into the liver substance.

Opacification of the Liver

Thorotrast. In the past thorotrast was used for cerebral angiography but it persisted, particularly in the liver, spleen and para-aortic lymph nodes, showing as multiple small opacities of metallic density which remained throughout the patient's life.

Haemochromatosis. In this condition iron is deposited in the liver. As the liver is slightly denser than normal there is a double shadow at the level of the diaphragm particularly on the right side. The more translucent narrow upper one is, of course, the diaphragm. The spleen is usually also enlarged. A similar appearance results from deposits of iron following multiple blood transfusions.

Tumours of the Liver

The liver is enlarged but unless it is of appreciable size the movements of the diaphragm are not affected. Enlargement may cause displacement of the stomach, duodenum or colon (pp. 44 and 196). Rarely a tumour is calcified.

Arteriography may be of value in demonstrating tumour staining, arterial displacement, arterial obstruction, etc. In some instances splenic venography is even more helpful.

RECOMMENDED READING

McNULTY, M. R. (1968). High dose percutaneous transplenic portal venography. *Br. J. Radiol.*, **41**, 55-58.

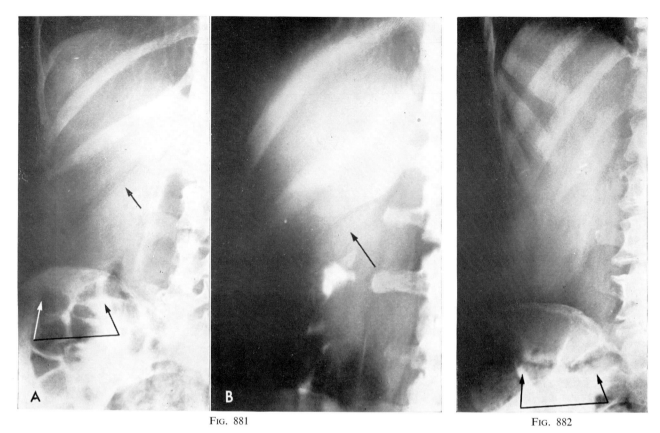

FIG. 881   FIG. 882

Fig. 881. Two films (of same patient) showing the different levels of the anterior and posterior margins of inferior surface of liver. A: Antero-inferior border opposite the iliac crest indenting the gas-filled bowel (lower double arrow). Postero-inferior margin (top single arrow) at a higher level. B: Tomogram of kidney area shows clearly the postero-inferior border of liver just below 12th rib.

Fig. 882. Riedel's lobe (arrowed) causing a smooth soft-tissue shadow extending to below the level of iliac crest. Incidental finding.

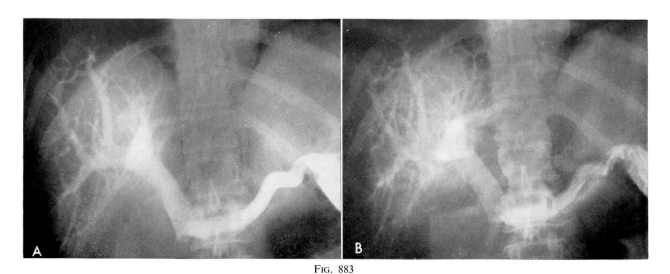

FIG. 883

Fig. 883. Normal splenic venogram. A: The large number of branches in the liver and their uniform distribution and diminishing calibre are seen. Four seconds after injection. B: Three seconds later. Increased filling of smaller branches.

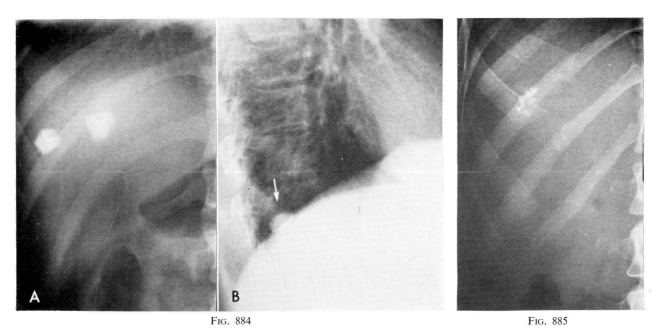

FIG. 884   FIG. 885

Fig. 884. Calcification at right costo-phrenic angle. A: Postero-anterior view shows two areas of calcification which might be in the liver. B: Lateral view of chest shows one area (arrowed) clearly to be in the lung. The other was also in the lung, seen on fluoroscopy.

Fig. 885. Dense calcification in the liver. Nature uncertain, but might be in a dermoid cyst. Incidental finding.

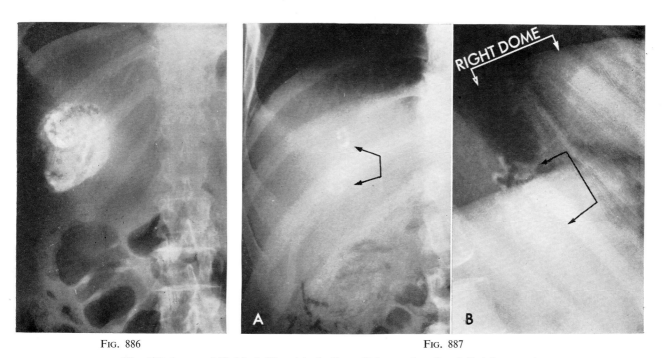

FIG. 886   FIG. 887

Fig. 886. Large calcified hydatid cyst in the liver. It is more heavily calcified than usual.

Fig. 887. Sinuous calcification (arrowed) in the liver of a soldier who had served many years in the tropics: ? ascaris, ? guinea worm. A: P.A. view. B: Lateral view.

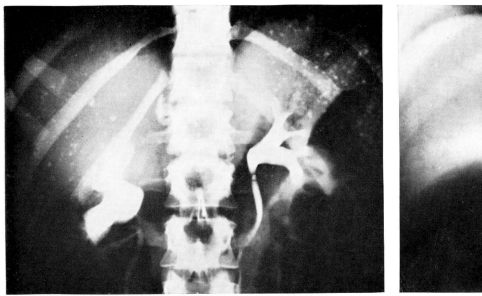

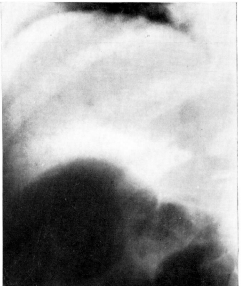

FIG. 888   FIG. 889

Fig. 888. Multiple calcified spots in the liver and spleen from old healed miliary tuberculosis noted during the course of an I.V.P.

Fig. 889. Gas in the portal circulation—a grave sign. Case of severe necrotising enteritis. Typical branching translucencies extending far out almost to the periphery of the liver.

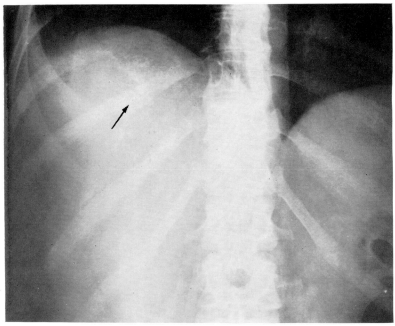

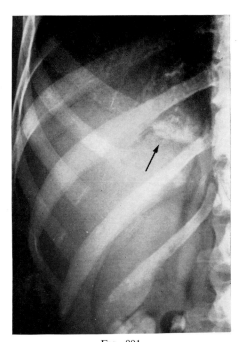

FIG. 890   FIG. 891

Fig. 890. Gumma of the liver causing mottled calcification (arrowed). Case of congenital syphilis.

Fig. 891. Calcification in a cyst (arrowed) in the liver. The cyst was discovered at a previous laparotomy and contained pure bile. It is presumably congenital.

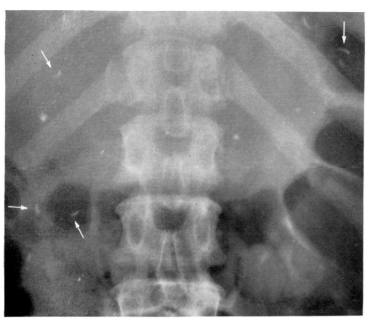

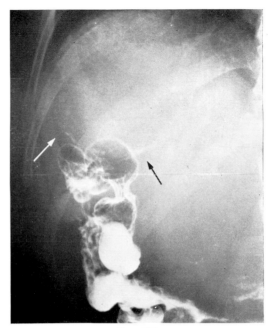

FIG. 892   FIG. 893

Fig. 892. Armillifer armillatus infestation. Typical calcified spots (arrowed), some circular, some crescentic in liver and abdomen.

Fig. 893. Chronic amoebic abscess of the liver with peripheral calcification (arrowed). The liver is also moderately enlarged. Autopsy confirmation. The patient unfortunately died of a massive pulmonary embolus following an abdominal operation. This patient had lived all his life in a rural district of south-west Scotland. (Same case as Fig. 656.)

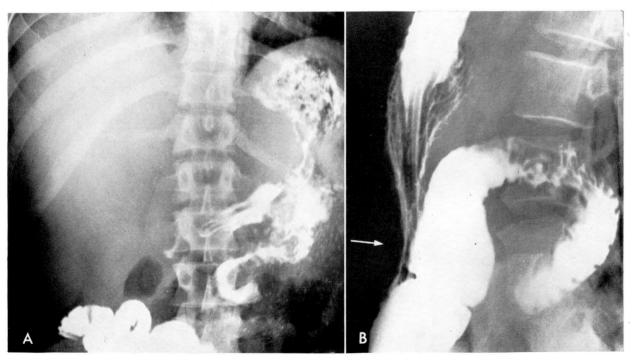

FIG. 894

Fig. 894. Grossly enlarged liver due to liver abscesses following *E. coli* septicaemia. A: The stomach and small bowel (outlined by barium), and the hepatic flexure of colon (outlined by gas) are displaced downwards and to the left. B: Lateral view with the patient lying on his right side and the head of the X-ray table slightly raised. Slight backward displacement (arrowed) of body of stomach.

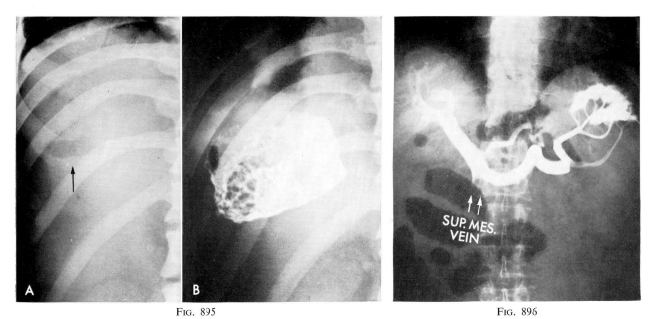

FIG. 895   FIG. 896

Fig. 895. Amoebic abscess of liver. A: Gas in the abscess cavity (arrowed) following drainage. B: The cavity is clearly
outlined following injection of Hypaque directly into the cavity and rolling the patient from side to side.

Fig. 896. Alcoholic cirrhosis with portal hypertension. Splenic pressure 450 mm of water. Splenic venogram shows a patent
duct system but a small liver with narrowing and distortion of the intrahepatic veins. A little filling of the left gastric vein
with evidence of varicosity.

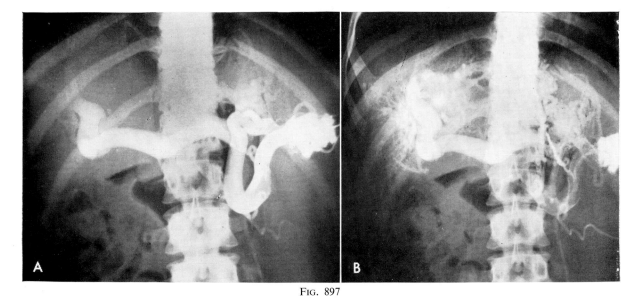

FIG. 897

Fig. 897. Cirrhosis of the liver. Splenic venogram. A: The splenic and portal veins are patent. The branches within the
liver filled slowly and are narrowed. Extensive gastric varices also present with some collateral vessels. B: Five seconds later.
The narrowing of the veins in the liver is now more obvious. Collateral channels are now well filled. Varices also clearly seen.

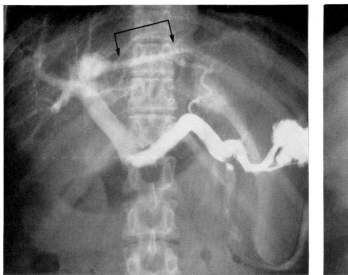

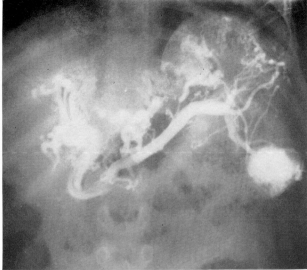

FIG. 898

FIG. 899.

Fig. 898. Cirrhosis of the liver. Splenic venogram shows obvious stretching of left hepatic vein (arrowed). The liver is small.

Fig 899. Cirrhosis of the liver in a child following pyaemic abscesses—arising from peritonitis. Splenic venogram shows a patent splenic vein but distortion and narrowing of many of the branches of the portal vein in the liver. Well marked gastric varices.

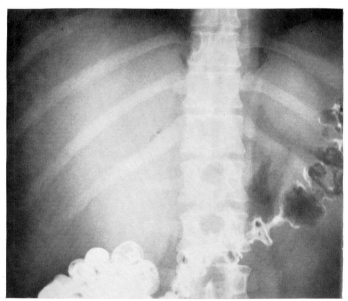

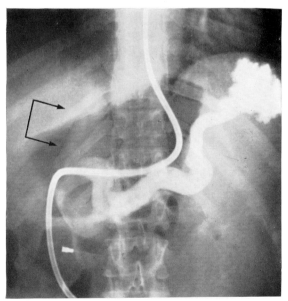

FIG. 900

FIG. 901

Fig. 900. Cirrhosis of the liver which is markedly enlarged causing displacement of hepatic flexure and transverse colon. Operative confirmation. Chronic alcoholic.

Fig. 901. Well functioning porto-caval anastomosis. Normal splenic vein and commencement of portal vein. No medium has entered the branches of the portal vein in the liver. The inferior vena cava (arrowed) is only faintly opacified as the dye is diluted by the large volume of blood in the inferior vena cava.

U

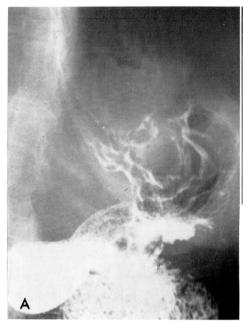

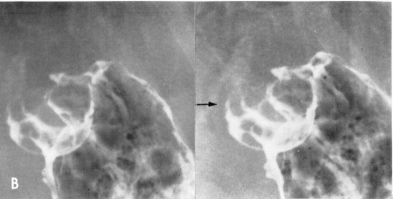

Fig. 902

Fig. 902. Deformity of fundus of stomach from transection and ligation of varices a year previously. Case of cirrhosis of liver. Gross deformity which could be mistaken for a carcinoma. Recurrence of varices in fundus and lower oesophagus. A: Large prone film. B: Stereoscopic pair showing recurrence of varices (arrowed).

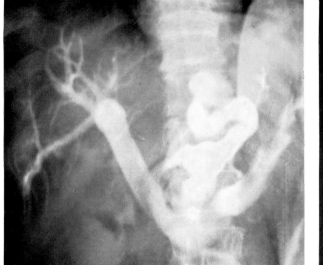

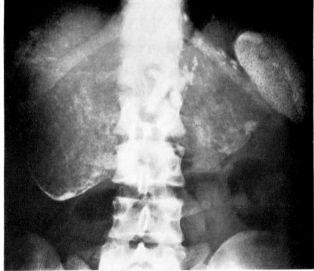

Fig. 903   Fig. 904

Fig. 903. Severe portal hypertension with enlargement of spleen and very high splenic pulp pressure up to 480 mm. of water. Large gastric varices. Narrowing of the portal vein at the porta hepatis. Delayed filling of the branches within the liver which are narrowed. Provisional diagnosis of partial nodular transformation of the liver. First liver biopsy normal. Patient admitted with massive haematemesis.

Fig. 904. Thorotrast in the liver, spleen and adjacent lymph nodes. Cerebral angiogram 20 years previously.

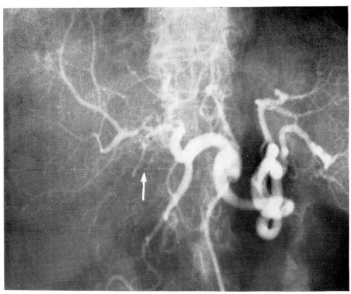

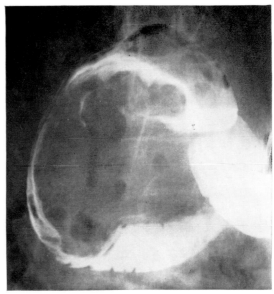

Fig. 905

Fig. 906

Fig. 905. Highly malignant tumour (a primary carcinoma of liver) at porta hepatis. Ill patient with deepening jaundice. Selective coeliac angiogram shows grossly abnormal vessels (arrowed) with distortion and irregularity at porta hepatis. The percutaneous transhepatic cholangiogram prior to this was unsatisfactory and the barium meal was negative.

Fig. 906. Cholangioma of liver arising from its lower border causing gross displacement of second part of duodenum. The appearances radiologically are indistinguishable from a large carcinoma of head of pancreas.

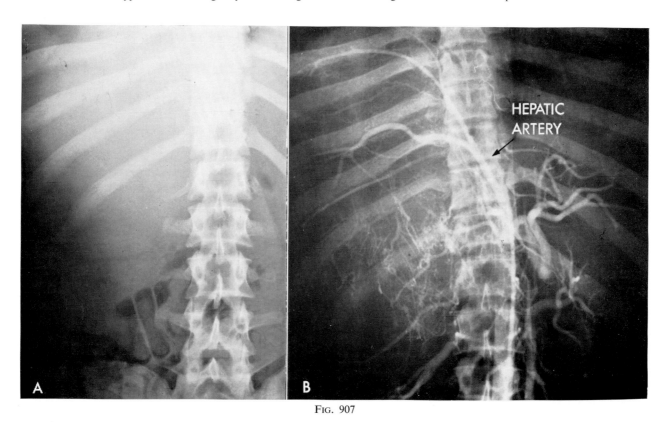

Fig. 907

Fig. 907. Retroperitoneal sarcoma. Laparotomy confirmation. A: Large mass on right side initially suggesting a tumour of liver. B: Aortogram shows the hepatic arteries to be normal apart from some displacement. There is a large tumour with an abnormal circulation which is derived from the right upper lumbar and lower intercostal arteries. This indicates that this is not a tumour of the liver.

CHAPTER X

THE PANCREAS

RADIOLOGICAL METHODS OF INVESTIGATION

Plain Films. Erect and supine views of the abdomen and a film of the chest are required in acute cases. In chronic disease the erect film can usually be omitted.

Barium Meal and Gastrografin Meal. A barium meal is the standard method of examination except in suspected acute pancreatitis when Gastrografin is used.

Intravenous Cholangiography. The method is the same as for the investigation of disease of the biliary tract (p. 261). In the early stage of jaundice excretion of Biligrafin may be adequate for diagnostic purposes. Once jaundice is established the investigation is pointless. In acute pancreatitis intravenous cholangiography is generally of little or no value because of inadequate excretion of Biligrafin.

Percutaneous Transhepatic Cholangiography. See Biliary Tract (p. 262).

Angiography. Aortography is of limited value because of the diffuse nature of the blood supply to the pancreas. Simultaneous coeliac and superior mesenteric angiography have been employed in some centres with varying degrees of success.

Splenic Venography. This is employed when a tumour or cyst of the pancreas is suspected to have caused splenic vein thrombosis.

Operative Pancreatography. Following opening of the second part of the duodenum a fine catheter is threaded into the pancreatic duct and 1 to 2 ml. of 60 per cent. Urografin* injected. It is used in cases of chronic pancreatitis and suspected duct obstruction.

Pancreatic Scanning. By the use of an appropriate radioactive isotope the pancreas can be scanned and its shape and function demonstrated. This investiga-tion is still being evaluated but promises to be more accurate than conventional radiology in the detection of small tumours and other abnormalities.

CLINICAL RADIOLOGY

NORMAL APPEARANCES

The normal pancreas cannot be identified on a plain film of the abdomen.

On a barium meal examination the retrogastric space is normally no greater than the depth of the body of a lumbar vertebra. However in stout or thick-set individuals the space is larger. Since also in these patients the duodenal loop is relatively wide especially in the prone position a tumour of the pancreas might erroneously be suspected.

During operative pancreatography the medium may opacify the substance of the pancreas either locally or diffusely, but this is quite normal. Very rarely this examination causes an acute pancreatitis.

At post-operative cholangiography the terminal portion of pancreatic duct fills in approximately 5 to 10 per cent. of cases.

During splenic venography occasionally the splenic vein does not fill when, in fact, it is patent. The cause of the apparent blockage is uncertain but an error in diagnosis should be avoided as in such cases there is no evidence of varices or of abnormal communicating veins.

CONGENITAL ANOMALIES

There are few congenital anomalies of radiological importance.

Annular pancreas is rare and causes narrowing of the second part of the duodenum.

* Manufactured by Schering A. G., Berlin.

Pancreatic rests in the stomach or duodenum produce small filling defects indistinguishable from simple tumours.

Occasionally the wall of a *congenital cyst* calcifies and is usually easily recognised on a plain film by its position. A barium meal or intravenous cholangiogram may occasionally be necessary for precise localisation.

CALCIFICATION

Calcification of the pancreas is uncommon in Britain, but much more common in America, South Africa and in tropical countries. It is usually associated with chronic pancreatitis and in some cases diabetes is also present. It may follow congenital cystic fibrosis. The calcification may be uniformly scattered throughout the gland or may be localised, especially to the head of the pancreas.

The wall of a congenital cyst or of a pseudo-cyst may become partially calcified.

Pancreatic calculi may be single or multiple and are usually situated near the end of the duct in the head of the pancreas. They are usually densely calcified, laminated and lenticular in shape. Calcification within the gland is usually also present.

INFLAMMATORY DISEASE

Acute Pancreatitis

Radiology has much to offer in the investigation of this condition. Plain films show appearances which, though not diagnostic, indicate the necessity for further examination.

THE MOST SIGNIFICANT SIGNS ARE AS FOLLOWS:

(*a*) Stuart's sign, i.e. gas in hepatic and splenic flexures of the colon with its absence in the middle of the transverse colon. This usually indicates a fairly severe attack and is presumably due to spasm of the middle of the transverse colon. It is usually associated with oedema of the transverse mesocolon.

(*b*) Gas in the hepatic flexure alone—even earlier than Stuart's sign. This is sometimes present, however, in acute cholecystitis.

(*c*) Gas in the splenic flexure tailing off towards the middle of transverse colon—uncommon.

(*d*) Ileus of the jejunum and sometimes the duodenum—the so-called sentinel loop. It must be remembered that a similar appearance can be due to

Buscopan or Probanthine. A generalised ileus indicates a more widespread peritoneal exudate.

(*e*) Ileus of the transverse colon—uncommon.

(*f*) A soft-tissue swelling may be detected causing downward displacement of the transverse colon immediately distal to the hepatic flexure. In other cases the body of the stomach is displaced upwards and less commonly downwards. Sometimes there is blurring of the left psoas shadow.

(*g*) Calcification may be present suggesting an underlying chronic pancreatitis. The films should also be scrutinised for gall-stones since disease of the biliary tract commonly exists.

(*h*) Small effusion at the left costo-phrenic angle with elevation of the left dome of diaphragm.

(*i*) Absence of gas in the bowel producing a ground-glass appearance in the abdomen. This is only rarely seen and in the acute abdomen is more commonly due to other conditions (p. 332).

The next stage in the radiological investigation is a Gastrografin meal. Gastrografin is used because a perforation of a peptic ulcer has not been excluded at this stage.

THE FOLLOWING RADIOLOGICAL SIGNS MAY BE PRESENT:

1. *When the head of the pancreas is involved:*

(*a*) Enlargement of duodenal loop, local indentations of its concave border, or the reversed '3' sign of Frostberg.

(*b*) Coarsening of mucosa of duodenum.

(*c*) Upward displacement of the pyloric antrum.

(*d*) Narrowing of the junction of the first and second parts of the duodenum and sometimes the distal duodenum.

Acute pancreatitis may follow an operation on the biliary tract especially for the removal of stones from the lower end of the common bile duct. The head of the pancreas is usually involved and the appearances are as described above.

2. *When the body and tail of the pancreas are involved:*

(*a*) Upward and forward displacement of the body of the stomach. Downward displacement is uncommon.

(*b*) Impaired movement of the left dome of diaphragm on fluoroscopy.

(*c*) Some distortion, mucosal swelling and irritability of the adjacent loops of jejunum.

Acute pancreatitis affecting mainly the body but sometimes the whole gland may occur due to injury especially at partial gastrectomy. Radiologically it is impossible to differentiate from a local inflammatory mass.

Subacute Pancreatitis

This may follow acute pancreatitis or the disease may be subacute from the start. The radiological appearances are similar to those of the acute form although not so severe. A barium meal is safe and thus preferable to Gastrografin because it gives better detail. Some narrowing of the common bile duct is sometimes seen on intravenous cholangiography.

If operative pancreatography is carried out the main pancreatic duct may be distorted or blocked or may show local dilatation between stenosed segments.

A pseudo-cyst may develop, i.e. a localised collection of pancreatic fluid and exudate outside the gland itself. Depending on its position and size it displaces neighbouring organs sometimes to a gross degree. Adjacent bowel is distorted, narrowed and the mucosa may be swollen due to oedema. A pseudo-cyst may also occur following trauma and as a rare complication of gastric surgery.

Enlargement of the spleen is present if the splenic vein becomes thrombosed—an infrequent complication.

If a cysto-gastrostomy has been performed for treatment of either a pseudo-cyst or other form of cyst it is unusual for it to be outlined following a barium or Gastrografin meal. The reason for this is uncertain.

Chronic and Relapsing Pancreatitis

In some cases calcification is present and occasionally also densely calcified elliptical and sometimes laminated opacities representing stones in the pancreatic duct. Sometimes intermittent swelling of the pancreas occurs which is obvious clinically and radiologically.

In all cases the biliary tract must be investigated. The common bile duct is occasionally narrowed especially when pancreatic calcification is present. The narrowing can be shown by intravenous cholangiography especially with tomography, and also by operative or post-operative cholangiography.

An operative pancreatogram may show a stricture at the ampulla of Vater with dilatation of the pancreatic duct proximally. The stricture may follow impaction of a gall-stone at the lower end of the common bile duct.

DUODENAL DIVERTICULA

These are usually embedded in the substance of the pancreas The pancreatic duct and common bile duct may enter a diverticulum at the ampulla of Vater. Occasionally such a diverticulum predisposes to obstruction of the pancreatic duct resulting in severe pain. In rare instances the diverticulum becomes chronically inflamed causing jaundice.

MALABSORPTION IN PANCREATIC DISORDERS

Chronic pancreatitis, congenital atrophy, lipomatosis and congenital fibrocystic disease of the pancreas may cause malabsorption. The changes noted on a barium follow-through, viz. dilatation, coarsening of the mucosa, segmentation and flocculation, etc., are similar to those found in idiopathic steatorrhoea except that they are less pronounced. Thus even with moderate steatorrhoea no abnormality may be detected.

In lipomatosis—a rare condition—the general signs and symptoms of malabsorption are usually severe with osteomalacia, Looser's zones, weakness, anaemia, etc. Obvious enlargement of the pancreas is also present on barium meal.

CYSTS OF THE PANCREAS

The wall of a cyst may be calcified but otherwise is indistinguishable from a tumour (see below).

TUMOURS OF THE PANCREAS

Simple Tumours

Small tumours cannot be detected on plain films or by barium meal. When sufficiently large these tumours may cause displacement and indentation of the stomach and duodenum similar to a carcinoma but without infiltration or mucosal destruction. They may sometimes be demonstrated by selective angiography.

Malignant Tumours

A carcinoma is by far the commonest malignant tumour but occasionally a tumour of the reticulosis group may be found. A barium meal and occasionally an intravenous cholangiogram are the methods used and the findings depend on the site of the tumour.

A carcinoma of the head of the pancreas, even at the stage of causing jaundice, may cause no abnormality on a barium meal. Commonly the first sign is narrowing at the junction of first and second parts of the duodenum. Occasionally, indentation of the duodenal bulb from behind may be noted particularly on compression or palpation. Local indentations of the concave border may be seen, and when they occur above and below the ampulla of Vater, cause the reversed '3' sign of Frostberg.

When the tumour is large it causes enlargement of the duodenal loop, sometimes with infiltration and mucosal destruction. The antrum is displaced upwards and sometimes the right half of the transverse colon is displaced downwards. The hepatic flexure of colon however remains in its normal position.

At an early stage of a tumour of the head of the pancreas, even if jaundice is present, excretion of Biligrafin may be adequate. In a classical case there is obstruction of the common bile duct distal to the origin of the cystic duct with dilatation proximally but with absence of stones. The gall-bladder fills and may be enlarged. It does not opacify when there is a low insertion of the cystic duct into the common bile duct in the head of the pancreas.

Percutaneous transhepatic cholangiography is seldom performed since a laparotomy is indicated. When carried out in selected cases it shows the characteristic appearance of an obstruction in the common bile duct usually just distal to the point of junction of the common hepatic duct and the cystic duct.

A carcinoma of the body of the pancreas cannot be detected by a barium meal unless it is of moderate size. The tumour usually displaces the stomach downwards and to the left. There is an increase in the retrogastric space—more than the depth of the body of a lumbar vertebra. However the build of the individual must be taken into consideration as this distance is normally increased in stout or thickset individuals. In some cases there is an unusually sharp angle between the body and the fundus of the stomach.

In the supine position a crescentic indentation convex to the left may be noted on the posterior wall of the body of the stomach. Palpation during fluoroscopy is most important as an impression of fullness behind the stomach may be obtained.

A lateral view with the patient lying on his right side and the head of the table slightly elevated is helpful. In this position the stomach is displaced forwards and a 'wedge' effect is produced—the thin end of the wedge being posterior. Enlargement of the liver, if anything, displaces the stomach backwards.

Occasionally the spleen is enlarged due to thrombosis of the splenic vein.

Adenomata secreting Pharmacologically Active Substances, e.g. Polypeptides

These tumours may be simple but many are of low grade malignancy and are usually too small to be detected radiologically. Metastases may be present in the liver causing enlargement.

Depending upon the nature of the substance secreted there are three main types with different radiological features:

(*a*) *Carcinoid Type.* In these cases there is dilatation of the duodenum but without ulceration. In other instances intestinal hurry may be present.

(*b*) *Zollinger-Ellison Syndrome.* Peptic ulcers, often multiple, are present. They are most common in the first part of the duodenum but are not infrequent in the second part and are even occasionally seen in the jejunum. Severe peptic oesophagitis may also occur with an associated hiatus hernia. The mucosa of the stomach, duodenum and jejunum is coarse and hypertrophic. Segmentation and flocculation of the barium occur in the small bowel as the result of the high acid output. After a Polya gastrectomy jejunal ulceration is almost invariable.

(*c*) *Verner-Morrison Type.* In these cases profuse watery diarrhoea with hypokalaemia are prominent features. A plain film of the abdomen shows a large amount of gas in the small and large bowel.

The mucosal pattern in the stomach and duodenum is coarse but ulceration is usually absent. Coarsening of the mucosal pattern with flocculation and segmentation of the barium may also occur in the small bowel.

RECOMMENDED READING

BROWN, P. W., SIRCUS, W., SMITH, A. N., DONALDSON, A. A., DYMOCK, I. W., FALCONER, C. W. A. and SMALL, W. P. (1968). Scintillography in the diagnosis of pancreatic disease. *Lancet*, **1**, 160.

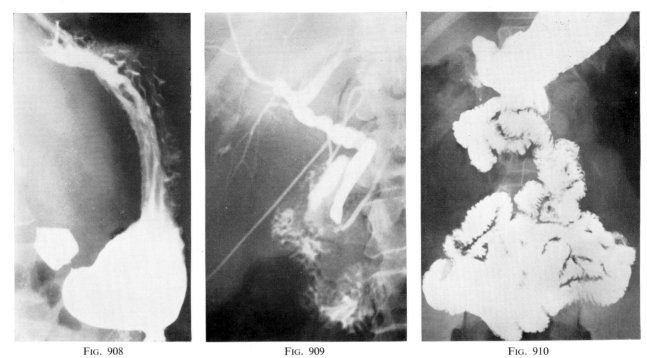

Fig. 908　　　　　　　　　Fig. 909　　　　　　　　　Fig. 910

Fig. 908. Normal pancreas. Increased retrogastric space in a broad, thick-set patient. No clinical history of pancreatic disease. **Fig. 909.** Normal pancreatic duct incidentally outlined at post-operative cholangiography—an occurrence in a small proportion of cases. Some dilatation of the common bile duct. At original operation a cholecystectomy had been performed and stones removed from the common bile duct. **Fig. 910.** Congenital atrophy of pancreas—confirmed at laparotomy. Normal jejunal biopsy. Marked steatorrhoea up to 40 grams faecal fat per day. Follow-through shows coarsening of the mucosal pattern in the small bowel with a little dilatation—the changes of the disordered X-ray pattern being less prominent than a similar degree of steatorrhoea of non-pancreatic origin. Patient initially presented with diabetes.

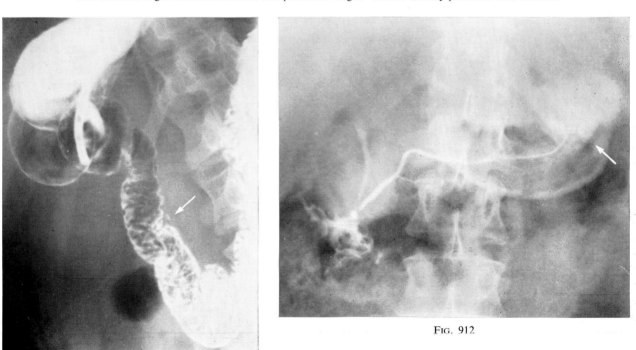

Fig. 912

Fig. 911

Fig. 911. Normal pancreas. Investigation by hypotonic duodenography. The normal ampulla of Vater (arrowed) is clearly seen as a small indentation of medial wall of second part of duodenum. **Fig. 912.** Normal pancreatogram. Laparotomy performed for diagnostic purposes because of history suggestive of chronic pancreatitis. Some medium has infiltrated the substance of the tail causing a diffuse opacity (arrowed). This is a fairly common occurrence. The pancreas felt normal. Biopsy of the pancreas including the tail was normal. A little medium has entered the lower end of the common bile duct.

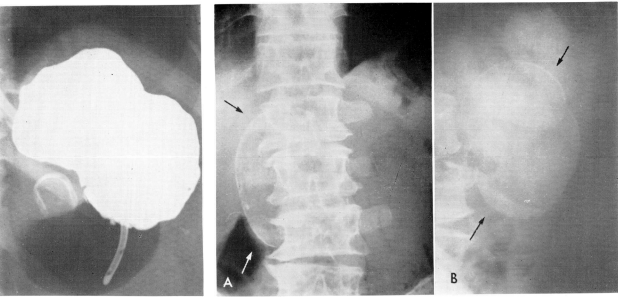

FIG. 913   FIG. 914

Fig. 913. Calcified cyst in tail of pancreas—confirmed at laparotomy which was carried out for a carcinoma of prepyloric region of stomach. Incidental finding during a barium meal.

Fig. 914. Calcified cyst of pancreas (arrowed) probably of traumatic origin. Partial gastrectomy two years previously following which a mid-line swelling developed. A: P.A. view. B: Lateral view.

(By courtesy of Dr. Sheila Kenny, Armagh, Northern Ireland.)

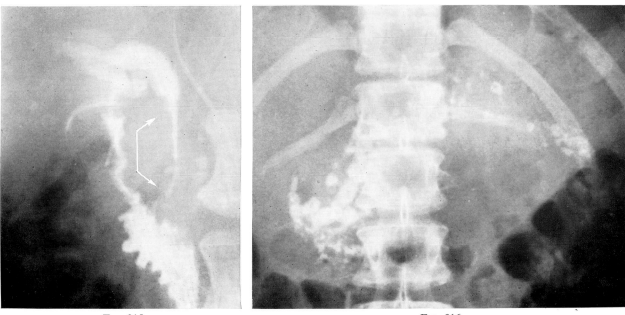

FIG. 915   FIG. 916

Fig. 915. Chronic calcific pancreatitis. Considerable narrowing of lower end of common bile duct (arrowed) in head of pancreas with some dilatation proximally. Post-operative cholangiogram. Extensive calcification also present in head of pancreas. Some narrowing of second part of duodenum due to spasm and oedema following duodenotomy and sphincterotomy.

Fig. 916. Multiple calculi in pancreatic duct shown as well calcified and mostly elliptical opacities in the line of the main pancreatic duct. Extensive pancreatic calcification also present. Case of chronic pancreatitis.

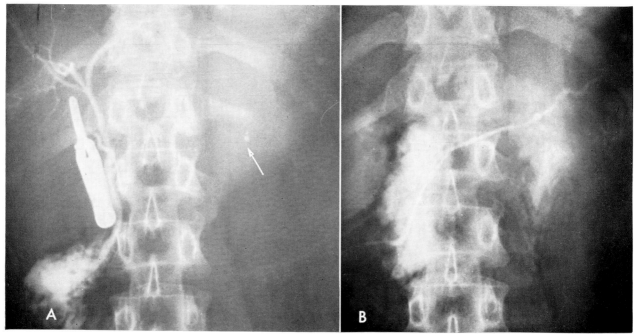

Fig. 917

Fig. 917. Chronic pancreatitis with stone in pancreatic duct. A: Operative cholangiogram. Normal bile ducts. Calculus in pancreatic duct (arrowed). B: Operative pancreatogram. The stone is obscured by medium of the same density in the duct. Proximal to the stone, i.e. towards tail of pancreas, the pancreatic duct is slightly dilated. Local dilatation also at point of impaction of the calculus. At laparotomy, well marked evidence of chronic pancreatitis. (By courtesy of Mr. A. A. Gunn and Dr. R. Saffley.)

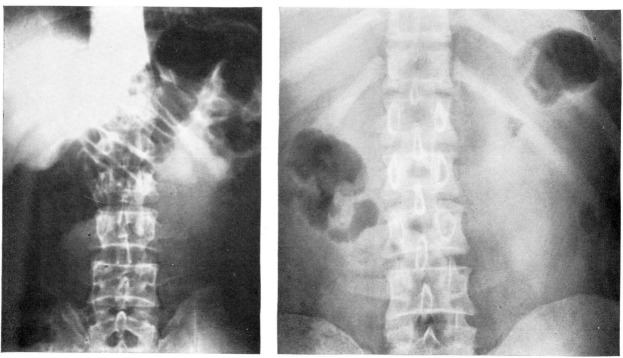

Fig. 918   Fig. 919

Fig. 918. Acute pancreatitis. Plain film shows dilatation and atony of transverse colon—a relatively uncommon sign. It is similar to the sentinel loop of the jejunum. **Fig. 919.** Acute pancreatitis. Plain film shows Stuart's sign, i.e. gas in the hepatic and splenic flexures, tailing off towards the middle of the transverse colon where it is absent.

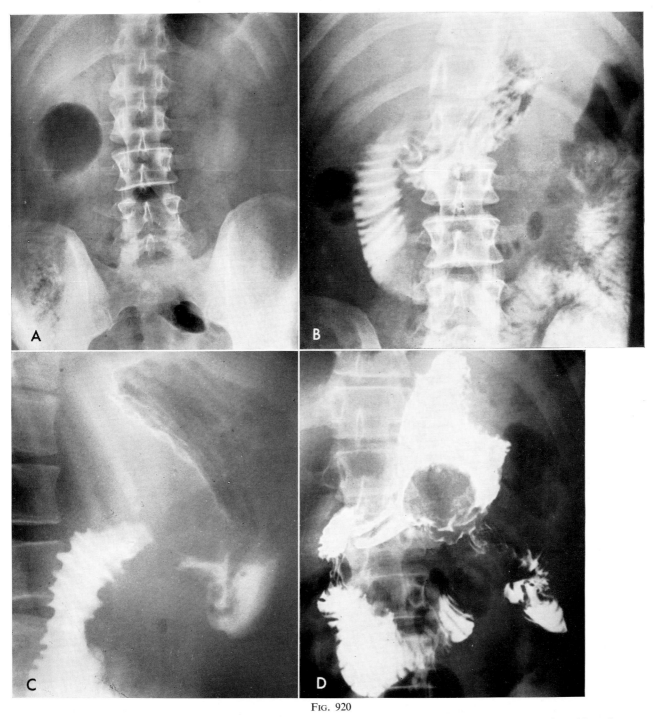

FIG. 920

Fig. 920. Acute pancreatitis involving the entire gland.   A: Plain film at commencement of illness.   Distension of hepatic flexure with gas—an infrequent but characteristic sign (sometimes also seen in acute cholecystitis).   B: Gastrografin meal. Upward displacement of body of stomach and downward displacement of jejunum—a common finding when the body and tail of pancreas are involved.   Coarse mucosal pattern in duodenum with indentation and displacement of third and fourth parts by the swelling of the pancreatic head.   Classical Stuart's sign in transverse colon, i.e. gas in the hepatic and splenic flexures, tailing off towards the middle of the transverse colon where it is absent.   C: Lateral view.   Upward displacement of antrum and indentation of duodenum with coarsening of mucosal pattern.   The body of the stomach is also displaced forwards by the enlarged body of the pancreas.   D: Post-operative barium meal two months later.   Marked clinical improvement.   Still some distortion with localised narrowed areas of duodenal loop.   Indentation of body of stomach by a localised abscess.   Another abscess arising from the tail of the pancreas and indenting the fundus of the stomach contains two or three small bubbles of gas.

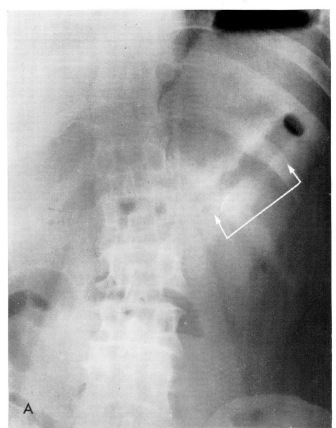

Fig. 921. Acute pancreatitis.   A: Plain film shows gas in splenic flexure tailing off towards middle of transverse colon (arrowed).   This is an unusual but characteristic appearance and less common than the classical Stuart's sign.   B: Ten days later with some clinical improvement. Stuart's sign now present.   Barium meal shows upward displacement of the stomach by a large pseudo-cyst.   Some irritability and coarsening of mucosal pattern of adjacent loops of jejunum due to the adjacent inflammatory mass.   C: Lateral view shows pseudo-cyst displacing the stomach upwards, the jejunum downwards, and the gas-filled splenic flexure of colon (arrowed) upwards and backwards.

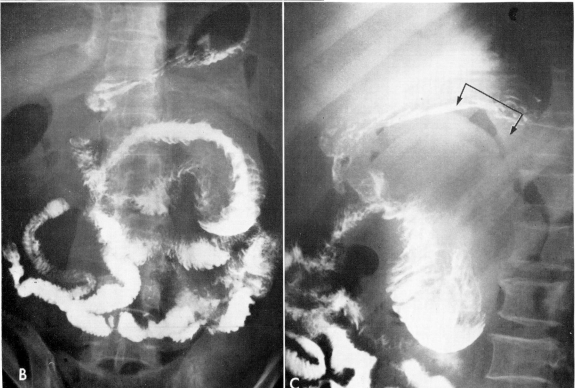

FIG. 921

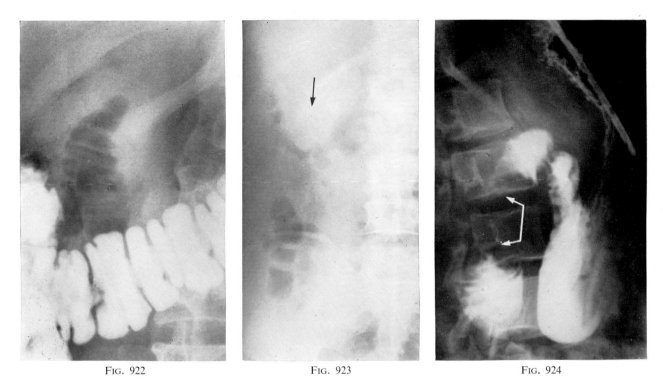

FIG. 922   FIG. 923   FIG. 924

Fig. 922. Acute pancreatitis. Ileus of second part of duodenum which is moderately distended with gas—the sentinel loop. Coarsening also of mucosal pattern.   Barium in colon from a previous barium meal. **Fig. 923.** Acute pancreatitis involving head of pancreas causing a large soft-tissue shadow which displaces the right half of transverse colon (arrowed) downwards. Some generalised adynamic ileus due to the presence of a peritoneal exudate. **Fig. 924.** Acute pancreatitis following cholecystectomy and the removal of a stone from lower end of common bile duct.   Displacement with marked narrowing of second part of duodenum (arrowed) due to swelling of head of pancreas. Gastrografin meal. Prone view. (Print reversed.)

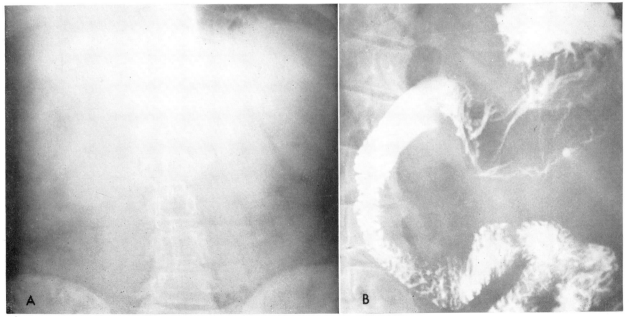

FIG. 925

Fig. 925. Acute haemorrhagic pancreatitis. A : Plain film shows ground-glass appearance of abdomen—a rare appearance and in cases of acute pancreatitis only seen when the disease is severe and extensive.   Enlargement of the spleen due to splenic vein thrombosis. B : Barium meal two weeks later.   Enlarged duodenal loop and downward displacement of duodeno-jejunal flexure.   Deformity and indentation of pyloric antrum and body of stomach—proved at laparotomy to be due to a large haemorrhagic effusion in lesser sac.

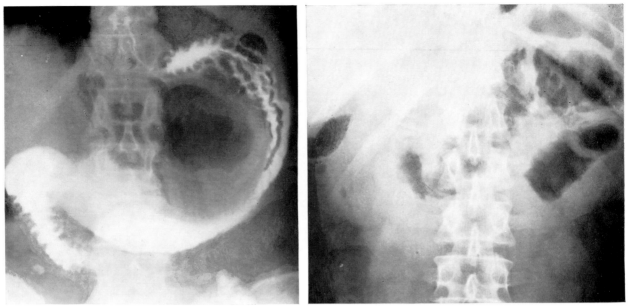

FIG. 926   FIG. 927

Fig. 926. Large pseudo-cyst involving body of pancreas following a severe acute pancreatitis.   Marked displacement of body of stomach downwards and to the left.   The cyst contains a large amount of gas but no Gastrografin.   Patient presented as an acute abdomen suggesting perforation of a peptic ulcer. **Fig. 927.** Adynamic ileus of duodenum and jejunum following Probanthine (for biliary colic) stimulating the sentinel loop of acute pancreatitis.   In such cases the information of any drugs the patient has been given should be made available to the radiologist.

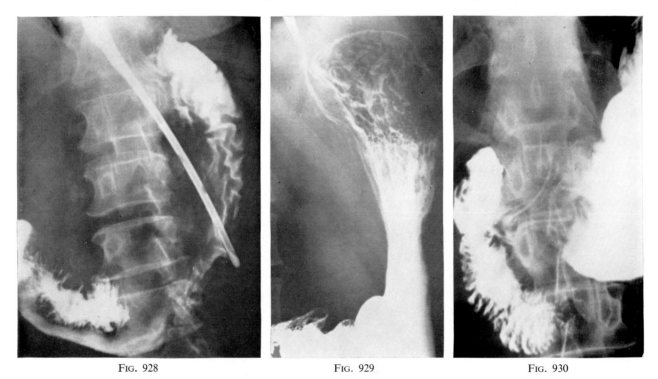

FIG. 928   FIG. 929   FIG. 930

Fig. 928. Subacute pancreatitis following an acute attack.   Downward and lateral displacement of body of stomach due to enlargement of body of pancreas.   During the acute stage there was obvious impairment of movement of left dome of diaphragm. Barium and not Gastrografin was used in this case to obtain better detail and since there was no question of a perforation. **Fig. 929.** Pancreatic cyst involving body and tail of pancreas following acute pancreatitis.   Barium meal shows lateral and forward displacement of fundus and upper part of body of stomach.   Splenic vein thrombosis and splenic infarct subsequently developed. **Fig. 930.** Subacute pancreatitis due to a small carcinoma of head of pancreas.   Distortion of mucosal pattern with rigidity on concave border of second part of duodenum.   A little displacement also of the pyloric antrum.   At laparotomy subacute pancreatitis of head of pancreas present but no tumour detected.   Six months later at a second laparotomy an obvious tumour of head of pancreas was present.

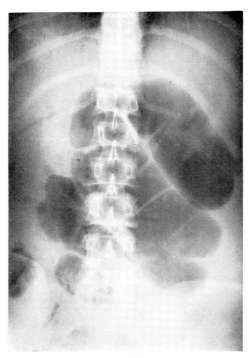

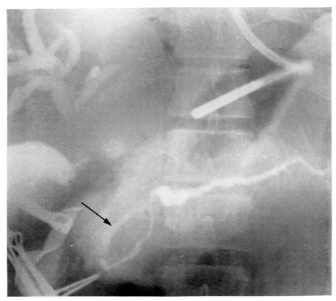

FIG. 932

FIG. 931

Fig. 931. Retro-peritoneal infection (following an operation on right kidney) causing dilatation and atony of transverse colon. Similar appearances can be caused by an acute pancreatitis. **Fig. 932.** Subacute pancreatitis. Operative pancreatogram shows narrowing, and downward and medial displacement (arrowed), of pancreatic duct by a large mass in head of pancreas. Dilatation of pancreatic duct proximally, especially in body of pancreas. An operative cholangiogram done immediately prior to the pancreatogram shows dilatation of the bile ducts and the gall bladder due to obstruction of the common bile duct. It was subsequently proved that the pancreatitis had been caused by a small carcinoma in the head of the pancreas.

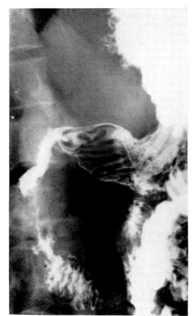

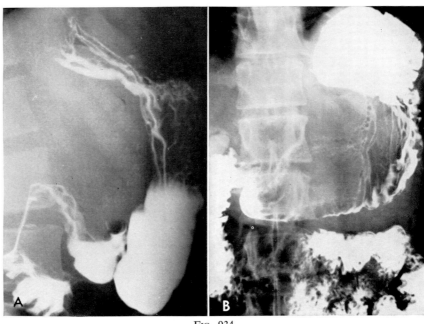

FIG. 933   FIG. 934

Fig. 933. Subacute pancreatitis causing irregular deformity of second part of duodenum with a little enlargement of duodenal loop. **Fig. 934.** Subacute pancreatitis with considerable enlargement due to a pseudo-cyst. A: Erect. Indentation and forwards displacement of body of stomach. Fine punctate calcification in body of pancreas. B: Supine. Well marked indentation of body of stomach and pyloric antrum. Downwards displacement of duodeno-jejunal flexure. History of repeated attacks of subacute pancreatitis. Intermittent abdominal swelling which subsided from time to time, coinciding with an acute attack of diarrhoea.

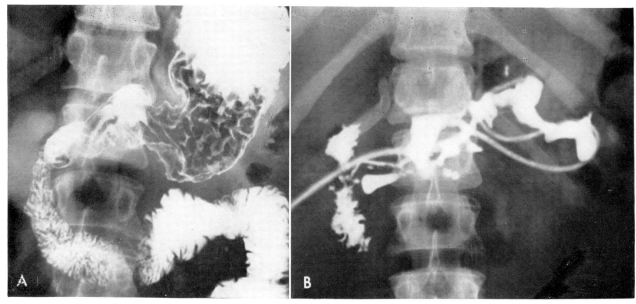

FIG. 935

Fig. 935. Subacute pancreatitis with a pseudo-cyst. A: Enlargement of duodenal loop with upward displacement of antrum.
The gall-bladder is opacified as a cholecystogram was performed at the same time. B: Post-operative sinogram. Extensive
dilated ramifications throughout the pancreas. In spite of the widespread destruction of pancreatic tissue the patient made an
almost complete recovery.

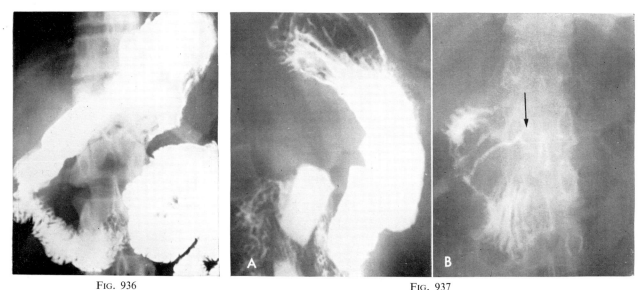

FIG. 936   FIG. 937

Fig. 936. Subacute pancreatitis involving mainly its body and tail causing irregular indentation of greater curvature aspect of
stomach and its posterior wall. Downward displacement of the duodeno-jejunal flexure. This is more common in enlargement
due to pancreatitis than from a tumour.

Fig. 937. Subacute pancreatitis following an acute attack. A: The posterior wall of body of stomach is rigid and angular with
forward displacement due to an increased retrogastric space. B: Operative pancreatogram. Obstruction (arrowed) in
pancreatic duct in neck of pancreas. Part of the duodenal loop is outlined with medium.

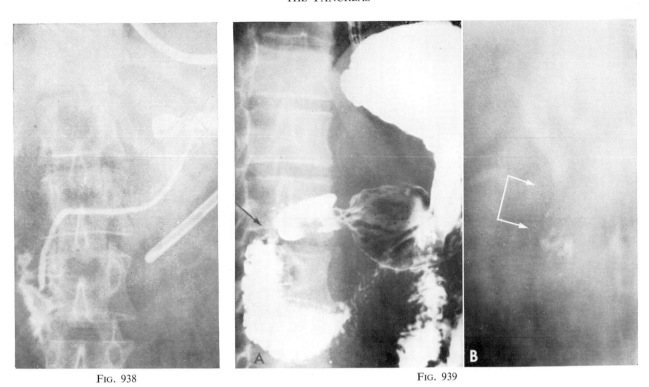

FIG. 938   FIG. 939

Fig. 938. Mild subacute pancreatitis (diagnosed at laparotomy) due to a stricture at distal end of pancreatic duct. Previous cholecystectomy with removal of stones from common bile duct. Pancreatogram at operation shows a little narrowing of the termination of the pancreatic duct with slight dilatation proximally. **Fig. 939.** Subacute relapsing pancreatitis with calcification in head of pancreas. A: Barium meal shows deformity of inferior aspect of bulb, some irregular narrowing at junction of first and second parts (arrowed), and narrowing of third and fourth parts of duodenum. B: Intravenous cholangiogram (tomogram). Dilatation of common hepatic duct and proximal part of common bile duct with narrowing of terminal 3 cm. (arrowed). The calcification in the head of the pancreas is well seen at the same level as the common bile duct on this tomographic cut. No Biligrafin in the duodenum. Sphincterotomy performed and the presence of chronic pancreatitis confirmed.

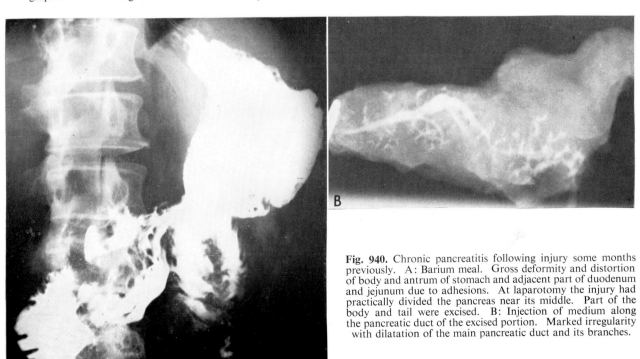

Fig. 940. Chronic pancreatitis following injury some months previously. A: Barium meal. Gross deformity and distortion of body and antrum of stomach and adjacent part of duodenum and jejunum due to adhesions. At laparotomy the injury had practically divided the pancreas near its middle. Part of the body and tail were excised. B: Injection of medium along the pancreatic duct of the excised portion. Marked irregularity with dilatation of the main pancreatic duct and its branches.

FIG. 940

X

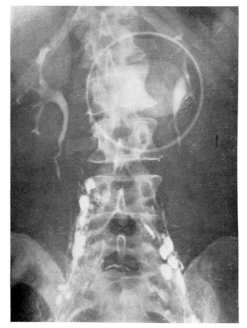

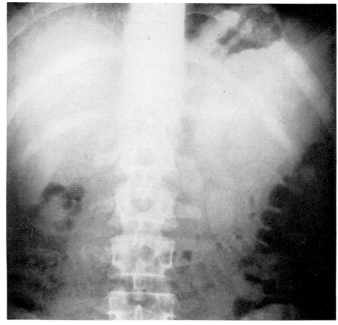

FIG. 941

FIG. 942

Fig. 941. Chronic pancreatitis with diffuse fibrosis causing lymphatic obstruction and chylous ascites. Lymphogram four days previously showed obstruction of lymphatic channels opposite L.V. 4. Sclerosis of L.V. 2 due to metastatic deposits. Previous transverse colostomy for treatment of diverticulitis of pelvic colon. At autopsy a small carcinoma was found in the pancreas. The cysterna chyli was involved with adhesions.

(By courtesy of Dr. Eric Samuel and Dr. A. Byrne.)

Fig. 942. Large pseudo-cyst of pancreas causing a soft-tissue shadow displacing the stomach upwards and the colon downwards (both outlined by their gas content). Repeated attacks of acute pancreatitis. Cysto-gastrostomy performed.

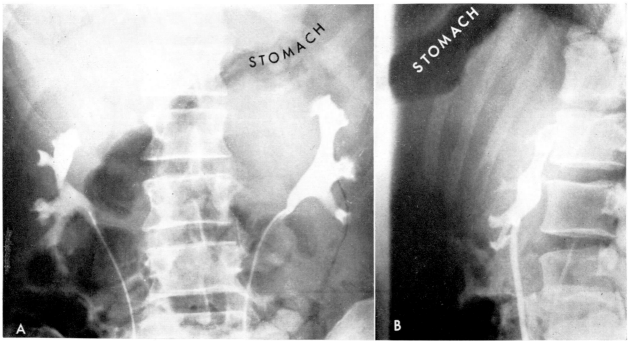

FIG. 943

Fig. 943. Pseudo-cyst of pancreas following relapsing pancreatitis. Large soft tissue swelling displacing the left kidney laterally and the stomach (outlined with gas) upwards. Retrograde pyelogram performed owing to clinical suspicion of enlargement of left kidney. A: A.P. view. B: Oblique view.

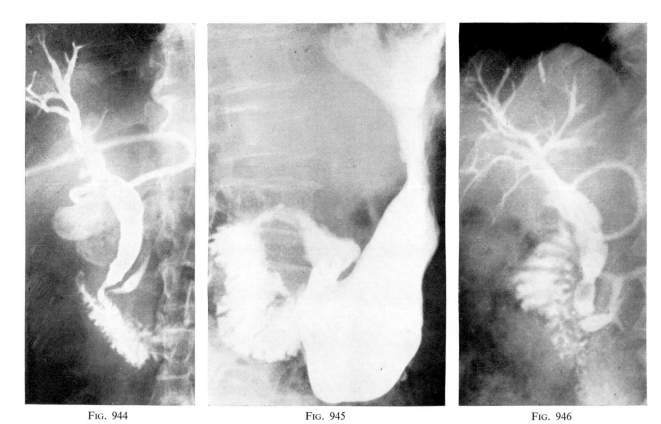

FIG. 944　　　　　　　FIG. 945　　　　　　　FIG. 946

Fig. 944. Chronic pancreatitis with dilatation of pancreatic duct in head of pancreas. Stricture also present at ampulla of Vater with dilatation of bile ducts. Post-operative cholangiogram. At the time of the cholecystectomy, stones were removed from the common bile duct. **Fig. 945.** Insulinoma of body of pancreas causing forward displacement of body of stomach with some irregularity of its posterior wall. History of blackouts and personality change. **Fig. 946.** Dilatation of terminal portion of pancreatic duct. Considerable irregular dilatation also of common bile duct with residual stone at its lower end. At the time of the cholecystectomy a stone impacted in the ampulla of Vater had been removed. Evidence of chronic pancreatitis also present. Post-operative cholangiogram.

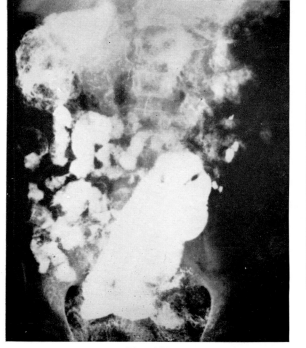

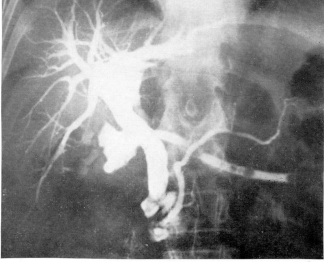

FIG. 948

FIG. 947

Fig. 947. Congenital fibrocystic disease of the pancreas. Child aged 12 with gross steatorrhoea. Moderately disordered X-ray pattern with segmentation and flocculation. A similar degree of steatorrhoea in coeliac disease would have caused more gross changes. **Fig. 948.** Pancreatic duct and common bile duct entering duodenal diverticulum. Dilatation of the common bile duct and to a lesser degree the pancreatic duct. A little medium has extravasated into the gall-bladder bed along the side of the T tube—a comparatively common occurrence. A stone had been removed from the lower end of the common bile duct at the time of the cholecystectomy. Post-operative cholangiogram.

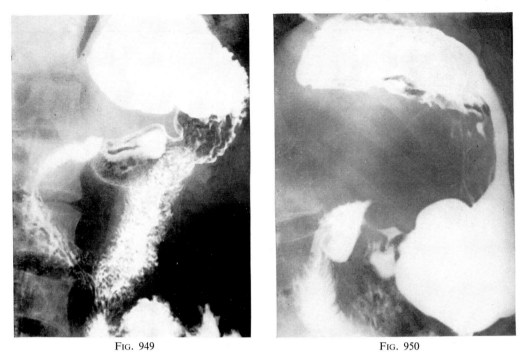

FIG. 949   FIG. 950

Fig. 949. Lipomatosis of the pancreas. Barium meal shows stretching of duodenal loop due to enlargement of head of pancreas. Patient extraordinarily weak and thin with steatorrhoea, osteomalacia and multiple Looser's zones. At laparotomy the pancreas was enlarged due to massive infiltration with fat. Marked clinical improvement on substitution therapy. **Fig. 950.** Large cystadenoma mainly affecting body of pancreas. The body of the stomach is compressed and displaced forwards. Irregularity and distortion also of prepyloric region of stomach.

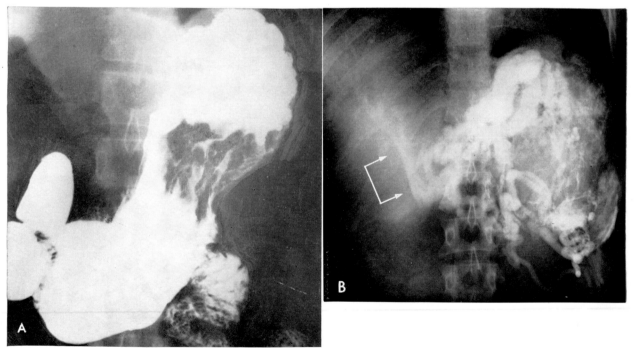

FIG. 951

Fig. 951. Large adenoma of tail of pancreas. A: Barium meal showing filling defect of greater curvature aspect of body of stomach. Some enlargement also of the spleen. B: Splenic venogram. Gross gastric varices with enlarged communicating veins subsequently feeding into the portal vein (arrowed). The splenic vein did not fill as the adenoma had caused local thrombosis. Operative confirmation.

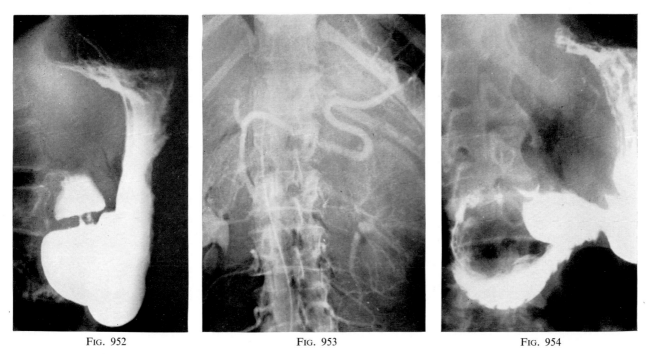

FIG. 952   FIG. 953   FIG. 954

Fig. 952. Carcinoma of body and tail of pancreas. Forward displacement of body of stomach with sharpening of angle between fundus and body, causing tendency to formation of a shelf. Erect film. On fluoroscopy sense of fullness behind the stomach on palpation.

Fig. 953. Large cystadenoma of pancreas which had undergone malignancy. An aortogram was carried out in order to find out if the splenic artery was obstructed. Some displacement of the splenic artery, but no obstruction.

Fig. 954. Carcinoma of head of pancreas. Indentation of second and third parts of duodenum with only minimal enlargement of duodenal loop. The mucosal pattern has been 'ironed out' on the concave border as compared with normal pattern on the convex border.

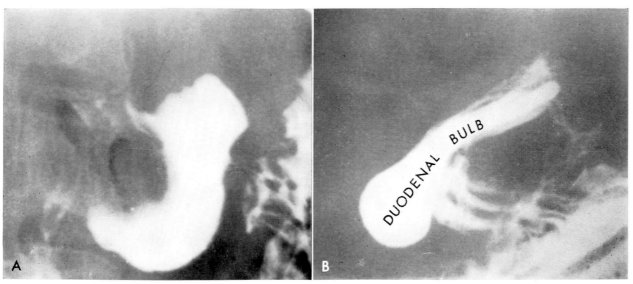

FIG. 955

Fig. 955. Carcinoma of head of pancreas. A: P.A. view. Indentation with finger-printing of duodenal bulb when compression is applied. B: Oblique view, supine, with left side raised. The duodenal bulb is displaced forwards and compressed by the tumour.

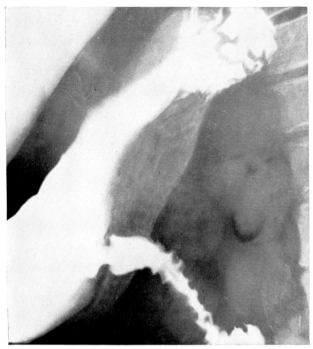 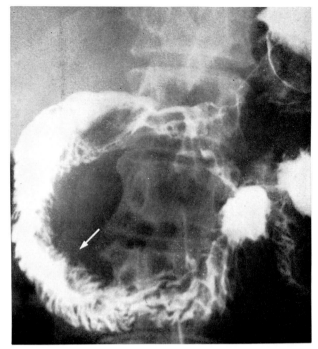

FIG. 956   FIG. 957

Fig. 956. 'Wedge' effect i.e. forward displacement of body of stomach with compression and narrowing towards its posterior wall. This was due to enlargement of body of pancreas—caused by a pseudo-cyst following acute pancreatitis. To demonstrate the wedge effect the stomach is well filled with barium, the patient lies on his right side, and the head of the table is moderately raised.

Fig. 957. Large carcinoma of head of pancreas causing (a) enlargement of duodenal loop, (b) upward displacement of the pyloric antrum, (c) indentation of the duodenal bulb, (d) reversed '3' sign of Frostberg due to displacement of duodenum above and below the ampulla of Vater (arrowed).

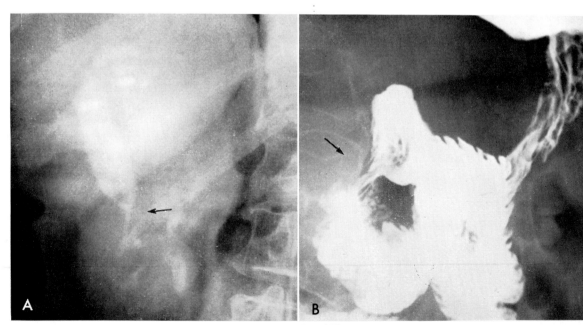

FIG. 958

Fig. 958. Carcinoma of head of pancreas with only recent development of jaundice. Operative confirmation. A: Intravenous cholangiogram one hour after injection of Biligrafin showing narrowing (arrowed) of lower 2 cm. of common bile duct with dilatation proximally. B: Barium meal. Characteristic narrowing (arrowed) at junction of first and second parts of duodenum. The duodenal loop is not enlarged.

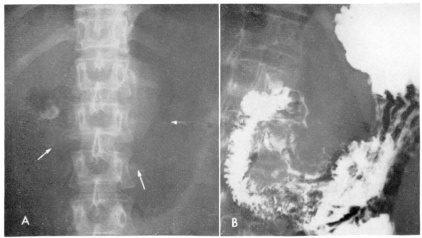
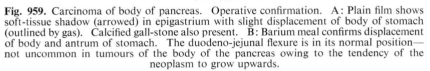

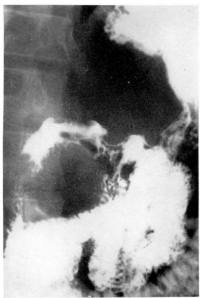

Fig. 959

Fig. 959. Carcinoma of body of pancreas. Operative confirmation. A: Plain film shows soft-tissue shadow (arrowed) in epigastrium with slight displacement of body of stomach (outlined by gas). Calcified gall-stone also present. B: Barium meal confirms displacement of body and antrum of stomach. The duodeno-jejunal flexure is in its normal position—not uncommon in tumours of the body of the pancreas owing to the tendency of the neoplasm to grow upwards.

Fig. 960

Fig. 960. Carcinoma of head of pancreas. Indentation with narrowing of middle of second part of duodenum, and slight upward displacement of the first part.

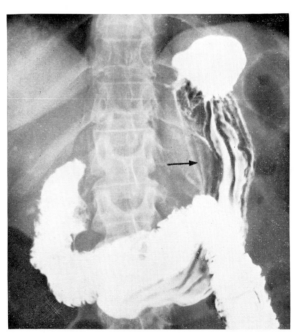

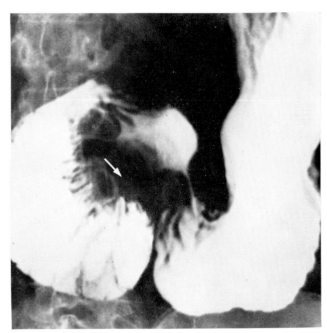

Fig. 961   Fig. 962

Fig. 961. Carcinoma of body of pancreas causing a crescentic indentation (arrowed) of body of stomach. Supine film. The duodeno-jejunal flexure is not displaced—a not infrequent finding—since the tumour commonly grows upwards and forwards.

Fig. 962. Carcinoma of uncinate process of pancreas causing obstruction of third part of duodenum (arrowed) with dilatation proximally. A little indentation also of inferior aspect of duodenal bulb.

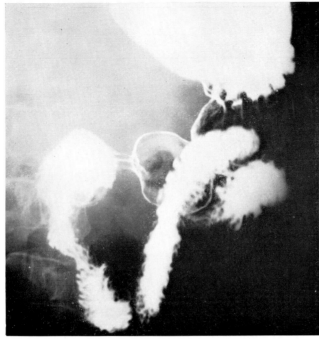

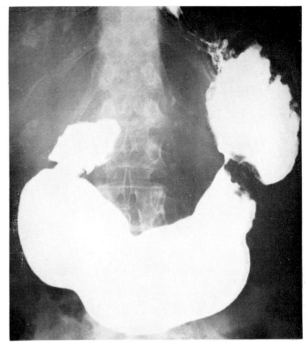

Fig. 963

Fig. 964

Fig. 963. Normal barium meal indicating the difficulty in diagnosis of small tumours of pancreas. Pancreatic carcinoma 5 cm. in diameter in middle of body of pancreas opposite duodeno-jejunal flexure—discovered at laparotomy. Even retrospectively no abnormality detected. **Fig. 964.** Carcinoma of body of pancreas. Laparotomy confirmation. A little downward displacement of body and antrum of stomach, but this could readily be overlooked. Some fullness in the epigastrium on palpation. Hour-glass deformity of upper part of body of stomach also present from a chronic gastric ulcer.

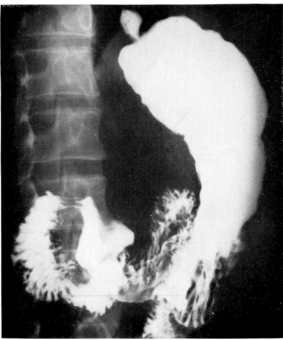

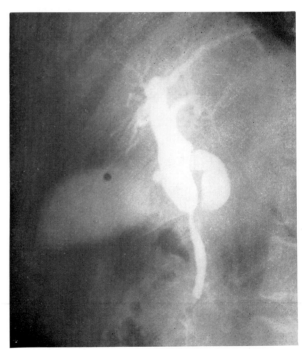

Fig. 965

Fig. 966

Fig. 965. Carcinoma of body of pancreas. Displacement of body and antrum of stomach downwards and laterally. The duodeno-jejunal flexure is in its normal position because the tumour grew upwards and forwards. **Fig. 966.** Carcinoma of head of pancreas demonstrated by percutaneous transhepatic cholangiogram. Characteristic high narrowing of common bile duct in head of pancreas with dilatation proximally. The cystic duct is also markedly dilated and passes behind the common hepatic duct entering the latter on its medial aspect. A little filling of the gall-bladder which is faintly opacified.

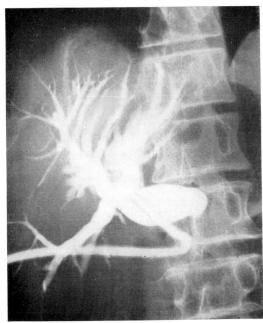

FIG. 967

Fig. 967. Carcinoma of head of pancreas causing obstruction and displacement of common bile duct and dilatation proximally. Post-operative cholangiogram.

Fig. 968. Hodgkin's disease of body of pancreas—found at laparotomy to have infiltrated the wall of the stomach. A: Supine view. Displacement of body of stomach with irregularity of medial aspect of fundus suggesting malignant infiltration. B: Lateral view with patient lying on his right side and X-ray table slightly raised. Large filling defect with irregularity high up on postero-medial wall due to indentation by the tumour.

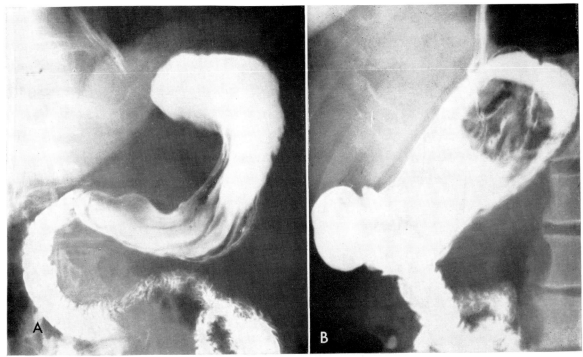

FIG. 968

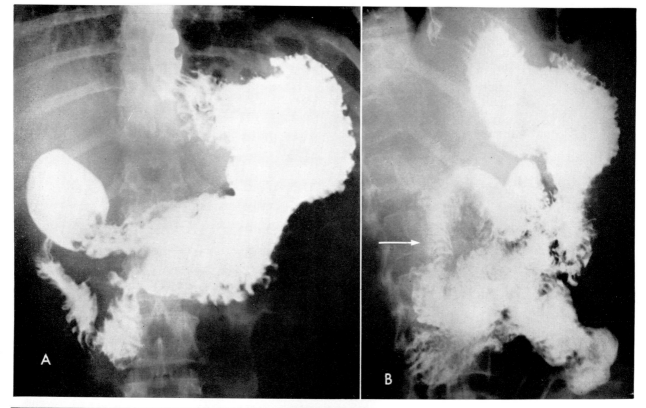

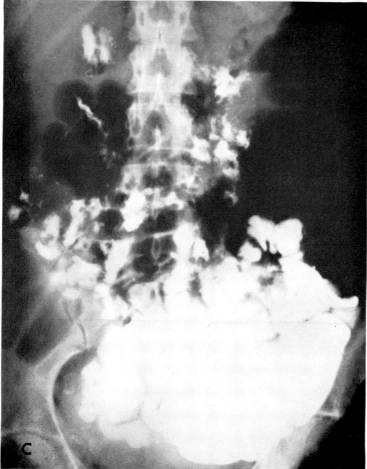

Fig. 969. Peptide secreting adenoma of pancreas (Verner-Morrison type). History of profuse watery diarrhoea resulting in gross hypokalaemia. A: Gross coarsening of mucosal pattern of stomach. No ulcer seen in stomach or duodenum. B: Indentation of convex border of second part of duodenum (arrowed). The coarsening of the mucosal pattern in the stomach is also very obvious. C: One-hour follow-through film. Some flocculation and segmentation with dilatation of loops of small bowel. After fluid and electrolyte replacement the basal acid output was 14 mEq/hr, having previously been normal. At laparotomy a tumour of the pancreas, mainly posterior and lateral to the second part of the duodenum, was removed with subsequent complete recovery.

CHAPTER XI

THE ABDOMEN AND PERITONEUM

LITTLE remains to be discussed, as many of the diseases and abnormalities have been described in previous chapters.

CLINICAL RADIOLOGY

NORMAL APPEARANCES

Extraperitoneal fat causes a thin line of relative translucency. In the flanks this is easily recognised, but occasionally under the diaphragm on the lateral aspect it can be mistaken for gas and can simulate a perforation.

ASCITES

A large ascites causes bulging of the flanks indicated by displacement of the extraperitoneal fat. The fluid causes a ground-glass appearance and initially tends to collect in the pelvis. In the erect position the loops of bowel float upwards and are situated at a high level in the abdomen. In the supine position the fluid separates translucent gas-filled loops which appear very obvious by comparison. If infection supervenes the distension of the bowel is considerably increased.

INFECTION

A localised abscess causes a soft-tissue swelling usually containing gas with a fluid level or levels in the erect position. In some cases there is one large collection of gas and in others multiple bubbles are present. There is usually distension with gas of adjacent loops of small bowel, which show a thickened mucosal pattern due to oedema.

When the abscess is subphrenic there is impaired movement of the adjacent dome of diaphragm with inflammatory changes at the base of the lung. A lateral view is important as the abscess which is commonly situated anteriorly may not show on a P.A. view.

Normally gas under the diaphragm following an operation is completely absorbed in 10 days. Any gas after that period suggests infection or a leak. Gas may be absent from one side if adhesions are present, e.g. from a previous operation.

A pelvic abscess generally causes a diffuse opacity with ileus of adjacent loops of ileum. Occasionally the abscess is localised and as it is not usually exactly in the midline differentiation from a full urinary bladder rarely causes difficulty.

CALCIFICATION

Tuberculous Nodes. These are the commonest calcifications and are readily recognised by their granular appearance. Mesenteric nodes can be displaced by palpation but para-aortic nodes are fixed.

Peritoneum. Calcification is most commonly seen in the subphrenic region due to an old healed subphrenic abscess and shows as dense linear or curvilinear opacities.

Hydatid Cysts. Occasionally a hydatid cyst, e.g. of the liver, ruptures into the peritoneal cavity, causing multiple cysts which may become calcified with a fine egg-shell type of calcification.

Talc Granuloma. In the past when talc was used as a glove powder granulomata occasionally formed. These sometimes become calcified causing multiple small circular or curvilinear opacities.

Appendix Epiploica. The most common site for calcification is at the hepatic flexure and this closely simulates a gall-stone on a plain film. It may become detached and thus be situated anywhere in the peritoneal cavity. It tends to gravitate into the pelvis where it could be mistaken for a stone at the lower end of a ureter.

Uterine Fibroids. These have a granular appearance when calcified and may be large.

SOFT-TISSUE SHADOWS

The rounded soft-tissue shadow caused by a colostomy or ileostomy should not be confused with an intra-abdominal mass.

THE ACUTE ABDOMEN

Reference should be made to previous sections where individual conditions are more fully described (perforation, p. 95; acute appendicitis, p. 186; acute cholecystitis, p. 265; acute pancreatitis, p. 309). It must be remembered that in cases where there is doubt the clinical findings are more important than the radiological features.

Torsion of a mesenteric or ovarian cyst, or a ruptured ectopic pregnancy in the early months causes a soft-tissue shadow with marked distension of the small and large bowel. There are however no specific diagnostic radiological features.

METHODS OF INVESTIGATION AND CLINICAL RADIOLOGY

Plain Films. Erect and supine views which must include the diaphragm are essential. A lateral decubitus view is of value if the patient cannot sit. A P.A. view of the chest is also necessary as a pulmonary lesion such as pneumonia or infarct may be demonstrated. In addition, gas under the diaphragm indicating a perforation is more clearly seen on this film than on the erect view of the abdomen. The gas is sometimes even more obvious on a right lateral view of the chest.

After consideration of the clinical findings the diagnosis may be established beyond reasonable doubt by the radiological appearances on plain films.

The ground-glass appearance in a very ill patient with acute abdominal symptoms may be due to:

(*a*) a large strangulated segment of bowel;

(*b*) profuse watery diarrhoea such as is caused by a fulminating viral infection;

(*c*) superior mesenteric occlusion with extensive gangrene of small bowel;

(*d*) the late stage of disseminated lupus erythematosus;

(*e*) rarely acute pancreatitis.

Gastrografin Meal. This is the next procedure when the diagnosis is uncertain, in particular between acute cholecystitis, acute pancreatitis and perforation of a peptic ulcer. It must be remembered that Gastrografin is sometimes excreted in the urine in intestinal atony, in dehydrated patients and in children.

Intravenous Cholangiography. In cases where doubt persists following a Gastrografin meal and where an acute cholecystitis is a likely diagnosis, an intravenous cholangiogram may be helpful (p. 265).

Intravenous Pyelogram. This is of great value in diagnosing or excluding renal colic. On the affected side there is delayed excretion, swelling of the kidney, a dense nephrogram and commonly a stone, often tiny, in the ureter. A film after 12 or even 24 hours may be of value showing the ureter dilated down to the level of the obstruction.

TUMOURS

(a) *Cysts.* A mesenteric cyst lies more anteriorly than other intra-abdominal cystic swellings. It is smooth, mobile and causes displacement of the bowel, and can usually be differentiated from an ovarian cyst which obviously arises out of the pelvis.

(b) *Malignant tumours* involving the peritoneum are usually secondary and are associated with ascites.

ABDOMINAL INJURIES

Plain films show a variable degree of adynamic ileus. The psoas shadow on the injured side may be absent but its presence never excludes injury or rupture of an adjacent organ. The ribs and lumbar transverse processes should be scrutinised for fractures. If found, the suspicion of injury to a neighbouring organ is increased.

In rupture or suspected rupture of the liver precious time must not be wasted on complicated radiological procedures.

The films should be carefully inspected for the following:

(a) Gas below the liver or diaphragm indicating a perforation of the stomach or bowel.

(b) A soft-tissue shadow especially with bulging of a flank suggesting a haematoma.

(c) Evidence of rupture of the spleen. This may cause a soft-tissue shadow and bulging of the left flank with elevation of the left dome of the diaphragm. Diaphragmatic movements are impaired on the left side. A Gastrografin meal usually shows displacement of the stomach.

(*d*) Evidence of rupture of a kidney. In most cases a soft-tissue shadow is present with bulging of the flank on the affected side. An intravenous pyelogram provides the diagnosis, showing distortion of the calyces and sometimes extravasation of contrast medium.

(*e*) Evidence of rupture of the liver. A soft-tissue shadow may be present on the right side of the abdomen due to a haematoma. The stomach, if identified by its gas shadow, may be obviously displaced to the left and sometimes downwards.

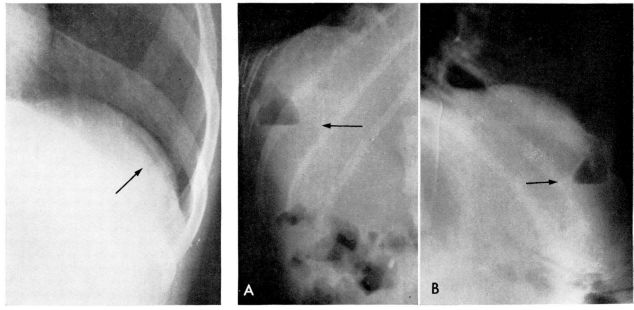

FIG. 970   FIG. 971

Fig. 970. Translucency (arrowed) under dome of diaphragm due to extraperitoneal fat. This must not be mistaken for gas which would indicate a perforation.

Fig. 971. Subphrenic abscess on right side. Erect films two weeks after partial gastrectomy. A: P.A. view. Abscess (arrowed). B: Lateral view. The abscess (arrowed) is anterior—the common site.

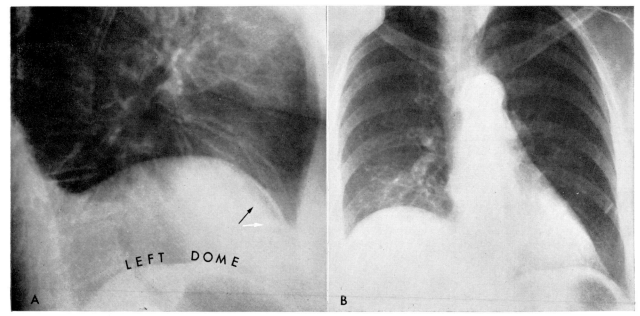

FIG. 972

Fig. 972. Small subphrenic abscess on right side. Three weeks after laparotomy. A: Lateral view. Erect. The small abscess cavity (arrowed) is seen anteriorly. Trace of fluid at right costo-phrenic angle. B: P.A. view of chest. The right dome of diaphragm is elevated, but no actual abscess seen as it is obscured by the dense liver shadow.

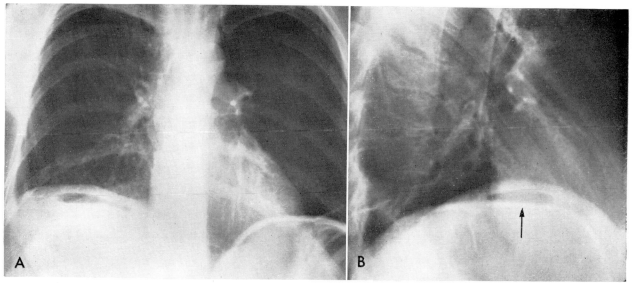

FIG. 973

Fig. 973. Subphrenic abscess on right side—eighteen days after laparotomy. Residual gas with a fluid level and subdiaphragmatic thickening. A: P.A. view of chest. B: Lateral view. Abscess (arrowed).

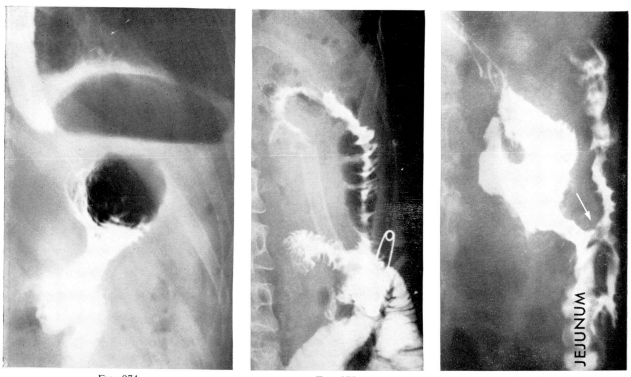

FIG. 974   FIG. 975   FIG. 976

Fig. 974. Subphrenic abscess on left side with subdiaphragmatic thickening. Two weeks following repair of hiatus hernia. Film taken following the swallowing of a small amount of barium. The patient had been supine in order to coat the fundus of the stomach. The film was then taken in the erect position. On a plain film the abscess could be mistaken for the gastric fundus.

Fig. 975. Large subphrenic abscess containing a number of small bubbles of gas. Drainage tube down to the abscess cavity. Gastrografin meal shows irritability of jejunum and coarsening of its mucosal pattern due to adjacent inflammatory mass.

Fig. 976. Large subphrenic abscess on left side which had ruptured into jejunum. The abscess followed resection of the tail of the pancreas. Gastrografin meal shows a fistula (arrowed) leading into the abscess cavity.

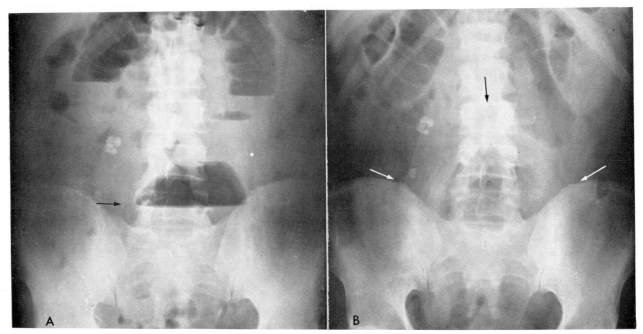

FIG. 977

Fig. 977. Large thick-walled abscess in peritoneal cavity situated in lower abdomen. Some dilatation of small bowel partly due to adynamic ileus, partly to mechanical obstruction. A: Erect. Large fluid level (arrowed) in the abscess. B: Supine. Vague soft-tissue shadow (arrowed) with some gas in its centre, in lower abdomen. The abscess was drained, but its cause could not be determined at laparotomy.

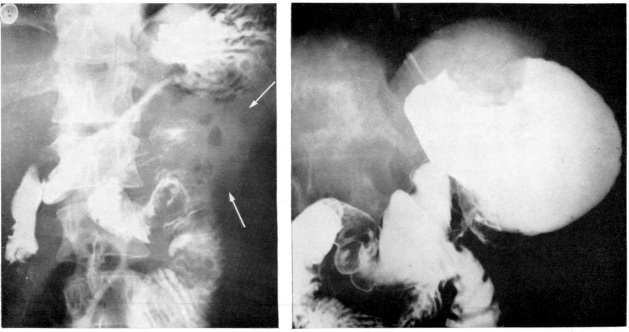

FIG. 978   FIG. 979

Fig. 978. Abscess in peritoneal cavity following a procto-colectomy. Soft-tissue shadow (arrowed) containing three or four bubbles of gas but no barium. Some distortion also of upper jejunum due to the adjacent inflammatory mass. Half-hour barium follow-through.

Fig. 979. Subphrenic abscess following an abdominal operation three months previously with a stormy post-operative course. Barium meal shows indentation of fundus of stomach simulating a carcinoma. Considerably increased distance between fundus of stomach and base of lung due to the inflammatory mass. Operative confirmation.

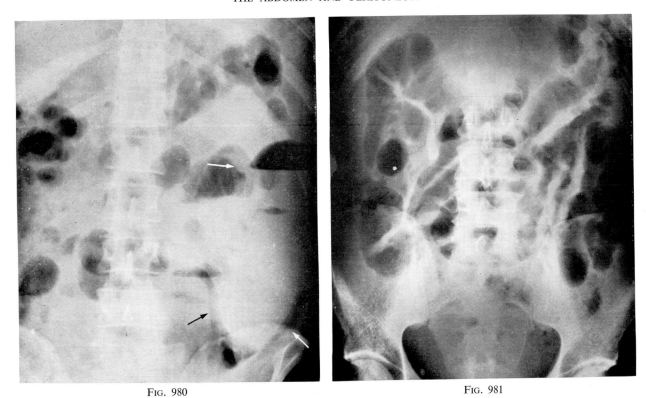

Fig. 980   Fig. 981

Fig. 980. Large abscess containing a fluid level (top arrow) following myotomy of colon for diverticular disease. The lower part of the abscess is indicated (lower two arrows). Bulging of the left flank. Some generalised distension of small bowel due to widespread peritonitis. Erect film. **Fig. 981.** Diffuse peritonitis causing generalised adynamic ileus. Fluid present resulting in separation of loops of bowel and bulging of the flanks. Fluid is also present in the pelvis displacing the bowel upwards. At laparotomy suppurative peritonitis was present but its cause could not be determined. Supine film.

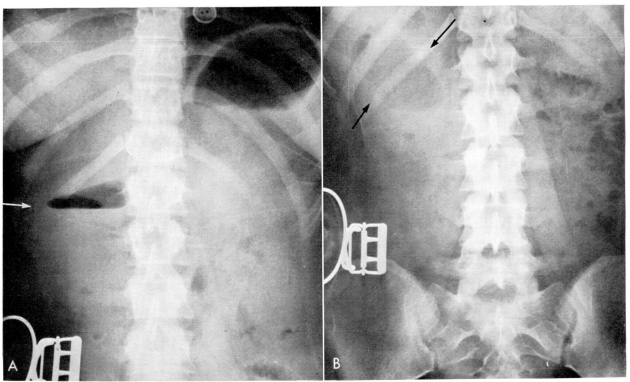

Fig. 982

Fig. 982. Subhepatic abscess on right side. Total procto-colectomy two weeks previously. A: Erect film. Large abscess with air-fluid level (arrowed). Elevation of right dome of diaphragm. B: Supine film. The abscess (arrowed) is not so obvious.

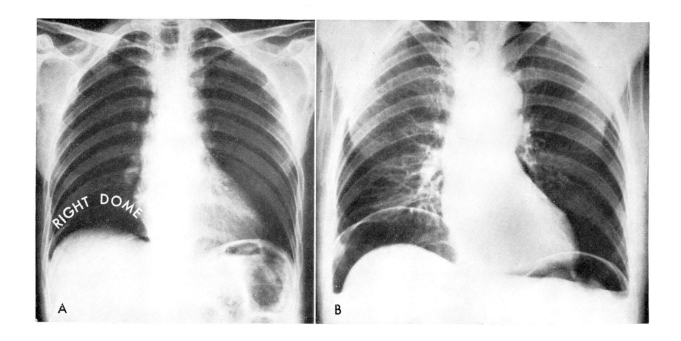

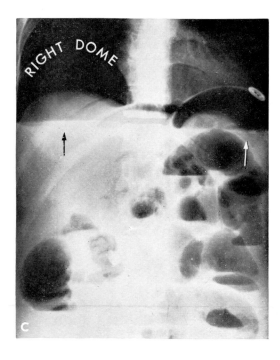

Fig. 983. Post-operative leak indicated by marked increase in sub-diaphragmatic gas. A: Chest film. Second day after operation. Normal amount of gas under right diaphragm. B: Chest film on tenth post-operative day. Markedly increased amount of gas which is now present on left side as well. C: Erect film of abdomen same day as B., i.e. tenth post-operative day. Large amount of subdiaphragmatic gas terminating inferiorly in horizontal lines (arrowed). This does not necessarily indicate actual subphrenic loculations in the case of recent leaks, perforations, or abdominal operations. It is then merely due to approximation of the visceral and parietal layers of peritoneum with sometimes only a trace of fluid. Operative confirmation of leak and absence of localised subphrenic abscesses. Generalised distension also of loops of small bowel due to widespread peritonitis.

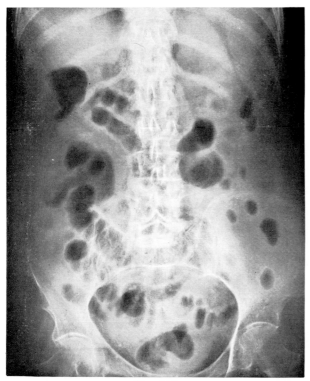

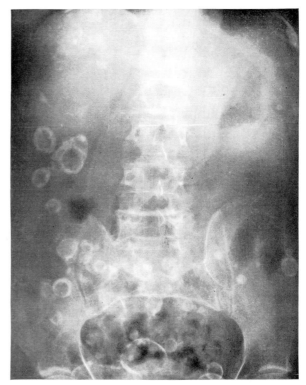

FIG. 984   FIG. 985

Fig. 984. Peritonitis causing adynamic ileus with moderate distension of small bowel with gas. Appearances clinically indistinguishable from acute appendicitis. The peritonitis was due to perforation of the ileum by a sharp foreign body. **Fig. 985.** Multiple hydatid cysts scattered throughout the peritoneal cavity. Large calcified hydatid cysts also present in the liver. Presumably one of the cysts in the liver had ruptured into the peritoneal cavity. (By courtesy of Dr. Eric Samuel.)

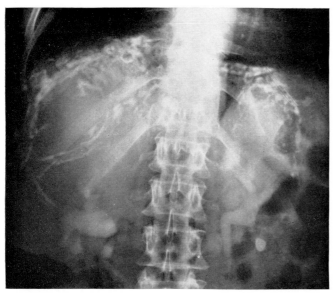

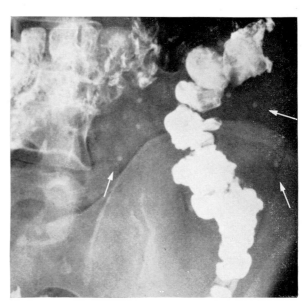

FIG. 986   FIG. 987

Fig. 986. Extensive calcification under both domes of diaphragm from old subphrenic abscesses following childhood appendicitis with peritonitis. Calcification discovered at the time of an intravenous pyelogram. **Fig. 987.** Talc granulomata in lower abdomen causing a number of small calcified opacities (some of which are arrowed). A laparotomy had been performed many years previously. Barium in colon from barium meal two days beforehand.

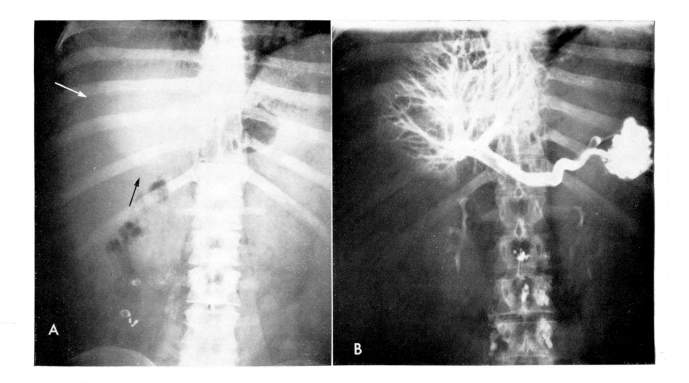

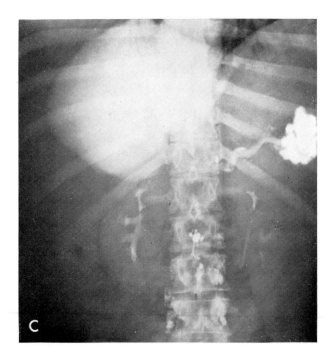

Fig. 988. Cirrhosis of liver with gross chylous ascites. A: Plain film. Large ascites present. The liver (arrowed) is small and its margins are seen since it is surrounded by chylous fluid which is more translucent than other soft tissues. B: Splenic venogram three seconds after injection showing patent splenic and portal veins. Grossly shrunken liver. C: Splenic venogram, nine seconds after injection. The liver is uniformly opacified by the medium.

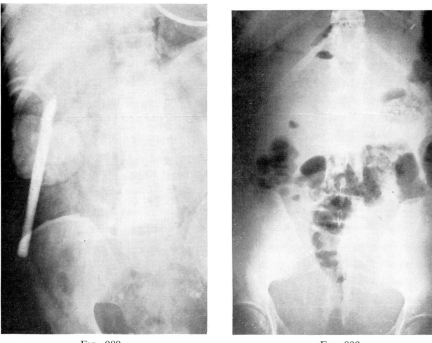

FIG. 989   FIG. 990

Fig. 989. Circumscribed opacity on right side caused by a colostomy loop.

Fig. 990. Gross ascites. The translucencies in the bowel due to gas content are very clear, being thrown into relief by the surrounding fluid. Considerable amount of fluid has gravitated to the pelvis causing some compression of the pelvic colon. Case of diffuse peritoneal metastases.

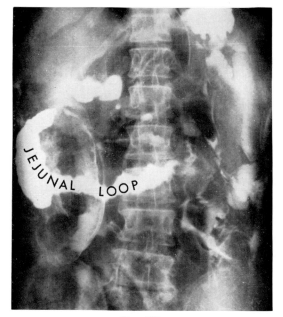
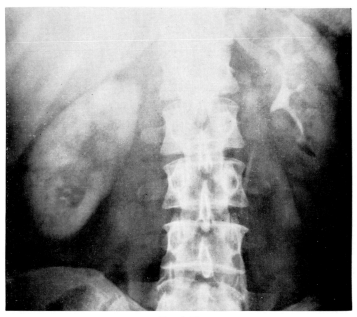

FIG. 991   FIG. 992

Fig. 991. Barium in peritoneal cavity causing streaking and smearing of bowel loops. Case of oesophageal and gastric varices with a large gastric ulcer which perforated during the course of the barium meal.

Fig. 992. Right renal colic in a patient sent to hospital as an acute abdomen. Twenty-minute intravenous pyelogram film shows dense nephrogram on the right side with a swollen right kidney. A tiny stone was present at the lower end of the right ureter.

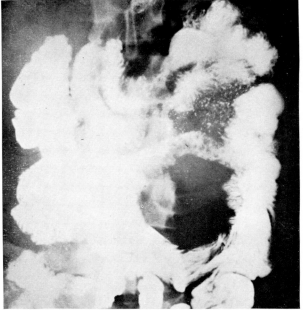

FIG. 993

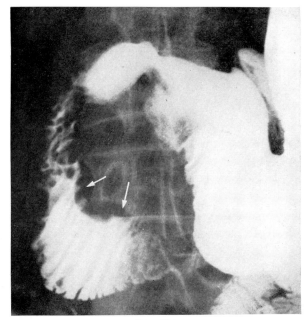

FIG. 994

Fig. 993. Simple tumour in the mesentery. The loops of small bowel are displaced by a smooth round mass proved at laparotomy to be a fibroma. Some stretching of the loops but no infiltration. The tumour could readily be palpated and displaced during fluoroscopy.

Fig. 994. Crescentic filling defect (arrowed) on concave border of duodenum, caused by enlarged mesenteric lymph nodes. No jaundice, suggesting that this is not a carcinoma of pancreas. Case of reticulosis.

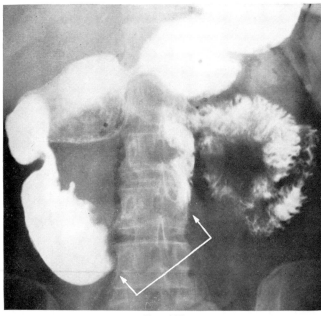

FIG. 995

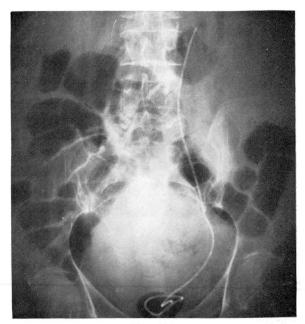

FIG. 996

FIG. **995**. Mesothelioma of peritoneum involving third part of duodenum. Barium meal shows an irregular filling defect (arrowed) with obstruction. Laparotomy proof.

Fig. 996. Sarcoma of great omentum causing a large soft-tissue shadow in pelvis. Ureteric obstruction present shown later on a retrograde pyelogram. Supine film of abdomen. The gas shadows of the small bowel are clearly seen as they are surrounded by fluid (malignant ascites present). The bladder is contracted and just accommodates the coiled loop of the ureteric catheter. Gas in the bladder introduced during cystoscopy.

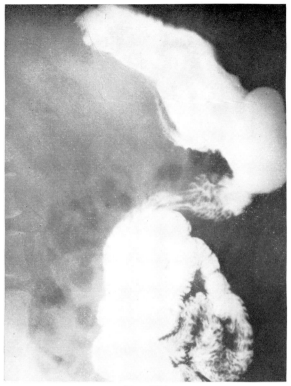

FIG. 997

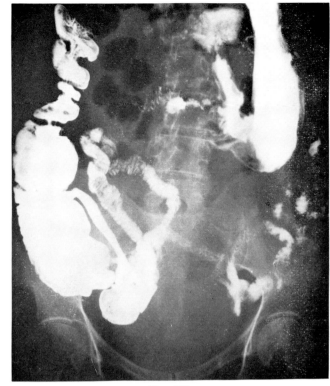

FIG. 998

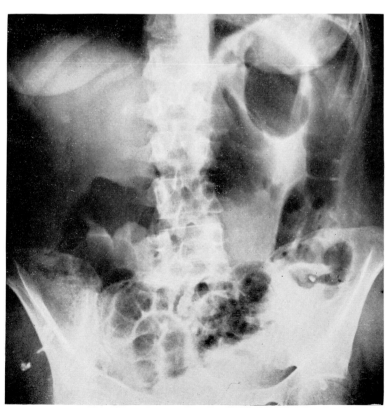

FIG. 999

Fig. 997. Marked forward displacement of stomach and small bowel by grossly enlarged para-aortic lymph nodes. Case of seminoma of testis.

Fig. 998. Mesenteric cyst in lower abdomen. Large soft-tissue shadow displacing small bowel but without infiltration.

Fig. 999. Adynamic ileus particularly affecting the small bowel due to a retroperitoneal haemorrhage. Complaint of severe back pain. Bleeding also from the renal and alimentary tracts, and subcutaneous bruising. Patient under treatment with anticoagulants. Erect film.

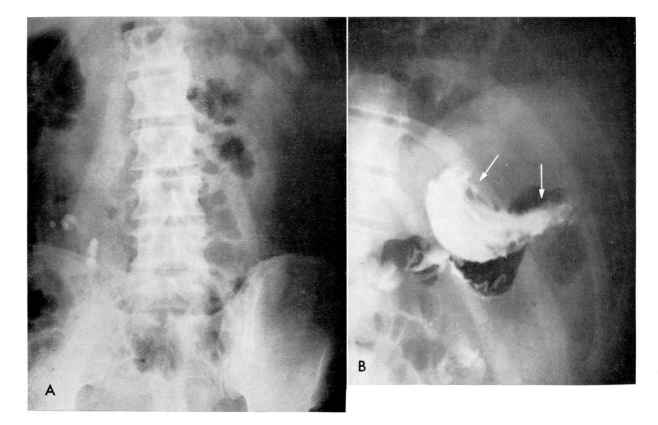

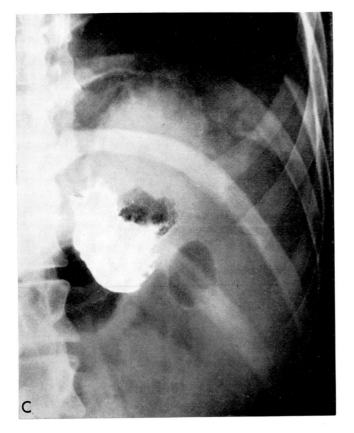

Fig. 1000. Rupture of the spleen. A: Plain film of abdomen shows faint soft-tissue shadow in left hypochondrium. Adynamic ileus of small bowel. The psoas shadow is present—a common finding. B: Gastrografin meal. Marked indentation of fundus of stomach (arrowed) due to a large haematoma. C: The stomach is displaced medially and indented as in B by a large soft-tissue shadow. History of a minor injury to left side of chest with complaint of severe pain on left side three days later. Laparotomy confirmed a ruptured spleen (of normal size) with a large haematoma.

INDEX

INDEX

Page numbers in heavy type indicate illustrations

Printed in Great Britain by
T. & A. Constable Ltd.
Edinburgh